Home Remedies and Healing Techniques

PREVENTION®

SENIOR HEALTH LIBRARY

Home Remedies and Healing Techniques

By the editors of

PREVENTION
Health Books™

Rodale Press, Inc.
Emmaus, Pennsylvania

The information in this book is excerpted from *The Doctors Book of Home Remedies for Seniors* (Rodale Press, 1999) and *The Doctors Book of Home Remedies II* (Rodale Press, 1993).

Cover and Book Designer: Diane Ness Shaw

ISBN 1-57954-219-0 paperback

2   4   6   8   10   9   7   5   3   1   paperback

— OUR PURPOSE —

We inspire and enable people to improve their lives and the world around them.

Contents

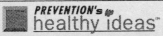

PREVENTION's
healthy ideas™
For the best interactive guide to healthy active
living, visit our Web site at **www.healthyideas.com**

Introduction

Beating the Little Things

Older Americans are bombarded with news about heart disease, stroke, cancer, and other catastrophic ailments. Yet these probably aren't the problems that you and your friends talk about when someone mentions aging.

You're concerned about the things you're facing now—the hundreds of little things that make getting older so difficult. Things like arthritis, morning aches and pains, dry mouth, forgetfulness, and cold feet and hands. You're concerned about the things that nip away at your self-reliance, independence, and self-confidence and threaten to make you feel older than your years.

In the pages that follow, scores of doctors and other health care practitioners nationwide who specialize in the treatment of older Americans share tips and techniques that can help you care for yourself and remain robust for years to come. You'll find tips to help you stay mentally sharp, eat well, get enough exercise, prevent accidents, and get the best possible care from your doctors.

You'll also find hundreds of doctor-recommended remedies that can help you prevent, relieve, and even self-treat more than 100 ailments that commonly affect older Americans. From aches and pains to yeast infections, you'll find the solutions to many of your most vexing health problems. Many chapters also offer advice about managing your medications. And we'll tell you when it's best to seek professional advice rather than treat yourself.

From the first page to the last, *Home Remedies and Healing Techniques* truly is a comprehensive guide to beating the little things that make you feel older. But much more than that, we sincerely hope reading it will allow you to live well and bask in that time of life that famed choreographer Martha Graham called "the glory of years."

Aches and Pains

Between arthritis and the hard-knock experiences of a life well-lived, aches and pains seem to be an inevitable part of aging. But they're not.

In fact, everyday aches and pains in your joints aren't necessarily due to arthritis. Sometimes, pain can simply occur from an afternoon of really brisk walking or a morning spent out in the garden. Those are the pains that you can alleviate or easily prevent.

First, you have to know your trouble zones. Men and women over 60 tend to be most prone to pain in the lower joints—the hips, knees, ankles, and feet—according to Dale L. Anderson, M.D., coordinator of the Minnesota Act Now Project in Minneapolis and author of *Muscle Pain Relief in 90 Seconds*. These are the areas that you'll especially want to protect and pamper.

If you have occasional joint pain and inflammation, you can do a number of things to feel better and prevent them from returning. If your pain frequently returns, it could be the result of arthritis.

Make it right with RICE. If you have joint pain, then RICE might be the answer, says William Pesanelli, a physical therapist and director of Boston University's rehabilitation services. In this case, we're not talking about Uncle Ben's latest concoction. RICE is an easy way to remember the pain-relieving sequence of rest, ice, compression, and elevation.

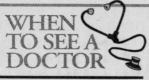

WHEN TO SEE A DOCTOR

Everyday minor aches and pains are just a part of life for most people. But if the aches and pains in your joints worsen after three or four days or if you have pain that doesn't subside at all after proper rest and other home remedies, then it's time to see a doctor, says David Richards, M.D., orthopedic surgeon at the Lexington Clinic Sports Medicine Center in Lexington, Kentucky.

1. Until you notice that the pain has decreased, rest the affected area and avoid the activity that caused the pain, Pesanelli says.

2. Put ice on the injured area to help narrow the blood vessels and limit swelling. Keith Jones, trainer for the Houston Rockets basketball team, recommends applying ice wrapped in a towel or cloth to the area at least three times per day for 20 minutes.

3. Use compression, which means wrapping an elastic bandage, such as an ACE bandage, around the injured area to help limit the swelling and to allow you to resume your everyday activities, recommends Pesanelli. However, remove the bandage at once if the area below the bandage feels numb or tingles like it is falling asleep, if it changes color, or if it feels cooler than the rest of your body. Wait for those symptoms to subside and then rewrap it more loosely.

4. Elevate the affected area above the level of your heart. This will prevent blood and other fluids from collecting at the injury, thereby reducing the swelling, says Pesanelli. If you have a history of impaired circulation in the injured area, however, skip the elevation step because limiting blood flow to an area of the body with impaired circulation can be dangerous, says Dr. Anderson.

Mix RICE with peas. An ice pack is good, but frozen peas are better, at least when it comes to icing a sore joint, says Pesanelli. A bag of frozen peas won't leak the way some ice packs do, he points out. "And because the peas are so small, you're able to bend the package to conform to the painful area, whether it's your shoulder or your kneecap." He suggests applying the bag of peas wrapped in a thin towel every couple of hours as part of the RICE sequence.

After you've used the peas once, you can toss them back in the freezer compartment, get them iced, and use the same bag again. But since bacteria can quickly multiply in food that has been thawed and refrozen, make sure to clearly label the bag so that you don't accidentally try to serve the peas for dinner.

Lose some weight. "If people lose five to 10 pounds, it considerably lightens the load on all of their lower joints—hips, knees, ankles, and feet," according to Dr. Anderson. "One of the main causes of these joint-related pains is that people are simply overweight. They're carrying a Mack truck frame on Volkswagen tires, and eventually their joints wear out from the stress."

Alter your walking style. If your ankles, feet, or knees are aching, you may be walking too hard. Hard walkers suffer from more aches and pains in their feet, ankles, and knees because their heels strike the ground with greater force than soft walkers' heels do,

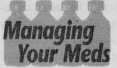

Managing Your Meds

Taking 600 milligrams of a non-steroidal anti-inflammatory drug (NSAID), such as ibuprofen or aspirin, four times per day for a week to 10 days should help ease inflammation pain in your joints.

But if you have certain pre-existing abdominal conditions, these medications can make them worse, says David Richards, M.D., orthopedic surgeon at the Lexington Clinic Sports Medicine Center in Lexington, Kentucky. Ask your doctor for another kind of pain relief if you've been previously diagnosed with ulcers or any inflamed bowel disorder. And of course, you never want to take aspirin if you know you're allergic to it.

says Dr. Anderson. But he points out that it's never too late to alter your walking style.

Just try this exercise: Imagine that you're a puppet with threads lifting you up at the head and shoulders. Visualize yourself lightening up and walking on a layer of air, with your feet gliding as though on imaginary ice skates.

Shoe away the pain. If you do a lot of walking, boot out any hard leather-soled shoes or high heels that are in your closet, recommends Dr. Anderson. "Opt instead for a shoe with a cushioned sole and heel and proper arch supports to save some wear and tear on your legs, ankles, feet, and hips."

Stand up straight. It turns out that your mom—or your drill sergeant—was right all those years ago when she told you to stand tall like a soldier. Stand up straight, push your shoulders back, arch your back slightly, and keep your chest out when sitting and walking. If you walk with your shoulders slouched, your chin forward, and your back rounded, it can lead to back, shoulder, or neck pain.

Stay active. To prevent joint aches and pains, get yourself on an exercise program, says Pesanelli. Joint surfaces naturally wear down over time, and this is complicated by the fact that your body usually produces less lubricating fluid as you get older. Since movement helps get vital nutrients into your joints, you can keep the joints better lubricated if you keep them warm and moving, he adds.

Pesanelli suggests a thorough warm-up routine with plenty of gentle stretching, followed by low-impact activities such as brisk walking or lap swimming for at least 20 minutes at a time three or four times per week. This is a sound form of exercise for seniors, he says, not only to keep your joints in good shape but also to keep your heart and lungs in working order. Just be sure to check with your physician before you begin an exercise regimen.

Age Spots

Talk about a spotty reputation! Heck, most people can't agree on what to *call* these unappealing but otherwise harmless dark spots that usually occur on the forehead and the back of the hands and arms.

Some folks think age spots are caused by old

age—an understandable mistake, since the spots are extremely common *after* age 55 and rarely appear before middle age. Others know them as liver spots.

The appearance of these dark, blotchy spots can be scary—resembling the early forms of skin cancer to the untrained eye. But genuine age spots are really nothing more than "adult freckles" that result from overexposure to the sun. (However, if you notice an increase in size or "bizarre" color changes, see your doctor immediately.)

"Age spots should really be called sun spots, because they are caused by being out in the sun," says D'Anne Kleinsmith, M.D., a cosmetic dermatologist at William Beaumont Hospital in Royal Oak, Michigan. "They have absolutely nothing to do with your liver and little to do with your age, other than the fact that they usually occur on older people."

Still, they *are* unbecoming. Sometimes they may be raised and look like tiny moles. Usually, though, they're just like dark, smooth freckles. If you've had them, you've probably noticed that they seem to appear suddenly on sun-exposed skin areas (usually areas *not* protected with sunscreen). So here's what to do about liver spots . . . er, age spots, uh, *lentigines* (their medical name).

Get help from hydroquinone. This safe "lightening agent" is found in products such as Porcelana and Esoterica that you can obtain without a prescription. Hydroquinone helps lighten age spots until they become unnoticeable. "Dab it on the individual spots with a cotton ball," says Dr. Kleinsmith.

But don't expect overnight success: This therapy usually takes a month or two before you see any results. Follow the directions on the package and try to

Sunscreen Each Day
Keeps Age Spots Away

The best way to avoid *ever* having age spots is to use a good-quality sunscreen each time you go outdoors, including when it's overcast. And if you already have age spots, sunscreen will keep them from darkening and will help prevent new ones.

Either way, remember the "15" rules.

Look for a sun protection factor (SPF) of at least 15. Unprotected, the average person's skin turns red—a signal of overexposure—after just 30 minutes. But with SPF 15 sunscreen, you can stay out 15 times as long, or seven hours, with the same effect (although it's not recommended).

Apply sunscreen at least 15 minutes before going outdoors. That way, the skin has a chance to absorb it.

dab the medication right on the spots, so you don't "bleach" the pigment in nonaffected skin.

Shed away "spotted" skin. Lac-Hydrin Five lotion, another nonprescription remedy, contains lactic acid. "The acid can help bleaching agents work faster by enhancing the normal shedding of upper, 'dead' skin layers," says Michael Ramsey, M.D., clinical instructor of dermatology at Baylor College of Medicine in Houston. This leaves a lighter layer of skin underneath.

Reach for lemon aid. "The juice of a fresh lemon is acidic enough to safely peel off the upper layer of skin, which will remove or lighten some age spots," says Jerome Z. Litt, M.D., assistant clinical professor of dermatology at Case Western Reserve University School of Medicine in Cleveland. "Rub it on with a cotton ball twice daily where the age spots are, and in six to eight weeks, they should begin to fade away."

How about an onion rub? Rubbing a piece of sliced *red* onion on age spots can have the same fading effect, "since it has the same peeling acid as fresh lemon juice," adds Dr. Litt.

Use castor oil for smooth relief. "If the surface of individual lesions appears rougher than surrounding skin—which often occurs with age spots—applying castor oil twice daily with a cotton swab will sometimes bring about improvement," says Dr. Ramsey. On larger lesions, a bandage applied with the castor oil at nighttime may speed improvement.

Be a shady character. "Since age spots are caused by excessive sun exposure, avoid the sun and you'll avoid age spots," suggests Albert M. Kligman, M.D., Ph.D., professor of dermatology at the University of Pennsylvania School of Medicine in Philadelphia. "You will never see an age spot on someone who stays in the shade." If you already have age spots, limiting sun exposure will help prevent them from darkening and will minimize a recurrence or the appearance of new ones.

Cover 'em up. If all else fails in trying to remedy them, hide them. "Many types of makeup can cover the spots," says Edward Bondi, M.D., a dermatologist who is affiliated with the University of Pennsylvania Hospital in Philadelphia. "If they are really dark spots, a heavier-based makeup will work, but if they're not so bad, then many water-based types will do the trick. A product called Covermark has routinely been used to hide age spots." *Note:* If you suffer from adult acne, avoid heavier oil-based makeups, because they can worsen blemishes.

Aging Eyes

It happens to a lot of people around age 40. You begin to realize it takes a Herculean effort to read the newspaper or the tiny type on a food package or an aspirin bottle. As for threading a needle or removing a splinter—forget it! These simple tasks have become impossible feats.

That's because anything closer than an arm's length from your eyes is now one big blur.

If that happened to you, you're not alone. If your faraway vision is fine (with or without corrective eyewear) but your close-up vision is fuzzier than a teddy bear's coat, blame it on an inflexible lens. And it's a problem as common as crow's feet and silver hair.

After age 40, you may find it's more difficult to focus on near objects, particularly printed words when you're reading. Doctors call this presbyopia.

But before you shell out the green stuff for special prescription glasses, these tips may help you fine-tune your focusing.

Do the fine print sprint. "Part of the problem of the aging eye is that the lens becomes less flexible," says Bruce Rosenthal, O.D., professor and chief of low vision services at the State University of New York College of Optometry in New York City. "If you exercise the muscles that control the shape of the lens, it may be possible to delay near-point fuzziness to some degree."

9

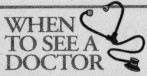

WHEN TO SEE A DOCTOR

Gradual changes in vision as you age are normal, but a sudden change in your vision—no matter what your age—isn't, says Bruce Rosenthal, O.D., professor and chief of low vision services at the State University of New York College of Optometry in New York City. "Blurred vision can be a first sign of eye diseases such as glaucoma, macular degeneration, or cataracts, which can seriously impair your vision."

Other conditions that can cause cloudy vision include diabetes, side effects of medications, anemia, kidney disease, and optic nerve disease. So it's important to see a doctor as soon as possible if there's any sudden blurriness in your near or distant vision.

One exercise involves cutting headlines of decreasing size out of the newspaper and affixing each one to a pencil. Then hold the largest headline about a foot away from your face. Gradually bring it in toward your nose, trying to keep the print in focus. Move the headline back out again. Repeat with the next smaller headline, then the rest, until you have looked at all the headlines.

"With practice, you may be able to read even the tiniest labels on medicine bottles with no difficulty," says Dr. Rosenthal.

Follow the bouncing thumb. To keep your eye muscles fully flexed, hold out your thumb at arm's length. Move it in circles, then in figure eights, closer and farther away. Follow it with your eyes. This helps keep the fine motor system of your eyes in working order, says Dr. Rosenthal.

Switch frequently from near to far. If you keep your eyes fixed for long periods on a computer screen, for example, your eye muscles can temporarily become stuck. This slows focusing when you try to zoom from near to far and back again, says Dr. Rosenthal. To keep your eye muscles loose, look up every 10 minutes and focus on a poster located about eight feet away. Then look back at the words on the computer screen. Shift your focus back and forth repeatedly for 30 seconds.

Invest in brighter bulbs. As your eyes age, you may begin to need more light for everyday activities. In fact, by age 60, you could need six times as much light as you did at age 20 to perform the same tasks, according to Dr. Rosenthal. "If you have better lighting, the pupils become smaller, and the amount of blur you experience may be less," says James Sheedy, O.D., Ph.D., associate clinical professor at the University of California, Berkeley, School of Optometry. You may find that high-wattage incandescent bulbs will help you see better than harsh fluorescent lights.

Check out off-the-rack reading glasses. All you may need to read and see close up are simple magnifiers, says Richard P. Mills, M.D., professor of ophthalmology at the University of Washington School of Medicine in Seattle. "The drugstore demi-glasses that come in about 10 different powers are medically acceptable," says Dr. Mills. "Just make sure they have no optical distortion."

To find out, hold the glasses at arm's length, then

How to Adjust to Bifocals

If you have trouble with both near and distant vision, you may eventually end up with bifocals. But getting used to bifocals can be a lot like stumbling through a fun house filled with wavy mirrors.

Be patient, says Joseph P. Shovlin, O.D., an optometrist at the Northeastern Eye Institute, with headquarters in Scranton, Pennsylvania, and chairman of the Contact Lens Section of the American Optometric Association. "It can take from a few days to several weeks to get used to multifocal lenses." Be prepared for possible return visits to the optometrist for adjustments, since a dual-prescription lens often requires more precise measurements than a single-vision lens.

Here are tips to focus on.

■ Wear the glasses all day for the first week or two until you're accustomed to them, even though you may not need them for all tasks.

■ Avoid looking at your feet when walking.

■ Hold reading material closer to your body and lower your eyes, not your head, so that you are reading out of the lowest part of the lens.

■ Fold the newspaper in half or quarters and move it, rather than your head, to read comfortably.

look through them as you move them in a circular motion. If there's some "swim," or distortion, get another pair. If you find that these reading glasses give you a headache or tired eyes, however, you're better off with prescription glasses.

Anal Fissures

When it comes to pain, embarrassment, and inconvenience, these painful tears in the sensitive skin around your anus are truly a thorn in your (back)side. Fissures are usually caused by trying to pass hard, large stools. Since more fiber in your diet means looser stools, anal fissures are a sharp reminder to eat shredded wheat with newfound gusto. But here's how to fizzle your anal fissures.

Go high on fiber. Maybe oat bran doesn't go down as easy as a thick, juicy steak, but consuming a high-fiber diet is the best way to soften stools. Besides eating more grains, you should also eat plenty of fresh fruits and vegetables, all of which are natu-

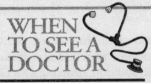

WHEN TO SEE A DOCTOR

If you've tried self-help measures and still have anal fissures, or if you notice blood in your stool or experience any bleeding while trying to pass your stool, see your doctor as soon as possible. While some bleeding occurs because of hemorrhoids or trying to pass hard stools, rectal bleeding may be a warning sign of colon cancer or another serious problem. But you'll need a doctor's examination to find out the cause.

Maybe a Spray Will Do

As anyone with anal fissures can tell you, wiping with dry tissues is no picnic. To make personal hygiene a little easier on your tender bottom, there's ClenZone. This small cleansing device hooks up to your bathroom faucet; just spray yourself clean with a narrow stream of water aimed at the anal area. There's no need for toilet paper, except to pat yourself dry.

It can be used for both fissures and hemorrhoids. It's available through Hepp Industries, 687 Kildare Crescent, Seaford, NY 11783.

rally high in fiber. "Fruits, vegetables, and whole grains are the best remedy and preventive measure for fissures," says J. Byron Gathright Jr., M.D., chairman of the department of colon and rectal surgery at the Ochsner Clinic in New Orleans and president of the American Society of Colon and Rectal Surgeons.

Drink a lot of water. Drinking six to eight glasses a day adds bulk to your system and softens stools, says Dr. Gathright. In addition, drinking a lot of water may help reduce some of the stomach discomfort you may experience when starting a high-fiber diet.

Try over-the-counter vitamin creams. To soothe the pain and help heal fissures, try over-the-counter ointments that contain vitamins A and D, suggests Marvin M. Schuster, M.D., chief of the department of digestive diseases at Francis Scott Key Medical Center in Baltimore. Hydrocortisone creams, available at drugstores, are also helpful, adds Dr. Gathright.

Soothe your sit-upon. You can also protect your anal canal by lubricating it before each bowel movement. A gob of petroleum jelly inserted about ½ inch into the rectum may help the stool pass without causing any further damage, advises Edmund Leff, M.D., a proctologist in Phoenix and Scottsdale, Arizona.

Wipe yourself with facial tissue. The best toilet paper isn't toilet paper at all. Facial tissues coated with moisturizing lotion offer the least amount of friction to your fissure-plagued anal area, says Dr. Leff.

Talc yourself up down there. Following each shower or bowel movement, dust yourself with baby powder. This will help keep the area dry, which can help reduce friction throughout the day, says Dr. Schuster.

Angina

When you have angina, your heart has to go begging for fresh oxygen—a task that it hates. This heart complaint occurs because your pumper isn't receiving enough blood and, therefore, is not getting all the oxygen it needs. If you have what doctors call stable angina, challenging activities like fast walking or digging in the garden may cause your overworked heart to start up the protests.

But there's another kind of angina, called unstable angina, in which the heart doesn't get enough blood even when you're doing something as simple as kicking back in a lounge chair or crossing the room.

If you're in your sixties or seventies, don't count on the usual type of chest pain if you have angina, says Gary Francis, M.D., director of the coronary intensive care unit at the Cleveland Clinic Foundation. Instead, you might just feel pressure. Or suddenly, for no apparent reason, you find you're short of breath. And some people experience angina in the form of a squeezing sensation in the chest, as if someone diabolical is tightening a belt around their ribs. Oddest of all, you might have pain in some area that seems completely unrelated to your heart, for instance, in your jaw or even one of your elbows.

The tips below are all about stable angina because the unstable variety is no candidate for home remedies. Here are some steps to stop the pain quickly or prevent it from starting at all.

Stop. If angina comes on during an activity, stop whatever you are doing. Sit down and prop up your feet, says Michael A. Brodsky, M.D., professor of medicine in cardiology at the University of California, Irvine, Medical Center. Don't try to work or push through the pain. Take a few minutes to relax.

"If you stop the activity, the pain should go away," adds Robert March, M.D., associate professor of cardiovascular surgery at Rush-Presbyterian–St. Luke's Medical Center in Chicago.

Don't take it lying down. If you are lying down or sleeping when you have angina pain, sit up or stand up. "Standing up takes the pressure off your heart," Dr. Francis says. When you take the pressure off, your body demands less from your heart, giving it time to recover from the angina episode.

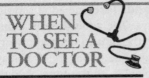

WHEN TO SEE A DOCTOR

If you've had angina pain before and are under a doctor's care, be alert to changes, says Robert March, M.D., associate professor of cardiovascular surgery at Rush-Presbyterian–St. Luke's Medical Center in Chicago. If the pain comes on more frequently with less activity, see your doctor.

Call for immediate medical help if you have pain that lasts more than 10 to 15 minutes and you get no relief from nitroglycerin.

If angina comes on in the middle of the night or when you haven't been doing anything active, you should call your doctor or go to the emergency room.

Breathe deeply. It's not a coincidence that many angina episodes get started when someone's in a tense situation. Stress often precedes a bout with angina, Dr. Francis says. When in the midst of an angina attack, calm down by taking slow, deep breaths. That may help control your stress and stop the pain. Deep breathing, experts explain, is when your abdomen expands outward as you inhale rather than your chest or shoulders rising.

Can the cigarettes. If you are a smoker, you are making it that much harder on your heart, Dr. March says. Cigarette smoke absorbs oxygen out of your blood, and nicotine constricts your blood vessels. That triggers angina because your arteries shrink, and less blood makes it to your heart.

Keep aspirin on hand. Take one adult aspirin tablet a day, Dr. March says. The adult dose is about 325 milligrams. Aspirin is thought to decrease heart damage during an angina episode. While the drug may not prevent an attack of angina all the time, studies show that men with angina who take aspirin are less likely to have heart attacks or die of heart problems than men who don't take aspirin.

Make it a slow morning. Take your time when you get up in the morning, Dr. Francis suggests. Don't hop right out of bed. Stretch, get acclimated to being awake, and give yourself enough time to eat a nice breakfast and read the paper.

Why the early morning slowdown? Because the early hours of the day are the most dangerous for your heart, Dr. Francis says. As people get older, their bodies can't handle the jump-out-of-bed-grab-a-quick-bite-rush-to-work routine, he points out. If you force it in the morning hours, you might put a lot of unnecessary pressure on your heart, and that additional pressure could jump-start an angina attack. "Get up a little more slowly and don't rush around," Dr. Francis says.

Put one foot in front of the other. Walk as much as you can every day. "Walking is the best exercise," Dr. Francis says. The activity keeps your heart healthy, which may help offset angina. Unlike other activities, walking won't put much strain on your heart. If you like other forms of exercise such as swimming or bicycling, go ahead as long as they don't bring on angina, Dr. Francis says. "I encourage physical activity as long as you feel good doing it." Strive for at least 20 minutes three times a week.

Eat light before exercise. Don't have a heavy meal before taking your walk. If you're hungry, munch

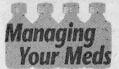

Managing Your Meds

The key medication for angina is nitroglycerin. It is available in two forms. One, such as the patch (Nitro Dur), reduces the number of attacks. The other, like the under-the-tongue tablet (Nitrostat), relieves an attack in progress. Your doctor may advise you to keep the tablet form of nitroglycerin with you at all times and may give you a list of a few precautions.

Nitroglycerin works by dilating blood vessels, which reduces the workload for your heart. But while it's doing this, the medication can also lower your blood pressure very rapidly. When that happens, you're at risk of fainting. So the medication should only be taken while you're sitting down, says Robert March, M.D., associate professor of cardiovascular surgery at Rush-Presbyterian–St. Luke's Medical Center in Chicago. If you feel dizzy or faint, there's no harm done as long as you're not standing or walking around.

Talk to your doctor before mixing nitroglycerin and any of the following medications.

✦ High blood pressure medication like beta-blockers such as metoprolol (Toprol-XL)

✦ Sildenafil (Viagra), a drug used to treat impotence

on a light snack such as an apple, Dr. Francis suggests. If you eat a big meal and then exercise, you are more likely to experience angina pain.

Leave heavy lifting to others. If you have to move something heavy, find someone else to do the job, Dr. March says. Heavy lifting is a common trigger for angina pain in many people, he adds. Even something as simple as lifting a suitcase and carrying it up a flight of stairs can cause angina pain.

Stay by the fireplace. When the weather is ice cold, make it a point to stay inside and stay warm. Below-freezing days provoke angina in some people, Dr. Francis says. "On extremely cold days, it's dangerous for people with angina to go out."

Identify your triggers. What triggers angina is different for each person. "People should learn to identify the activities that provoke angina, then they should avoid those activities," Dr. Francis says. If you can't see an obvious cause, write down the circumstances around each angina episode or just think about exactly what was happening. Over time, you will probably find a pattern, and once you're familiar with that pattern, you may be able to offset future angina attacks. "Listen to your body. It will tell you when angina is going to happen," he says.

Apnea and Snoring

If you snore, you're not alone. The National Sleep Foundation in Washington, D.C., estimates that 40 percent of adult Americans saw logs in their sleep.

But as people age, their sleep becomes lighter and more fragmented. Your spouse's snoring, which you may have been able to put up with 20 years ago, may be too disturbing now. And if you're the snorer, you may even be waking yourself up.

What's more, the snoring may actually be a signal of a more serious problem. If the snoring occurs in loud gasping snorts that may ultimately cause you or your bedmate to stop breathing for brief periods of time, then there's a good chance that snore isn't just a snore—it's sleep apnea.

To avoid confusion, let's define the two right here: Snoring occurs as you inhale during your sleep and the soft tissues of your throat—the uvula and soft palate— vibrate against the back of your throat or tongue.

Sleep apnea, however, occurs when the muscles in the back of your throat relax during sleep. With this relaxation, breathing passages become narrower and may completely obstruct the passage for as long as 60 seconds. This causes a gasping type of snoring that can be serious if it isn't controlled, says Nancy Collop, M.D., pulmonary/critical-care doctor specializing in

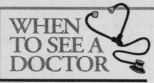

WHEN TO SEE A DOCTOR

Light snoring isn't a serious health problem, but see your doctor if you think you have apnea or if you are excessively sleepy in addition to snoring, says Peter Hauri, M.D., co-director of the Mayo Clinic Sleep Disorders Center in Rochester, Minnesota, and author of *No More Sleepless Nights*. When you have sleep apnea, you actually stop breathing, and this can cause your body to react in such a way that your blood pressure rises. That, in turn, can increase your risk of heart failure. If you do happen to have a severe case of apnea, a doctor can treat it, often with easy-to-use breathing devices.

sleep medicine and associate professor at the Medical University of South Carolina in Charleston.

Apnea puts you at risk for high blood pressure. During apnea, when you obstruct the breathing passage, the levels of oxygen in your blood decrease. Your body treats this as a panic situation and starts pouring hormones into your bloodstream to wake you up or get you breathing again. An unfortunate side effect of this strategy is that the hormones cause your blood pressure to climb. When people with apnea are monitored all night long in sleep labs, researchers have found that their blood pressures go up at a time when blood pressure is normally at its lowest. In fact, that's one way researchers can tell if you have apnea.

"It's clear from research that, in its severe form, apnea produces high blood pressure, heart failure, depression, and mental clouding," says Daniel Kripke, M.D., professor of psychiatry at the University of California, San Diego. For that reason, if you suspect that you have sleep apnea, it's important to see a sleep specialist to determine how serious the problem is.

If it turns out that you do have a less severe apnea or just a serious case of snoring, consider some of these tips to improve your slumber.

Sleep on your side or stomach. If you sleep on your back, your tongue will relax back toward your throat, making it harder to breathe and easier to snore. Try sleeping on your side in a half-sitting position so that doesn't happen, suggests Dr. Kripke. It helps to have your head propped up with thicker pillows or more of them—but the main thing is to sleep on your side or stomach. Sometimes, a well-placed pillow can help you maintain these positions.

Because people move around in their sleep, you might be turning over on your back even if you start out in another position. Dr. Kripke says the easiest way to keep yourself from rolling onto your back is to sew a tennis ball into the back of your pajamas; you'll feel it when you roll onto it. "It's a very inexpensive way to train people not to sleep on their backs," he observes.

Lose some weight. Excessive weight aggravates apnea and snoring. So give yourself an honest appraisal in the mirror: If you have more than one chin on the outside of your neck, Dr. Kripke says, you have fatty deposits on the inside that may be contributing to constricted airways. In fact, if your neck size is greater than 17 inches, you're at greater risk for

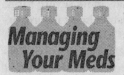

Managing Your Meds

The following types of drugs can all make snoring and sleep apnea worse, according to Daniel Kripke, M.D., professor of psychiatry at the University of California, San Diego. Talk to your doctor if you're taking:

✦ Sleeping pills (either prescription or over-the-counter) such as zolpidem (Ambien), flurazepam (Dalmane), temazepam (Restoril), or triazolam (Halcion)

✦ Sedatives such as diazepam (Valium) or lorazepam (Ativan)

---

apnea. So change to a lower-fat diet and incorporate some exercise into your life to help trim off some of that fat.

Clear the airways. Any type of congestion, from colds to allergies, can aggravate a snoring problem. "The more resistance there is in your nose, the more you have to suck in to breathe," says Dr. Kripke. And that action can cause apnea. You can treat a stuffy nose with a nonaddicting nasal spray that contains cromolyn sodium (Nasalcrom). Use this over-the-counter product before bedtime to help you breathe more easily.

Keep your nostrils spread. For some people, collapsing nostrils are a problem that can be helped with Breathe Right nasal strips. These strips, which are taped over the outside bridge of the nose to keep the nostrils from collapsing, are available at most pharmacies. There's a quick way to see if these strips might be helpful to you, Dr. Kripke says. Stand in front of a mirror, take deep breaths in through your nose, and observe whether the sides of your nostrils get sucked in as you breathe. If they do, you can probably benefit from using the strip since it will help force your nostrils to stay open.

Don't do the dinner drinks. Alcohol has an initial sedating effect, and this can worsen snoring and apnea by increasing muscle relaxation, Dr. Kripke says. So you may want to avoid alcohol in the evening.

Snooze without sleeping pills. If you take sleeping pills, the medication might be contributing to apnea or making snoring worse, Dr. Kripke says. The pills relax your muscles, including those around your tongue and throat.

Humidify the house. A lack of humidity can cause the membranes in your airways to dry out and swell, increasing the potential for one tissue to rub against another and vibrate, says Peter Hauri, M.D., co-director of the Mayo Clinic Sleep Disorders Center in Rochester, Minnesota, and author of *No More Sleepless Nights*. A humidifier in the bedroom can help you remain moist and may help you sleep more quietly.

Check for allergies. Allergies can cause swelling in the airway membranes, Dr. Collop says, leading to more friction, more snoring, and worse apnea. If you know you have allergies, take your medication regularly. If you suspect that allergies may be causing snoring, talk to your doctor about being tested for allergies.

Put down the cigarette. Besides all of the serious health consequences, smoking irritates the nose and throat, causing swelling that can make the vibrations of snoring more likely and make apnea worse, Dr. Hauri says. Kick the habit, and you'll snore less.

Get a good night's sleep. Most people, even seniors, need about eight hours of sleep a night. If you don't get enough, your body has a tendency to make up for a lack of rest by making your sleep deeper the next time you sleep, explains Dr. Collop. In deeper sleep, your muscles become more relaxed, setting the scene for increased snoring. So try to get your full night's rest. If you can't, try to take a nap during the day. You'll be better rested and less apt to snore.

Arthritis

Here's a disease that's so common that nearly one in seven Americans already has it—and a new case is diagnosed every 33 seconds. In fact, arthritis is *the* most widespread chronic disease in people over age 45, even when you consider the untold millions who never see a doctor about that blasted pain in their joints.

When you do see a doctor about that blasted pain, he will usually tell you what kind of arthritis you have. Although there are more than 100 different types, most fall into two broad categories.

Inflammatory arthritis (or rheumatoid arthritis) is best treated with anti-inflammatory drugs, though diet and lifestyle changes may help. Non-inflammatory arthritis (or osteoarthritis) results when cartilage in joints deteriorates from injury or excessive use. Weight control, proper exercise, and pain relievers are the key treatments here.

Although arthritis is potentially crippling, there are things you can do that may help control it. Here's what doctors recommend.

Eat your vegetables. Researchers at the University of Oslo in Norway discovered that people with rheumatoid arthritis who began a vegetarian diet saw dramatic improvements in their conditions within *one month* after cutting out meat, eggs, dairy products, sugar, and foods with gluten, such as wheat bread. "A vegetarian diet is good, because the goal for arthritis sufferers is to cut as much saturated fat from their diets as possible and replace it with more polyunsaturated fat," says Paul Caldron, D.O., a clinical rheumatologist and researcher at the Arthritis Center in Phoenix.

Try something fishy. One of the best sources of polyunsaturated fat is cold-water fish such as salmon, sardines, and herring. "They are rich in omega-3 fatty acids, which have been shown to have some minor beneficial effect on reducing the inflammatory aspects of arthritis," says Dr. Caldron.

Get hot on hot-pepper cream. Research shows you can ease the pain by rubbing the joint with an over-the-counter ointment called Zostrix, made from capsaicin—the stuff that puts the hot in hot peppers. "You need to apply it three or four times a day on the affected area for at least two weeks before you'll see any improvement. An initial burning sensation at the site is not unusual for the first few days, but this goes away with continued application," says Esther Lipstein

Remedies for Your Specific Aches

From head to toe, there are specific arthritis treatments for specific body parts, according to Paul Caldron, D.O., a clinical rheumatologist and researcher at the Arthritis Center in Phoenix.

Give your neck a break. Don't extend your neck by looking up for long periods. If you're painting, hanging curtains, or doing other work that requires you to look up for a long time, get a ladder and bring yourself to the same level as the work.

Support your shoulders. Don't sleep with your arms over your head, because that strains your shoulders. Dr. Caldron advises women to lighten their handbags so that they carry *only* what they need. And big-busted women are advised to get bras with more support to ease shoulder strain.

Glove your hands. Wear gloves with a thick palm padding—like work gloves—whenever you're holding

---

Kresch, M.D., an assistant professor of medicine at the Albert Einstein College of Medicine of Yeshiva University in New York City who has studied the effectiveness of capsaicin cream. "I also advise washing your hands immediately after you apply it—or even wearing gloves when you apply it—because it can sting, and you don't want to get it in your eyes." (Sorry, but eating hot peppers won't help relieve arthritis.)

Use a dehumidifier. If the humidity is kept constant in your house, it can help calm arthritis pain caused by weather changes, says Joseph Hollander, M.D., professor emeritus of medicine at the University of Penn-

something tightly. With thick gloves, you don't have to exert as much force on the hand joints to hold a heavy skillet, a broom, or a wrench. Also, you can build up handles of tools and garden supplies with foam rubber padding or terry cloth, so you're exerting less force on the joints.

Never squat or kneel. That's about the worst thing you can do to arthritic knee and hip joints.

Wear running or walking shoes whenever possible. To ease the pressure on aching feet, you want footwear that provides comfort and support. When shopping for dressier footwear, look for shoes that have a wide toe box and good, built-in arch support.

The best shoes have heels approximately one to 1½ inches high, and they come up high on the instep. For men, a lace-up oxford, as opposed to a slip-on, is the preferable dress shoe.

sylvania Hospital in Philadelphia. When rain is on the way, the sudden increase in humidity and decrease in air pressure can affect blood flow to arthritic joints, which become increasingly stiff until the storm actually starts. If you close the windows and turn on a dehumidifier—or run the air conditioning in summer—you may be able to eliminate this short-term but significant pain.

Stay active. "Probably the most important thing you can do for osteoarthritis is exercise as much as you're able to," says Halsted R. Holman, M.D., director and professor of medicine at the Stanford University Arthritis Center in Stanford, California. "You'll find that the better your physical condition, the less arthritis pain you'll have."

Dr. Caldron recommends low-impact aerobic exercises and, if tolerated, very light weight lifting with one- to two-pound dumbbells. "Build up the muscle and tissue surrounding the joint," he suggests. "You can exercise on a floor mat, in a chair, on a stationary bicycle, or in the water. The key is regularity, doing it no less than three times a week but preferably daily."

Learn your food "triggers." "Some people with rheumatoid arthritis seem to have flare-ups after eating certain foods—especially alcohol, milk, tomatoes, and certain nuts," says Dr. Caldron. "Although there's really no telling what your trigger might be, if you notice your condition worsens after eating a certain food, then listen to your body and avoid that food." The same goes for foods that improve arthritis, such as fish and fiber; try to eat them more regularly.

Take time to smell the roses. When you're tensed up, you hurt more. "Many people use relaxation as an effective way of diminishing arthritis pain," says Dr. Holman. "It really doesn't matter what you do—biofeedback, meditation, even listening to music—whatever helps you relax. The point is to practice a regular relaxation period and then also to use relaxation when pain is particularly severe."

Slim down. "Being overweight can enhance damage to joints by putting excess pressure on them, resulting in worsening osteoarthritis, so I advise losing any excess weight you're carrying," says Richard M. Pope, M.D., an arthritis researcher and chief of arthritis/connective tissue diseases at Northwestern University Medical School in Chicago. In fact, being overweight increases your risk of developing osteoarthritis, even if you don't have it now.

Try slow dancing. Dancing is a good way to combine weight loss, exercise, and stress reduction. "Many of my patients participate in easy dance routines created as part of an overall education and activity program that shows them how to exercise while protecting their affected joints," adds Dr. Pope. "Easy, slow dancing is perfect for those with inflammatory arthritis, or osteoarthritis, because it's low impact."

Reach for the "right" pain reliever. Not all pain relievers are the same—at least for those with arthritis. "People with inflammatory arthritis should get more relief from aspirin or ibuprofen (Advil) but may get more stomach irritation with these," says Dr. Caldron. For over-the-counter pain relief without stomach irritation, he recommends acetaminophen (Tylenol). Recommended doses of these drugs should not be exceeded nor should regular dosing be continued for more than three weeks without consulting your physician.

Immobilize the pain. "Splints, slings, cervical collars, and other protective devices are extremely useful when an area is particularly painful or inflamed," says Dr. Caldron. But he cautions that you can't leave these devices on for more than two days at a time. Even though these devices help reduce pain, your muscles can "rely" on them and weaken very quickly.

Use ice and heat judiciously. Although both ice packs and heat packs can provide some relief, don't use either for more than 10 minutes at a time, advises Dr. Caldron. Usually ice is used to prevent swelling but may also douse pain; heat in small doses may promote muscle relaxation and soothe pain.

Asthma

Of the 13 million Americans who have asthma, 1.5 million of them are 65 or older. Asthma in the over-60 set doesn't pose any more health dangers than it does for the rest of the population. In fact, when asthma is controlled with medication and lifestyle changes, people of any age should be able to lead full and active lives.

But the risk that asthma poses to older folks is that it can mimic and complicate other serious health problems. The symptoms of asthma—wheezing, coughing, shortness of breath, and chest tightness—are similar to symptoms of emphysema, bronchitis, and even heart disease, which may also cause breathing problems.

Without tests, it may be difficult for the doctor to diagnose asthma in people over 60. One tip-off is that the symptoms occur after someone is exposed to a trigger, says Henry Gong Jr., M.D., professor of medicine in the division of pulmonary and critical-care medicine environmental health service at the University of Southern California School of Medicine in Downey. A trigger is something that irritates the airways, causing them to get inflamed and swell, which narrows the air passages.

Know your enemy. Strong odors and exposure to chemicals tend to cause more problems for older people with asthma. Whatever aggravates your asthma, stay away from it, says Karin Pacheco, M.D., physician in the division of occupational and environmental medicine at the National Jewish Center for Immunology

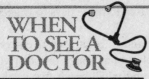

WHEN TO SEE A DOCTOR

People with asthma usually develop a sense of what is normal and what needs attention, says Joe W. Ramsdell, M.D., head of the general internal medicine and geriatrics division at the University of California, San Diego, School of Medicine. But get in touch with your doctor if:

■ Your symptoms become more intense or frequent than they used to be.

■ You wake up almost every night with attacks.

■ You find that you need to use your inhaler or any short-acting medicine more than four times a day.

■ Your inhaler doesn't seem to be working for you.

and Respiratory Medicine in Denver. Although every person may have a different set of triggers, some common potential problems include cold air, tobacco and wood smoke, perfume, paint, hairspray, room deodorizers, cleaning chemicals, and talcum powder.

Follow pollution reports. For older people with asthma, pollution is more likely to trigger an episode, explains Dr. Pacheco. Many television and radio stations now track pollution and air quality. Use these reports and then plan your day accordingly.

If the pollution is high, stay indoors and keep the air conditioner on (weather permitting), Dr. Pacheco recommends. You may not get asthma symptoms on the very day that pollution is high, she warns. Pollutants can take two to three days to trigger an asthma attack.

Roam the produce aisle. Eat at least five servings of fruits and vegetables a day. Have one or two servings with each meal, and you'll reach five easily. Fruits and vegetables are loaded with antioxidants including vitamins C and E, chemicals that may protect your lungs from an asthma attack, says Gary E. Hatch, Ph.D., researcher and pharmacologist in the U.S. Environmental Protection Agency Pulmonary Toxicology Branch in Research Triangle Park, North Carolina.

Seek supplements for extra protection. To be sure you keep those antioxidant levels up, take 500 milligrams of vitamin C and 400 international units (IU) of vitamin E a day, Dr. Hatch says. These supplements may be especially beneficial as you get older, especially if you have asthma, according to Dr. Hatch. Researchers at the University of Washington in Seattle found that taking 500 milligrams of C and 400 IU of vitamin E helped people with asthma breathe easier when exposed to pollutants. Although vitamin E is generally sold in doses of 400 IU, one small study showed a possible risk of stroke in dosages higher than 200 IU. Consult with your doctor if you are at high risk for stroke.

Deactivate the acid. When stomach acid backs up into the esophagus in a process called acid reflux, it causes heartburn. It may also cause an asthma attack. The esophagus contains nerves that connect to your lungs and airways. Researchers think that those nerves may send signals that unleash an asthma attack when the reflux triggers the symptoms. "If you take care of acid reflux, asthma gets better," Dr. Gong says. To keep acid reflux to a minimum, follow these simple tips.

◆ Eat smaller but more frequent meals throughout the day.

◆ Don't eat heavy late-night snacks before bed.

◆ Put bricks underneath the bed legs near your head so you lie at a 45-degree angle while sleeping. Lying flat causes acid to work its way back into your esophagus.

◆ Ask your doctor about over-the-counter acid-suppressing drugs such as famotidine (Pepcid AC) and ranitidine (Zantac).

Dust out dust mites. Among older people, allergies caused by dust mites aren't a common problem, yet they can still trigger asthma in some cases, Dr. Gong says. These barely microscopic bugs thrive on dust and humidity. To keep their numbers down, follow these basic tips.

◆ Clean often with a damp mop or cloth.

◆ Wash your bedding in water that is at least 130°F.

◆ Encase pillows and mattresses in airtight covers that keep dust mites out.

◆ Use window shades or blinds instead of curtains.

While you'll never be able to completely get rid of the dust mites, these practices can help keep them under control and may rescue you from an attack of asthma.

Vacuum into the light. When trying to figure out what triggered his own asthma, Dr. Hatch suspected that his old vacuum cleaner might be a culprit. So he turned his vacuum cleaner upside down under a strong light in a dark room and hit the power switch. Clouds of dust and irritants spewed out. "Under the

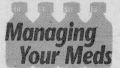

Managing Your Meds

Many medications can help treat asthma. The key approach to treatment of persistent asthma is the use of anti-inflammatory agents, especially corticosteroids. These include triamcinolone (Azmacort) and beclomethasone (Vanceril), drugs that prevent the asthma attack and the airways from closing up. But these medications have many possible side effects, says Michael S. Stulbarg, M.D., professor of clinical medicine and director of the clinical pulmonary center at the University of California, San Francisco.

For some people, the medications may speed up the onset of osteoporosis—bone loss—and also glaucoma. Two other classifications are leukotriene antagonists such as zafirlukast (Accolate) and mast cell inhibitors such as cromolyn (Intal). These medications do not have significant side effects and may be used over the long term to manage asthma. But they are not useful to stop an asthma attack.

Another group of medicines are inhaled bronchodilators such as albuterol (Proventil) and salmeterol (Serevent), which are used during an asthma attack to open the airways by relaxing the bronchial muscles. Some people may experience nervousness or trembling with these medications.

Other kinds of medications can actually make asthma worse. Talk to your doctor before taking the following:

✦ Aspirin

✦ Blood pressure medications known as beta-blockers, such as propranolol (Inderal)

✦ Beta-blocker eyedrops such as betaxolol (Betoptic) and carteolol (Ocupress) that are used to treat glaucoma

light, you can see all of the dust blowing out into the air," he says.

Try this light test with your own vacuum. If you see dust spurting out, change the bag. If that doesn't help, it may be time to invest in another vacuum cleaner. Look for one that has anti-allergenic features like special bags or a HEPA filter, says Dr. Hatch.

Backache

Considering all the grief and bother it causes people, back pain ranks right up there with the common cold. And like the common cold, which responds just as well to chicken soup as to antibiotics, "treating chronic low back pain effectively requires the consistent use of seemingly simple remedies, not rocket science methods," says Brent V. Lovejoy, D.O., an occupational medicine specialist in Denver and a medical consultant to the construction industry.

Only about 20 percent of acute back pain can be traced to some obvious cause, such as a herniated disk. So most back pain is considered a "mechanical" problem. And it's not all that easy to diagnose.

"Check with 10 different doctors and you will get 10 different opinions as to exactly where in the back this pain originates," says Scott Haldeman, M.D., D.C., Ph.D., associate clinical professor in the department of neurology at the University of California,

Irvine, and adjunct professor at the Los Angeles Chiropractic College. Muscle spasms, jammed back joints, and stretched ligaments have all been implicated.

What is known for sure is that in addition to having a medical evaluation, there are lots of things you can do for yourself, both to ease flare-ups and to ward off future backaches. In fact, a few of these things are so important that doctors who treat back pain successfully consider them *essential*, not optional!

Raise your fitness level. "If you have a back injury that does not require surgery, studies indicate your aerobic capacity level is the single most important predictor of getting better," Dr. Lovejoy says. In other words, if you're physically fit, you're much more likely to recover.

That's why daily aerobic exercise is the "treatment of choice" in the view of Dr. Lovejoy and many other doctors. "For the construction workers I treat, I recommend brisk walking with hand weights and strength training with free weights," Dr. Lovejoy says. Adds Dr. Haldeman: "Do anything and everything that you can do comfortably and continuously."

Cushion your dogs. The pounding stress that running, and even just walking, normally produces is transmitted right up your back. And for a weak back, that can mean pain.

"Shoes designed specifically to absorb shock, such as running shoes, or special shock-absorbing inserts available at sporting goods stores may reduce back pain," says researcher Arkady Voloshin, Ph.D., professor of engineering in the department of mechanical engineering and mechanics at Lehigh University in Bethlehem, Pennsylvania. In one study, Dr. Voloshin found that 80 percent of back pain sufferers reported rapid and significant relief when they switched from basic street shoes to lightweight, flexible-soled shoes with simple shock-absorbing cushions.

Get horizontal—then get going. Rest, not exercise, is what most doctors recommend *initially* for acute back pain. "But we tell people that in order to get their circulation going, they need to be up and walking around for 45 minutes of every three hours," Dr. Lovejoy says. "Otherwise, they stiffen up like a board, and everything they do hurts."

Don't overdo a rest stop. More than two days' bed rest may not be helpful, according to Richard A. Deyo, M.D., D.P.H., professor in the departments of medicine and health services at the University of Washington in Seattle.

He found that back pain sufferers who were advised to stay in bed just two days missed 45 percent fewer days of work during the following three months than patients advised to rest for a full week. Muscles may weaken quickly with bed rest, and weak muscles can perpetuate an aching back.

Turn to aspirin, Advil, or Tylenol. Any over-the-counter painkiller that contains aspirin, ibuprofen (Advil), or acetaminophen (Tylenol) could ease your back pain, according to Dr. Haldeman. But don't use painkillers before the fact. "If you know you are going to have back pain if you do something such as running, it's better not to do the activity than to mask your pain with drugs," says Dr. Haldeman. And do not give aspirin to children because of the risk of Reye's syndrome.

Get a posture check. Neither a fence post nor a spaghetti noodle be. An erect but *relaxed* stance, both standing and sitting, puts the least stress on back muscles, experts say.

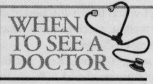

WHEN TO SEE A DOCTOR

"Seventy to 90 percent of back pain goes away either by itself or with some minor home treatment," says Scott Haldeman, M.D., D.C., Ph.D., associate clinical professor in the department of neurology at the University of California, Irvine, and adjunct professor at the Los Angeles Chiropractic College.

See a doctor if your back pain doesn't improve after three days—or if the pain is so bad you can't budge from the bed. You'll also need a doctor's advice if your legs are weak or numb or if back pain is accompanied by fever. Other call-the-doctor symptoms include stomach cramps, chest pain, and difficulty breathing.

In some cases, back pain may be associated with loss of bowel or bladder control. This demands immediate attention: It may indicate a severely herniated disk or spinal cord or nerve damage.

Find your most restful position. Is your lower back acting up? Try this relaxation tactic: Lie on the floor with your knees bent at a 90° angle and your calves resting on the seat of a chair. "This position reduces pressure in your back more than anything else," Dr. Haldeman says. "Most people find it very comfortable."

Warm up your muscles before you hit high gear. Like old rubber bands, stiff muscles can fray when they're stretched by sudden movement. So warm up first with a few minutes of relaxed walking. Swing your hips and arms as you walk, then try a few slow side-to-side twists. If you're planning a specific activity, such as a golf swing, go through the motion several times, slowly, before you add speed and force.

Try some aqua- and yoga-laxation. Water exercises, especially an arthritis range-of-motion program, are a safe and effective way to knock the rust off back muscles that haven't been stretched for a while, says Dr. Haldeman.

Check with your doctor, hospital, or health center to find out where these programs are offered. Many people with back problems benefit from yoga, too, according to Dr. Haldeman—provided they begin slowly and advance according to their tolerance and ability.

Roll on a tennis ball. It's possible to relieve pain with acupressure or "trigger point" treatment using a tennis ball, says Robert King, co-director of the Chicago School of Massage Therapy and a nationally certified massage therapist. (He also recommends some of the wooden "pain relievers" designed for people who have aches and pains—such as a Backnobber.)

For the tennis ball treatment, lie on a hard surface and position the tennis ball under you so that it is pressing against a tender spot. Roll onto the ball gradually, utilizing your body weight until the pain and tenderness subside.

To decrease back pain, don't smoke. Experimental work has shown that smoking reduces the amount of oxygen that travels, via osmosis, to spinal disks at night while you sleep. "If you smoke a pack of cigarettes a day, you'll probably double the amount of back pain you would have if you didn't smoke," Dr. Lovejoy says.

Ice it up. To get ready for a gentle icing, first freeze some water in a small paper cup. When you're ready to use it, Dr. Haldeman says, peel back the side of the cup to expose about ½ inch or so of ice. Lie on your stomach with a towel on your back and have a friend or spouse massage your aching spots with the ice. (The ice should not be applied directly to the skin.) You can also lie down on your back with your knees bent and slide a bag of crushed ice (wrapped in a wet towel) under the sore spot, Dr. Lovejoy says.

Warm up the ache. A heating pad or hot water bottle can help. Or simply curl up in front of a hot wood stove to ease your aches. How do you decide whether your aching back needs heat or cold? "You pick one or the other, try it for a while and see if it helps," Dr. Haldeman says.

Bedsores

A bedsore, otherwise known as a pressure ulcer, starts as just a red spot on the skin. It occurs when you sit or lie in a single position for so long that the sheer weight of your body pinches off blood flow to a certain area.

Usually, the danger spots are bony areas of the body, especially the hips, buttocks, and heels. If blood flow is cut off long enough, the affected skin can blister, deteriorate, and die. Left untreated, the sore can break through the skin and then extend through fat, into muscle, and finally expose bone.

Anyone who is confined to a bed or wheelchair, especially someone who has suffered paralysis or a stroke, is in danger of developing a pressure ulcer, says Mitchell Kaminski Jr., M.D., staff surgeon at Thorek Hospital and Medical Center and clinical professor of surgery at the Finch University of Health Sciences/The Chicago Medical School. But you can minimize that danger.

Get a good pressure-relieving mattress. Try to keep the person on a mattress or cushion that distributes his weight more evenly, such as an air mattress, says Dr. Kaminski. "There are many kinds available, but a regular air mattress that you use at a lake or the beach can be used to help support a person who is bedridden." Be sure it's thickly covered with an airy cotton blanket and sheets to prevent sweating. Sponge mattresses and waterbeds are also good choices.

Other experts recommend using cotton padding or wool to soften the mattress. The extra padding should be evenly distributed, however, to prevent it from bunching and increasing the likelihood of pinched blood vessels.

Move around in bed. "You have to rotate the person's body throughout the day," says Dr. Kaminski. "The person should be shifted at least once an hour, just to relieve the pressure on any area of the body." Not only is this an essential way to keep bedsores from worsening once they start but it's also one of the best ways to prevent them. Be sure to reposition the person so that pressure is relieved from any reddened area on the body.

Maintain good nutrition. "In a scientific study of nursing home patients, we have never found a pressure ulcer in anyone who was well-nourished," Dr.

Kaminski said. "Along with pressure, malnutrition is the single biggest co-factor in the creation of bedsores."

Keep that from happening by getting your loved one the minimum daily requirement for protein, which is two to three servings of meat, poultry, fish, or eggs a day. A serving is two to three ounces of meat, poultry, or fish (which is a piece that's about the size of a deck of cards) or two or three eggs, says Dr. Kaminski.

In addition, doctors recommend that people eat six to 11 servings of unprocessed whole grains, two to four servings of fresh fruits, and three to five servings of vegetables a day.

Choose your oils wisely. If you're preparing food for someone who is bedridden, be careful about the kinds of oils that may be in the foods, according to

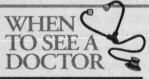

WHEN TO SEE A DOCTOR

Bedsores can develop into infection. Be alert to common signals such as odor, pus, drainage from the wound, or fever. If you note any of these, check with your doctor. He may want to prescribe antibiotics to assist healing. The doctor may also want to remove, or debride, dead tissue that surrounds a bedsore, says Mary Ruth Buchness, M.D., chief of dermatology at St. Vincent's Hospital and Medical Center in New York City and associate professor of dermatology and medicine at New York Medical College in Valhalla.

Dr. Kaminski. "Omega-3 oils, which are found in fish, canola oil, and flaxseed oil, lower blood cholesterol and support good circulation," Dr. Kaminski says. Avoid using corn or safflower oil in your cooking, because such oils can enhance inflammation, which decreases blood circulation and can increase bedsore risk, he adds.

Supplement against sores. Dr. Kaminski encourages people who are at risk for bedsores to take a multivitamin that contains vitamins C and E and beta-carotene. These are antioxidants that can speed healing.

Maximize blood flow to existing pressure ulcers. Make sure there is no pressure on any area where a pressure ulcer already exists, warns Mary Ruth Buchness, M.D., chief of dermatology at St. Vincent's Hospital and Medical Center in New York City and associate professor of dermatology and medicine at New York Medical College in Valhalla. If an ulcer appears on the heel, suspend the heel by raising the lower leg with pillows or soft blankets, she recommends. Once pressure is relieved, blood will flow to the existing wound and aid healing.

Make the wound moist. To help speed healing, cover any existing sores with gauze bandages coated in petroleum jelly or similar moist, thick ointment. This encourages tissues to grow rapidly, says Dr. Buchness. There are special dressings such as Duoderm and Vigilon, which are available through your pharmacist, that dissolve into the wound and create a good environment for healing.

Keep the healthy skin dry. "Keep the wound moist and the surrounding skin dry," suggests Dr. Kaminski. Healthy skin that is allowed to remain moist is more susceptible to developing a sore and an open wound. For patients who are incontinent, undergarments must be changed when needed in order to keep skin dry.

Keep the wounds clean. Pressure ulcers have to be kept clean in order to avoid infection and to heal properly. "Rinse the wound and surrounding skin with soap and water," says Dr. Kaminski. Do not use cleansing solutions containing disinfectants, such as povidone-iodine. Disinfectants generally slow the healing process.

Blisters

You've heard of body language? Well, consider blisters more like body *profanity*—the skin's response to getting too much friction. Don't believe it? Just try to break in a new pair of shoes and you'll end up with an (*expletive deleted*) friction blister on your heel. Or spend too much time raking leaves and you'll curse the fat blisters that show up on the palms of your hands.

But since there will always be new shoes to break in and lawns in need of care, there will always be blisters—unless you take some precautions. So here's how to banish that blister before it articulates new meanings for the nastiest four-letter word of all—pain. Let's start with the most prevalent kind—foot blisters.

Give your feet a lube job. "Blisters are the result of too much friction. To avoid some of that friction and prevent a blister, liberally rub Vaseline over your feet," says Robert Diamond, D.P.M., a Pennsylvania podiatrist affiliated with Muhlenberg Hospital Center in Bethlehem

The Right Way to "Pop" Blisters

Some doctors say that leaving a blister alone will reduce the risk of secondary infection. Others say that if a blister hurts, you should prick it with a pin to drain the water or blood that builds up under the "roof" of the skin. Draining it, they say, will ease the pain.

Since blisters usually hurt, most folks vote to pop—but often do it wrong and risk infection. Here's the proper procedure.

"One of the biggest mistakes people make is to pull off the skin from the top of the blister," says Rodney Basler, M.D., a dermatologist and assistant professor of internal medicine at the University of Nebraska Medical Center in Omaha. Instead, he suggests a specific procedure that has been proven to be most effective: After pushing the fluid to one end of the "bubble," prick the blister on the side containing the fluid, using a pin that's been sterilized with alcohol, a lighted match, or boiling water. The pin should prick the blister horizontally, just above the skin. Dr. Basler suggests doing it three times—when you first see the blister, again 12 hours later, and then 12 hours after that.

The buildup of fluid *does* cause pain, and by removing *all* the fluid, you reduce the pain. But remember: To avoid infection, always sterilize the needle with a flame, alcohol, or boiling water before lancing your blister, says Dr. Basler.

and St. Luke's Hospital of Allentown. "If the shoe doesn't fit correctly and your foot is slipping, the Vaseline will give you better glide, so there's less friction—and therefore less chance of developing a friction blister."

Quit the cotton. Sorry, but much-ballyhooed cotton sweat socks don't offer the best protection against blisters. In fact, sports podiatrists say that man-made acrylic socks are best for preventing blisters. "Cotton fiber becomes abrasive with repeated use, and it also compresses and loses its shape and 'cushion' when wet," says Douglas Richie Jr., D.P.M., clinical instructor of podiatry at Los Angeles County University of Southern California Medical Center in Los Angeles. According to Dr. Richie, "The shape of the sock is critical when it's inside a shoe." So a sock that loses its shape is just what your blister-vulnerable foot *doesn't* need.

Silken your skin. "Wearing a silk undersock can help prevent foot blisters and relieve the pain once you get them, since silk is less damaging to the skin than other fabrics," says Nicholas J. Lowe, M.D., clinical professor of dermatology at the University of California, Los Angeles, School of Medicine and director of the Skin Research Foundation of California in Santa Monica.

Use powder power. Rubbing baby powder on your feet *before* any blister-promoting activity is another good preventer. "Make powdering part of your daily routine," says Richard Cowin, D.P.M., director of Cowin Foot Clinic of Orlando, Florida. Reason: Like petroleum jelly, it helps reduce friction and eases glide.

Put new footwear in your handbag. "Probably the biggest cause of foot blisters in women comes from trying to break in a new pair of shoes," says dermatologist Joseph Bark, M.D., past chairman of the department of dermatology at St. Joseph's Hospital in Lexington, Kentucky. "My advice to women who get a new pair of shoes? Wear them for only 30 minutes at a time. It's all right to wear the shoes several times a day, but only for 30 minutes—at least for the first few days." (So carry an extra pair of broken-in shoes in your handbag and trade off a few times during the day.)

Pad it with moleskin. A moleskin pad (available at most drugstores) is the best *preventive* measure for the blister-prone, and it's also great for relieving pain once the blister forms. Cut the moleskin into a doughnut shape and place it over the blister (or the area where you're prone to get it). "Leave the central area open over the blister," advises Suzanne Tanner, M.D., assistant professor of orthopedics at the University of Colorado Sportsmedicine Center in Denver. The surrounding moleskin will absorb the shock and friction that cause or aggravate blisters.

Try a heel lift. Blisters on the back of the foot? They could be blamed on the heel counter—the tough shoe leather that covers your heel. If the counter rubs the wrong area of your foot, you'll have blister trouble fast. The fix? "All you usually have to do is put in a heel lift," says Dr. Cowin. Make sure to use the same size heel lift in both shoes unless advised differently by your doctor, even if only one heel is blistering.

Use an insole. To avoid blisters on the heel and other parts of the foot, many doctors recommend a Spenco insole. These store-bought inserts cut down on friction to prevent new blisters and help ease the pain of existing ones, says Dr. Diamond.

Soak 'em in Epsom. "If you perspire too much, you're more prone to getting blisters," adds Dr. Diamond. "If that's your problem, soaking feet in Epsom salts can help dry excessive sweating." Dissolve Epsom salts in warm water and soak your feet for about five minutes at the end of the day. Then dry thoroughly.

Give a double dose of healing gel. Research shows that triple antibiotic ointments can eliminate bacterial contamination after *two* applications. Neosporin and other nonprescription antibiotic ointments are sold in all drugstores. Avoid old standbys such as iodine and camphor-phenol, because they delay healing. After applying the antibiotic, you should cover the area with a gauze pad—but change that covering each time it gets wet to avoid contamination.

For hands—try a combination play. If your problem is hand blisters rather than foot blisters, the Epsom salts relief can be a big help. Also, wear heavy-duty work gloves whenever you have yard work to do. Another way to prevent blisters on your hands: Follow the advice of Dr. Cowin and rub some baby powder on your hands.

Bronchitis

It may produce some of the nastiest-looking phlegm you've ever seen, but bronchitis's bark is usually worse than its bite. Granted, it's quite a bark, as mucous membranes lining the air passages in your chest become irritated. To soothe the irritation, your body makes secretions to coat the airways. This produces a buildup of gunk in your lungs, which must be cleared by your coughing and sputtering more than a '67 Rambler in dire need of a tune-up.

Like the common cold, bronchitis affects most everyone sometime in his life. Acute cases are usually caused by a virus and will clear up on their own in a week or two. Chronic cases, however, are almost always caused by smoking—either your own habit or long-term exposure to secondhand smoke—and these cases may last for months. Bronchitis may also cause soreness, tightness, or wheezing in the chest as well as chills, fatigue, or a slight fever. But here's how to quiet all your symptoms.

Liquefy the problem. "Drinking fluids may help the mucus become more watery and easier to cough up,"

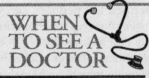

WHEN TO SEE A DOCTOR

Bronchitis is usually not a serious problem, but you should see your doctor if:

▧ Your cough doesn't improve, or it worsens after one week. (Sometimes the only way to distinguish bronchitis from pneumonia is with an x-ray.)

▧ You are coughing up blood.

▧ You are elderly and get a hacking cough on top of another illness.

▧ You are short of breath and have a very profuse cough.

▧ You have a very high fever (over 101°F) *or* one that lasts more than three days.

says Barbara Phillips, M.D., associate professor of pulmonary medicine at the University of Kentucky Medical Center in Lexington. Four to six glasses is probably plenty.

And while warm liquids like Mom's chicken soup may make you feel better, a cool glass of water, juice, or any other nonalcoholic beverage works just as well. "All beverages are the same temperature inside your body," says Douglas Holsclaw, M.D., professor of pediatrics and director of the Pediatric Pulmonary and Cystic Fibrosis Center at Hahnemann University Hospital in Philadelphia. To avoid losing fluids from your body, doctors advise staying away from booze, because it can actually cause dehydration. Also avoid caffeinated products such as coffee, tea, and cola, because they make you urinate more, and you may actually lose more fluids than you gain.

Reach for the red pepper. Hot peppers, curry, and other spicy foods that make your eyes water or nose run can help bring an early end to bronchitis. "Hot, spicy foods help mucous membranes all over, not just in your nose, to secrete more liquids, which can help thin mucus," says Varro E. Tyler, Ph.D., distinguished professor emeritus at Purdue University in West Lafayette, Indiana, and author of *The Honest Herbal*. The advantage of thinner mucus is that it's easier to cough up.

Get away from cigarettes. Even being near someone who smokes can make bronchitis worse or cause return episodes. "You need to avoid all tobacco smoke," says Dr. Phillips. "Even if you don't smoke but you're exposed to exhaled smoke, you are doing what's called passive smoking, and that can give you bronchitis."

If you do smoke, quitting is the most important thing you can do, since this habit has been linked to as many as 95 percent of all cases of chronic bronchitis. "Your bronchitis will improve when you stop smoking," says Gordon Snider, M.D., chief of medical service at Boston Veterans Administration Medical Center. Some new ex-smokers experience increased coughing and sputum production for a week or two after quitting, adds Dr. Phillips. This is actually a good sign—the airways are sweeping out a lot of accumulated secretions. Symptoms usually subside after two to four weeks.

Plug in the vaporizer. "If you have mucus that is thick or difficult to cough up, a vaporizer will help loosen the secretions," adds Dr. Phillips. If you don't have a vaporizer, either run a hot shower with the bathroom door closed or fill the sink with hot water, put a towel over your head and the sink to create a tent, and inhale the steam for five to 10 minutes every couple of hours, suggests Dr. Snider.

Don't rely on expectorants. Over-the-counter cough medicines may suppress your cough—the opposite of what you want. Besides, there's no evidence that they help dry up mucus. You'll get better—and cheaper—results by drinking lots of liquids.

Bruises

If you studied the history of your bruises over the last 60 years or so, it would be a book with many black-and-blue pages. And if you're somewhat older and somewhat more bruise-prone than you were in your youth, it may seem like you're adding a page a day. And maybe you are. That's because you tend to bruise more as you grow older.

When we start to get up there in years, we simply have less protection under the skin than we did in the past, says Mitchell Kaminski Jr., M.D., staff surgeon at Thorek Hospital and Medical Center and clinical professor of surgery at the Finch University of Health Sciences/The Chicago Medical School. "As we age, the layers of fat and connective tissues beneath our skin become thinner," he says. And that means those layers provide less of a cushion for blood vessels, making the vessels more susceptible to injury.

Most bruises do not pose a serious health risk and do not require any special treatment, says Dr. Kaminski. Still, there are ways to prevent bruising and several things you can do to promote healing once you suffer a bruise.

Curb the blues with RICE. The quickest way to control bruising is with a combination of four methods. RICE is an easy way to remember the pain-relieving sequence—rest, ice, compression, and elevation.

♦ Rest.

♦ Ice the injured spot.

♦ Apply compression.

♦ Elevate the limb.

Rest gives injured tissues a better chance to heal; ice constricts the blood vessels around the injury so less blood leaks into the tissues. Compression and elevation help drain blood from the injured area.

Apply ice as soon as possible after the injury occurs. Wrap the ice pack in a towel to keep it from contacting your skin directly and keep it in place for about 15 minutes. Then let your skin warm before you

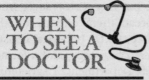

WHEN TO SEE A DOCTOR

Sometimes, bruises are indications of serious illnesses such as blood disorders, says Mitchell Kaminski Jr., M.D., staff surgeon at Thorek Hospital and Medical Center and clinical professor of surgery at the Finch University of Health Sciences/The Chicago Medical School. If you have bruises that appear without any seeming cause, you should talk to your doctor.

Also see your doctor if:

■ The bruise occurs at a joint and is accompanied by swelling.

■ The bruise occurs above the ear on the side of your head, which is an area that is susceptible to fractures.

■ The bruising is accompanied by a fever.

reapply the ice. You can ice the bruise four or five times the first day. After 24 hours, switch to heat to improve circulation to the bruised area, says Arthur K. Balin, M.D., medical director of the Sally Balin Medical Center for Dermatology and Cosmetic Surgery in Media, Pennsylvania, and co-author of *The Life of the Skin*.

Gently but securely wrap the bruise with an elastic bandage as soon after you injure yourself as possible, advises Dr. Balin. Then elevate your limb as much as possible for the first 24 hours. The pressure and elevation will help stop the blood from flowing into the tissues and will minimize the size of the bruise.

Sprinkle on some parsley. Crush some fresh parsley leaves, then spread them directly on the bruise, advises James Duke, Ph.D., botanical consultant, author of *The Green Pharmacy*, and a former ethnobotanist with the U.S. Department of Agriculture who specializes in medicinal plants. Parsley can promote healing and clear up black-and-blue marks within a day or so, he says. Hold the leaves in place with an adhesive bandage or with gauze and tape.

Reach for the citrus. Vitamin C and substances called bioflavonoids that are in oranges and other citrus fruits strengthen capillary walls. As the blood vessels get stronger, they're less prone to leakage, so there's less bruising, says Dr. Duke. Also, he says that both vitamin C and bioflavonoids promote more rapid healing of capillaries after they are damaged. To help prevent bruises, make sure you eat some citrus fruit every day.

Try a multivitamin. If bruises show up without much apparent cause, maybe you're just not getting enough vitamin C from your diet, says Dr. Kaminski. If so, be sure you get a supplement, he advises. "I recommend that people take a multivitamin to ensure that they're getting the basic requirements for the vitamins they need."

Go easy on aspirin. If you take aspirin for any reason, it could be contributing to the number of bruises you're getting, says Dr. Balin. "There is evidence that an adult aspirin, which is 325 milligrams, will thin the blood too much and cause blood to leak through the vessels. Among other things, that will lead to more bruises. It's good to take aspirin but only the smaller dose."

If you're taking aspirin to help reduce your risk of heart attack, as some doctors advise, you shouldn't stop taking it without talking to a physician. But your doctor might recommend another solution, such as switching

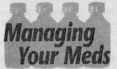

Managing Your Meds

Besides aspirin, there are several medications that can contribute to excessive bruising, says Arthur K. Balin, M.D., medical director of the Sally Balin Medical Center for Dermatology and Cosmetic Surgery in Media, Pennsylvania, and co-author of *The Life of the Skin*. These include:

✦ Anticoagulants like heparin (Heparin Flush) and warfarin (Coumadin)

✦ Nonsteroidal anti-inflammatory drugs such as ibuprofen (Advil)

✦ Certain antibacterials, including nitrofurantoin (Macrodantin)

✦ Certain heart drugs, such as verapamil (Isoptin)

Check with your doctor to see if a medication you are taking may be contributing to weakened blood vessels, excessive bleeding, or bruising.

to baby aspirin, which has only 81 milligrams. That much aspirin will not cause the same problems as the stronger adult dose, so it's safer and more appropriate for daily consumption, recommends Dr. Balin.

Try some special K. A deficiency of vitamin K can prevent normal blood clotting, says Dr. Kaminski, and you need some clotting action to help prevent bruising. "Some people who bruise excessively and have a lot of broken blood vessels below the skin should eat more vegetables rich in vitamin K," he says. Vitamin K is abundant in leafy greens and members of the cabbage family, such as broccoli, brussels sprouts, cabbage, and spinach, among others. "You might consider a supplement of K as well."

Protect your vulnerable spots. Be sure to wear protective clothing, especially over those areas where you tend to repeatedly bruise yourself, suggests Dr. Balin. Wear long sleeves and long pants, sweaters that fall below your waist and cover your hips, and shoes that protect your feet. If you repeatedly bruise your thighs or forearms, ask your pharmacist about protective pads that you can easily slip on to guard those areas.

Burns

Irons, microwaves, coffeemakers, stoves—our households are teeming with items that make life easier but that can also cause burns if you're not careful.

Every year, about two million Americans are burned or scalded badly enough to need some medical attention. Many of these burns occur in the home, the majority befalling children and older people, says Randolph Wong, M.D., plastic and reconstructive surgeon and director of the burn unit at Straub Clinic and Hospital in Honolulu.

If the burn is serious enough, you'll want a doctor to look at it. If you aren't sure whether you have a first- or second-degree burn, call your doctor. But minor singes and small burns are easily treated with these simple methods.

Cool it. As soon as you can, immerse the burned area in cool water and keep it there for five to 10 minutes, says Dr. Wong. Cool water stops the burning process and helps ease pain. Don't use ice to cool a burn, though. That's too cold and could further injure already-damaged skin.

If you're not near water, use whatever is convenient to cool a burn quickly—even a glass of milk or cold can of soda wrapped in a clean towel, says D'Anne Kleinsmith, M.D., cosmetic dermatologist at William Beaumont Hospital in Royal Oak, Michigan.

Deflame the pain. If you take an anti-inflammatory medication within an hour of getting the burn, you'll not only ease the pain but also prevent the burn from getting worse, says Evelyn Placek, M.D., dermatologist and doctor of internal medicine in private practice in Scarsdale, New York. Aspirin or ibuprofen (Advil) works best. Dr. Placek recommends taking two 200-milligram tablets or capsules of ibuprofen every six hours for one to two days to reduce inflammation and swelling and to help decrease the severity of the wound.

Cool with a compress. To further reduce pain, apply a washcloth or towel soaked in cool, not icy, water on and off for several hours, says Dr. Placek.

Use antibacterial ointments. Over-the-counter salves like Neosporin and Bacitracin will help kill germs and prevent infection, says Dr. Wong. Sealing the wound with greasy folk remedies such as butter or petroleum jelly can keep nerve endings from drying out, he says, but they do little to control bacteria that can get into a wound after a burn.

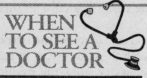
Bandage the burn. For small burns, place an adhesive strip over the antibacterial ointment, making sure the strip is large enough that it doesn't stick to the traumatized skin, explains Dr. Wong. For larger burns, you'll need a sterile piece of gauze dressing over the injured area, held down with medical adhesive tape. Be certain that it is loose enough to allow for some swelling and loose movement without compromising blood flow.

Say aloe. Aloe vera gel can speed the healing process, according to Dr. Wong. Whether fresh from the cleaned and sliced leaf of the plant or out of a tube, aloe vera gel seals and protects the burn, says Dr. Wong, and encourages healing with minimum scarring.

Take the sting out with honey. When applied as a lotion, raw honey, available in natural food stores as opposed to processed in the supermarket, can be spectacularly effective against burns. Recent Chinese research shows that honey has soothing antiseptic properties that help speed healing, according to Andrew T. Weil, M.D., director of the program in integrative medicine and clinical professor of internal medicine at the University of Arizona College of Medicine in Tucson.

Think zinc. To encourage healing from within, Dr. Wong suggests taking 220 milligrams of zinc sulfate in pill form once or twice a day until the burn dries up. But if you develop some gastrointestinal upset, discontinue its use immediately. This mineral helps the regeneration of new skin, he says, especially when taken with 10,000 international units of vitamin A or 10,000 international units of beta-carotene.

Keep it moist. Once the wound has healed over, keep it supple with a thin layer of moisturizing lotion. This will help restore elasticity to the skin and reduce dryness, itching, and scaling, according to Dr. Wong. Fragrance-free lotions are best, but anything that traps moisture will be effective, including vegetable shortening. However, don't use lanolin, he says, because it can cause a burning sensation.

Don't be a flame magnet. Something as innocent as putting a teakettle on the stove can have serious consequences if you're wearing a housecoat with dangling sleeves, which can easily catch fire. When you're cooking, don't wear loose-fitting clothing, especially garments with wide, dangling sleeves. Look for flame-retardant fabrics and avoid clothes made of cotton, cotton/polyester blends, rayon, and acrylic, which ignite easily and burn quickly.

Bursitis and Tendinitis

Bursitis and tendinitis sneak up on unsuspecting people all the time. Often, it happens something like this: After months of being trapped indoors because of frosty winter temperatures and snowstorms, you head outside as soon as the weather finally breaks. And suddenly you see 1,001 things to do: repaint the garage door, reseal the driveway, dig a new flower bed, or give the house a thorough spring cleaning.

Then after spending three to four hours doing chores on the to-do list, it happens. You may start to notice swelling in and around your joints, plus a pain that just won't quit. One of the all-too-common "-itises"—either bursitis or tendinitis—has claimed another victim.

But what exactly is going on? "With tendinitis, you get an inflammation that develops in your tendons, which connect muscle to bone," says David Richards, M.D., orthopedic surgeon at the Lexington Clinic Sports Medicine Center in Lexington, Kentucky. "And it can be quite painful."

Bursitis is equally painful but comes from different origins. It's caused by an inflammation of a bursa, a fluid-filled sac surrounding joints or tendons, says Keith Jones, head trainer for the Houston Rockets basketball team. These home remedies can help you ace either "-itis."

Give it a rest. This might sound obvious, but because bursitis and tendinitis are often triggered by using a body part in a way that it's not used to, rest is one of the first steps on the road to recovery. "Complete rest is necessary in order for the pain to subside," says Jones. Whatever activity triggered the bout of bursitis or tendinitis, avoid it for three to six weeks, if possible. Even multimillion-dollar athletes take a break when they have bursitis and tendinitis—you should, too.

Try some ice. In addition to rest, Jones recommends putting ice wrapped in a thin towel on the area that ails you. "If you suffer from bursitis or tendinitis,

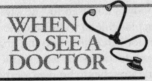

WHEN TO SEE A DOCTOR

If the pain from your bursitis or tendinitis worsens after three to four days, or if it doesn't subside at all after proper rest and other home remedies, then it's time to see a doctor, says David Richards, M.D., orthopedic surgeon at the Lexington Clinic Sports Medicine Center in Lexington, Kentucky. Besides ruling out serious injury, your doctor can prescribe medications and exercises that can alleviate pain and still give you some degree of mobility.

make sure you apply ice to the sore area for 20 minutes at least three times per day," says Jones. "The combination of the rest and the ice should pay noticeable dividends within days."

Beat the heat. If you're suffering from bursitis or tendinitis, avoid the urge to apply a heating pad to the affected joint, says William Pesanelli, physical therapist and the director of Boston University's rehabilitation services. "It's like pouring lighter fluid on an already existing fire," he cautions. "If you're suffering from bursitis or tendinitis, the tissues in the sore area are already inflamed and will feel warmer to touch than the rest of your body, so adding heat will only make matters worse." Instead, you'll find more relief by using ice until the inflammation is gone.

Limber up. To prevent bursitis and tendinitis, take time to stretch first, says Pesanelli. For example, if you are about to perform a task that your body is not used to, warm up that area of the body first. "Tendinitis or bursitis is often triggered when someone does something that his body is not used to," he says.

"If you've been playing pinochle all winter and then want to go out and garden for three hours on the first warm spring day, make sure to do some slow warm-up activities first, then a few gentle stretches to prepare for the activity," says Pesanelli. "And don't go out and do three hours' worth of activity if you've been inactive for a while. You need to gradually work up to that level of activity." To get an idea of what your body can handle (before you find out the hard way), it's a good idea to sign up for a stretching class at a senior citizen center or YMCA.

Elevate your injury. If the inflammation is in the knee, foot, or ankle, Jones recommends that you elevate the affected area above your heart level. "If you put two or three pillows below your sore ankle to

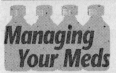

Managing Your Meds

Taking an anti-inflammatory for a week to 10 days, such as two to three ibuprofen (Advil) three or four times per day, depending on your weight, should help ease the pain and swelling that come with either bursitis or tendinitis, says Dale L. Anderson, M.D., coordinator of the Minnesota Act Now Project in Minneapolis and the author of *Muscle Pain Relief in 90 Seconds*. If the symptoms persist, a doctor might prescribe a different anti-inflammatory drug. All anti-inflammatory drugs should be taken with food or milk because they can cause your stomach to get upset if you take them on an empty stomach, says Dr. Anderson.

Because anti-inflammatory medicines like aspirin and ibuprofen may aggravate certain conditions, ask your doctor for another battle plan if you have ulcers or an inflamed bowel disorder, advises Dr. Anderson. Also, if you're planning to have surgery, make sure to stop taking the anti-inflammatory a week before your operation. These drugs can thin your blood, which can complicate surgery.

prop it up, it often can help reduce the swelling," Jones says. If you have a history of impaired circulation in the injured area, however, don't elevate it above your heart level, because limiting blood flow to an area of the body that has impaired circulation can be dangerous.

Wrap it up. If you need to continue to perform an activity that may cause a recurrence of the tendinitis in your knees, put on knee sleeves before you do anything else, says Jones. Available in pharmacies and many sports stores, the sleeves are flexible cylindrical bandages that you can pull into place over your knees.

"The knee sleeve serves two important purposes," says Jones. "First, it keeps the area warm, which helps maintain flexibility. And second, it keeps the joint from being bounced around and from causing another flare-up of the tendinitis." Similar devices for your ankles, elbows, and wrists are available at drugstores.

Keep active. To prevent injuries such as bursitis and tendinitis, get yourself on an exercise program, suggests Pesanelli. If you can get out for a brisk walk or swim three times or more per week all year round, you'll be able to keep your heart, lungs, and muscles in good condition. Many senior centers and YMCAs also offer exercise programs specifically tailored to older adults. Just be sure to consult with your physician before embarking on an exercise program, says Pesanelli.

Ease your way back into activity. After you've been treated for bursitis or tendinitis, don't jump head-first into the activities that you were doing before the attack. "You must ease yourself back into action after you start to feel better. Otherwise, it is a vicious cycle," cautions Dr. Richards. "You'll suffer an attack of bursitis, feel better, and then be in pain again quickly if you don't slowly ease your way back into things."

Canker Sores

Along with Zsa Zsa's *real* age and the location(s) of Jimmy Hoffa's grave, the mystery of the canker sore continues to baffle the experts. For some reason, those little white ulcers with red borders visit the mouths of some people quite frequently—while others get them rarely. And while some may have canker sores for just a few days, other people have them for weeks.

No one's really sure what causes these pesky and painful ulcers on the tongue or gums or inside the cheeks (although a predisposition for them seems to be hereditary). Luckily, doctors do have some answers on how you can cut short the usual 10- to 15-day life span of these annoying, although nonthreatening, lesions—or avoid them altogether.

Make yogurt a daily ritual. "Eat at least four tablespoons of unflavored yogurt every day, and you'll prevent canker sores," says Jerome Z. Litt, M.D., assistant clinical professor of dermatology at Case Western Reserve University School of Medicine in Cleveland. He adds that it's unclear why the yogurt works, but for some people, it can be very effective.

See the difference with vitamin C. "Vitamin C is very effective at preventing or healing canker sores, particularly for people who are under a lot of stress, consume a lot of alcohol, or smoke," says David Garber, D.M.D., clinical professor of periodontics and prosthodontics at the Medical College of Georgia in Augusta. And that's worth noting, since these are the very people most at risk for canker sores. Five hundred milligrams a day is sometimes recommended for a vitamin C supplement—but check with your doctor first. To introduce more vitamin C to your daily diet, go for broccoli, cantaloupe, red bell peppers, and cranberry juice. (Once you have a sore, however, the acidic juice may be more pain than gain.)

Squeeze on some vitamin E. Vitamin C isn't the only nutrient that can help heal canker sores. Craig Zunka, D.D.S., a dentist in Front Royal, Virginia, and chairman of the board of the Holistic Dental Association, says squeezing the oil from a vitamin E capsule onto your canker sore can bring relief.

Put some sore relief in your diet. Several studies show that one in seven people with canker sores is deficient in folate, iron, and B vitamins, and doctors believe that upping these nutrients can help prevent sores or quicken recovery from them. Peas, beans, and lentils are excellent folate sources; lean beef, tofu, and fortified cereals are high in iron; and meats and seafood are high in B vitamins.

Gargle with peroxide. "A solution of three parts water and one part hydrogen peroxide changes the pH of your saliva and makes for a harsh environment for the bacteria causing canker sores," says dentist Paul Caputo, D.D.S., of Palm Harbor, Florida. "Mixing this solution and gargling or swishing it around your mouth several times a day is very helpful when you have a canker sore. But don't swallow it."

Baste it with Orabase-B. This over-the-counter remedy gets thumbs up from all our experts as the best relief money can buy at your neighborhood drugstore. "It's a sticky substance you put directly on the sore to stop the pain and promote healing," says Dr. Caputo.

Another over-the-counter product that comes highly recommended is Zilactin, a medicated gel. And for those preferring a liquid form, there's Zilactol, says Dr. Garber.

Avoid sharp or spicy foods. And we mean that in both a culinary and a literal sense. "Many people know that you should avoid foods that are spicy or salty when you have a canker sore, because those foods increase the pain," says D'Anne Kleinsmith, M.D., a cosmetic dermatologist at William Beaumont Hospital in Royal Oak, Michigan. "But you should also avoid foods with sharp *edges*, such as potato chips. Anything with rough edges can puncture the skin and cause canker sores."

Besides spices and salt, it's best to avoid or limit citrus fruits and strawberries, cheeses, coffee, nuts, and chocolate if you're prone to canker sores.

Bag your pain with a tea bag. Rubbing a wet tea bag directly on the sore is another helpful home treatment, says Dr. Litt. Black tea contains tannin, an astringent with powerful pain-relieving qualities.

"If you're into herbal teas, drink chamomile tea, which cools canker sore pain and other mild skin irritations," says Varro E. Tyler, Ph.D., distinguished professor emeritus at Purdue University in West Layette, Indiana, and author of *The Honest Herbal*.

Ice it. Old cures are often the best, and there are few older (or better) than simply applying ice to the sore to help reduce pain and swelling.

Mylanta may be your healer. Swish a tablespoon of the antacid Mylanta or milk of magnesia around your mouth to coat the sore, advises Robert Goepp, D.D.S., Ph.D., professor of oral pathology at the University of Chicago Medical Center. But only use this technique if you are sure your ulcer is not infected. If you coat an infected ulcer, the coating will protect the bacteria causing the infection. An infected ulcer is usually marked by a red ring around its base and a grayish yellow color, Dr. Goepp says.

Cataracts

A cataract is a painless clouding of the normally clear lens of the eye. Left untreated, it can cause blindness. But this clouding has a silver lining: Surgery can restore lost sight in most cases.

While many people over age 60 do have some clouding of the eye lens and therefore some degree of cataracts, there are ways to help prevent cataracts from forming or getting worse. Here's how to help make sure your lenses stay clear.

Drink your orange juice. "Our research shows there's a lower risk of developing cataracts in people who consume a lot of vitamin C in their diets," says Allen Taylor, Ph.D., director of the Lens Nutrition and Aging Division of the U.S. Department of Agriculture Human Nutrition Research Center on Aging at Tufts University in Boston. "We're still trying to find out exactly how much is needed for protection against cataracts, but we know it's at least two times the Recommended Dietary Allowance." That amounts to one cup of orange juice, two oranges, or 1½ cups of strawberries.

Get your beta-carotene and vitamin E. "Vitamin E and beta-carotene also seem to offer some protection," adds Dr. Taylor. He recommends yellow and orange vegetables such as carrots, squash, and sweet potatoes as excellent sources of beta-carotene. Foods high in vitamin E include almonds, fortified cereals, peanut butter, and sunflower seeds.

Wear sunglasses or a hat. "The most credible evidence shows that the *best* way to prevent cataracts is to protect your eyes from the sun's ultraviolet rays," says Merrill M. Knopf, M.D., an ophthalmologist in Long Beach, California, and an officer of the California Association of Ophthalmology. "Be sure to wear sunglasses or a hat when you're outdoors. And there's no need to spend $100 or more for a pair of designer sunglasses, since all sunglasses sold in the United States offer UV protection. Putting a sticker on them to say that is simply a way to drive up the price. The kind sold at your drugstore will do as well as those sold by your eye doctor."

Look away when the microwave's in use. Even small doses of radiation make you more prone to developing cataracts, so limiting exposure to radiation sources—such as microwaves and x-ray machines—is recommended. "I know that all manufacturers say their ovens are safe, and maybe they are, but I make a point of turning my head away from my microwave and closing my eyes while it's in use," says Dr. Knopf. "I do the same when I'm at my dentist's office getting x-rays."

Control your vices. Occasional drinking won't affect you, but prolonged, problem drinking will. "Alcoholics are especially prone to developing cataracts, because alcoholism interferes with the nutritional pathway of food to the lens, making cataract formation more likely," says Dr. Knopf. Even in alcoholics who have good diets, essential nutrients intended for the eye are diverted.

Remember: Smoke gets to your eyes. Researchers at Johns Hopkins University in Baltimore report that cigarette smokers are more likely than nonsmokers to develop cataracts. That's because toxic substances in smoke damage the lens nucleus, causing cataracts. The good news is that by quitting smoking, you *halve* your risk of developing cataracts (compared with those who continue to smoke).

Take pain relievers. British researchers report that people who take aspirin, ibuprofen (Advil), and acetaminophen (Tylenol) are *half* as likely to develop cataracts as other folks. That's because cataract formation is related to blood sugar (one reason why people with diabetes are more susceptible to cataract formation), and there's some evidence that aspirin and aspirin-like products reduce the rate at which your body uses glucose.

Clumsiness

Everyone is occasionally fumble-fingered, less than graceful, or downright klutzy. In all probability, you are no more clumsy today than you were when you were in your twenties or thirties.

"Getting older doesn't necessarily mean that you'll drop more things or trip and fall more often," says Daniel Fechtner, M.D., assistant professor of rehabilitation medicine at Albert Einstein College of Medicine of Yeshiva University in New York City. "There are plenty of active people in their seventies and eighties who have never been tremendously clumsy and probably never will be." But if you do feel clumsier than usual, try these simple solutions.

Take a seat. Sit down at a table or on a counter-high stool when you do chores like peeling vegetables or washing dishes, Dr. Fechtner says. That should help you become less accident-prone, because you can concentrate on what your hands are doing without having to worry about tripping over your own two feet.

Tone up. The more physically fit you are, the less clumsy you'll be, says Jan I. Maby, D.O., director of the Geriatric Medical Home Care program at Mount Sinai

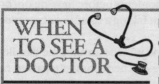

WHEN TO SEE A DOCTOR

Even if you have only an occasional clumsiness or balance problem, do not pass it off as a natural sign of aging, says Francis X. J. Bohdiewicz, M.D., specialist in physical medicine and rehabilitation at Youville Hospital and Rehabilitation Center in Cambridge, Massachusetts. "Let your doctor know about the problem and let him decide what the most appropriate next step is. A problem related to clumsiness, balance, coordination, or weakness could be a sign of treatable, underlying disease such as stroke, arthritis, complications of diabetes, or even cancer," he says.

Medical Center in New York City. Strong bones and muscles will help you maintain your balance and enhance your ability to reach and grasp.

Activities like gardening and walking that use the majority of your muscles are among the best exercises for older Americans, Dr. Maby says. Try to exercise at least 30 minutes a day three times a week, she suggests.

Eyeball your spectacles. Poor eyesight can make you seem more clumsy. Have your vision checked at least once a year or if you find yourself more fumble-fingered than usual, Dr. Maby suggests.

Take your time. You'll be more accident-prone when you are in a rush, Dr. Maby says. So allow yourself plenty of time to do chores, drive across town, or prepare for special occasions like Thanksgiving. If you feel more comfortable taking just a step or two at a time and pausing for a couple of moments before moving on, do it, she says. It's better than taking a tumble or bumping into a wall.

Make a grip. Wrap cork tape around the handles of your spoons, knives, and other eating utensils to reduce your risk of dropping these items, Dr. Maby says. A coarse, spongy material commonly used on bicycle handlebars, cork tape is available at most bicycle shops.

Select chunky handles. Thicker-handled coffee mugs and other specialized products also can make it easier for you to maintain a solid grasp on things, Dr. Maby says. Visit a medical supply store to see all the options available or check home health-care catalogs for major department stores.

Make nonskid fingers. Wear rubber gloves when washing dishes, Dr. Fechtner says. The rubber helps you grasp and hold slippery glasses and plates.

Spot your weakness. Often, clumsiness is

caused by poor depth perception, says Jim Buskirk, licensed physical therapist at Balance Centers of America in Chicago. But he says that you can learn to focus your eyes by moving your head toward a stationary object. The following exercise will help improve your depth perception and hand-eye coordination. Hand-eye coordination is dependent on good depth perception by the eyes and the ability to judge distances. Here are the steps.

1. Mark a dot on a wall at about eye level.

2. Stand opposite the dot with your hands pressed up against the wall.

3. Lower your upper body toward the wall as if you were doing a pushup. As you do this, keep your eyes focused on the dot.

4. Slowly push your body back to the starting position, again keeping your eyes focused on the dot.

Do this exercise for one minute three times a day, Buskirk advises. It may take a while, but gradually you'll be likely to notice an improvement in your ability to lay your hands on objects more quickly and smoothly.

Take time to melt down. Some people who are prone to stress or who are suffering from anxiety can become more fumble-fingered, says Marc L. Gordon, M.D., chief of neurology for the Hillside Hospital Division of Northshore–Long Island Jewish Health System in New Hyde Park, New York.

Movement meditation is a terrific stress buster that also may help you overcome clumsiness, says Eileen F. Oster, occupational therapist in Bayside, New York, and author of *The Healing Mind*. Here's how to do it.

Managing Your Meds

Virtually any drug that can cause drowsiness also can make you a bit more clumsy, says W. Steven Pray, Ph.D., R.Ph., professor of nonprescription drug products at Southwestern Oklahoma State University in Weatherford. In particular, be wary of over-the-counter (OTC) sleeping pills like diphenhydramine (Sominex) and prescription antianxiety medications known as benzodiazepines, including alprazolam (Xanax). In addition, consult your doctor or pharmacist if clumsiness develops when you are taking the following medications.

✦ OTC and prescription antihistamines that include diphenhydramine (Benadryl)

✦ Antipsychotics such as phenothiazines, including chlorpromazine (Thorazine)

✦ Diuretics and other high blood pressure medications, including prazosin (Minipress) and methyldopa (Aldomet)

---

1. Stand if you can or sit in a comfortable chair if you're concerned about falling. Take several deep, cleansing breaths.

2. Center yourself by visualizing your feet connected to the soil.

3. Visualize the center of the earth, from which we draw our energy.

4. Gently move your body in an undulating, snakelike, swaying motion.

5. See yourself as a flower opening up or as an animal gracefully moving through the brush.

6. If it pleases you, use music to focus your attention on the movement and on the vibration.

7. Allow yourself to get lost in the sense of movement and the beauty of your body as it moves. Feel the areas of your body that are tight and let the movement loosen them.

Practice movement meditation at least twice a day for five minutes a session, Oster suggests.

Cold Hands and Feet

At one time or another, everyone gets caught in the chilling grip of Old Man Winter. It's inevitable. However, some of us get the chills even after the winter months are in the rearview mirror. Believe it or not, some folks suffer from cold hands and feet just by setting foot in the frozen-food section of the supermarket or by entering an air-conditioned room.

If this happens to you, there's a good chance that you have Raynaud's syndrome. Raynaud's is a common disorder that causes your fingers and toes to become very cold and numb, says Jay D. Coffman, M.D., chief of peripheral vascular medicine at Boston University Medical Center.

A bout with cold fingers and toes is usually temporary and is mostly just uncomfortable. And if you do have this disorder, you aren't sentenced to a lifetime of cold hands and feet. Doctors have come up with things you can do to prevent rampant Raynaud's or even fight off the chilly numbness when it nips your fingers and bites your toes.

Get relief at arm's length. If you start to feel a chill and see your fingers begin to turn white, quickly place your cold hand in a warm place, Dr. Coffman says. Your armpit, for example. "By sticking your hand under your arm, you can stop the cold and numbing sensation of Raynaud's quickly," he says.

To reverse or help prevent the cold feet problem, try wearing thermal socks, using warming chemical packs obtained at a sports or ski shop, or purchasing boots that can be heated, suggests Dr. Coffman. "Remember not to stamp your feet when they are cold, to avoid injury to them," he says.

Freeze out your triggers. The next time your digits go cold, think about what might have triggered it. Were you holding a cold can of soda? Did you reach into the freezer? Now you know what to avoid. "Triggers can be everyday things like holding a frozen beer mug at a party, walking into an air-conditioned room from the sweltering heat, or emerging from a heated pool into a cooler environment," says Dr. Coffman.

Warm up to wearing mittens. Of course, if cold days are the trigger, you can't take a flight to the tropics every time winter sets in. But you can protect your hands. If gloves don't put your fingers in a tropical mode, try wearing mittens. "They do a better job of trapping the heat from your entire hand," Dr. Coffman says. Wear them whenever you go out on a cold winter day.

And you might need mittens inside the house,

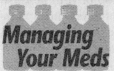
Managing Your Meds

The most commonly prescribed medication to treat Raynaud's is a vasodilator that acts as a calcium blocker, such as nifedipine (Procardia). Calcium blockers dilate the blood vessels in your body and allow blood to flow freely to your extremities, says Jay D. Coffman, M.D., chief of peripheral vascular medicine at Boston University Medical Center.

The most common side effect of taking calcium blockers is occasional headaches, but they are less common as your body adjusts to taking the medication, according to W. Steven Pray, Ph.D., R.Ph., professor of nonprescription drug products at Southwestern Oklahoma State University in Weatherford.

There are a number of medications that may *trigger* Raynaud's, except if you already have primary Raynaud's, in which case you won't be affected. Even if you aren't prone to cold fingers and toes, talk to your doctor before taking the following:

✦ Migraine headache medications such as ergotamine preparations (Wigraine)

✦ Heart and blood medications such as beta blockers, like propranolol, (Inderal)

too. "I have patients who wear mittens every time they reach into their freezer," says Dr. Coffman.

Wear a head-heating hat. When you warn your kids and grandchildren not to leave the house without a hat on, remember to take that advice yourself. You lose much body heat from the top of your head, so cover that head of yours with a hat, says Donald McIntyre, M.D., dermatologist in private practice in Rutland, Vermont. By keeping the heat in your body, you're protecting your hands and feet from a bout of Raynaud's.

Swing into action. Suffering from cold fingers? You can warm up those ice-cold digits with a simple arm-swinging exercise, says Dr. McIntyre. Pretend you're about to pitch a softball, but keep your fingers, wrist, and elbow straight while swinging your arm in a windmill fashion. "Living in Vermont, I borrowed this idea from people I watched up here on the ski slopes," says Dr. McIntyre. "I noticed that they kept their hands and arms warm by whirling them around when they were on top of the mountain. And I found out that it not only works on the mountain, it works in everyday life." Dr. McIntyre recommends a swinging speed of 80 whirls per minute but notes that any windmill speed will boost the blood flow to your cold digits.

Colds

The ancient Greeks thought leech-induced bleeding was the answer. More recently, Mom's answer was her chicken soup. And guess what? While we still spend more than $1 billion each year on cold remedies—nothing to sneeze at—we have yet to find a single way to make the common cold less common.

The good news is that the older you get, the less likely you are to fall victim to any of the 200 different viruses that can cause a cold. Children typically get six to 10 colds a year, because their immunity hasn't matured; adults usually get two to four.

While scientists are currently working on high-tech ways to stop cold viruses from spreading, here are some ways to cut down your risk—or at least reduce the time you spend suffering from America's most frequent health complaint.

Drink vitamin C–rich juice. Orange, tomato, grapefruit, or pineapple juice can help you get over a cold—but you need to drink at least five glasses a day. "Studies show it takes that much vitamin C (about 500 milligrams) to reduce sneezes and coughs in cold sufferers," says Jeffrey Jahre, M.D., clinical assistant professor of medicine at Temple University School of Medicine in Philadelphia and chief of the infectious diseases section at St. Luke's Medical Center in Bethlehem, Pennsylvania. If that amount seems like a bit much to swallow, you can take vitamin C supplements. But don't go overboard. Larger doses of vitamin C can cause stomach upset in some people.

Serve a steamy bowl of comfort. Any hot liquid helps cut through congestion, but chicken soup is probably best of all, according to Frederick Ruben, M.D., professor of medicine at the University of Pittsburgh and spokesperson for the American Lung Association. No study has shown *why* chicken soup seems to work so well, but it's certain that the soup is protein-rich, tasty, and a comforting way to get nutrients if you're not up to eating. "People who wouldn't drink hot water will readily eat chicken soup," says Dr. Ruben.

Keep a glass of water on your nightstand. "Taking sips of water during the night is another way to moisten the nose and help breathing," says Dr. Ruben. It also helps combat the dehydration that can result from fighting a cold.

Try a ginger brew. "For chills, I have patients drink tea made with a teaspoon of ground ginger in boiling water," says Charles Lo, M.D., a physician in Chicago and Oak Park, Illinois.

Eat south of the border. Break up congestion with a bowl of chili or other spicy foods containing horseradish, hot-pepper sauce, hot mustard, or curry, suggests Irwin Ziment, M.D., chief of medicine at Olive View Medical Center in Los Angeles. Hot Mexican or Indian foods are good congestion busters. As a rule of thumb, says Dr. Ziment, "if it makes your eyes water, it will also make your nose run."

Pump your legs. A daily 45-minute walk can help speed recovery from colds, according to studies conducted by David Nieman, Ph.D., a health researcher at Appalachian State University in Boone, North Carolina. "A daily walk helps shake up and spread out the natural killer cells—the Marine Corps of your immune system—making them more vigilant," says Dr. Nieman. But don't push yourself. Exhaustive exercise can actually impair the immune system. If you pace yourself so that you can comfortably talk while you walk, you're going at the right speed, according to Dr. Nieman.

Don't bother with antihistamines. Over-the-counter cold medicines that contain antihistamines do little more than make you sleepy. "New findings show that histamine is not produced when you have a cold," says Dr. Ruben, so the drugs designed to fight it won't help.

For headache, be selective. New evidence from Johns Hopkins University School of Hygiene and Public Health in Baltimore has shown that aspirin and acetaminophen (Tylenol) actually increase nasal blockage and reduce the level of virus-fighting antibodies. If you have a headache, ibuprofen (Advil) may be the better choice, says Dr. Ruben. If your child has a headache along with a cold, ask your doctor about child-size doses of ibuprofen. (Never give children aspirin without consulting a doctor, because it can contribute to Reye's syndrome, a life-threatening neurological condition.)

Snort salt water. For a stuffy nose, nasal sprays are safer and better than oral decongestants, says Herbert Patrick, M.D., assistant professor of medicine and medical director of the respiratory care department at Jefferson Medical College of Thomas Jefferson University in Philadelphia. But if you use them longer than three days, your nose will become stuffier than ever. So after you've used a nasal spray for a couple of days, switch to a commercial saline solution such as Ayr. Or make your own saline solution: Dissolve a teaspoon of salt in a pint of water, then use a nosedropper to drop it into your nose. Gently blow your nose on a tissue.

Sit in a sauna. There's no sure way to prevent a cold, but the Swedes may be on the right track. According to Dr. Jahre, researchers found that if you indulge in a sauna twice a week or more, you're less likely to catch a cold. Possibly, he says, the high temperature may block the cold viruses from reproducing.

Make your home tropical. "It's not the cold weather but the lack of humidity that is a major issue in catching colds," says Dr. Patrick. Overheated homes and offices are the perfect setup for a cold, he adds.

"When our nose and tonsils are dry, they cannot trap germs efficiently. It becomes difficult to sneeze and cough, so it's difficult to expel germs from the body." Turning down the thermostat and turning on a room humidifier keeps virus-laden mucus flowing out of your body, according to Dr. Patrick.

Chill out. In a study involving more than 400 people, researchers at Carnegie Mellon University in Pittsburgh and Britain's Common Cold Unit found that people who reported high levels of psychological stress were twice as likely to develop a cold as those reporting low stress levels. "We can only speculate that a change in stress hormones wears down the immune system," says Sheldon Cohen, Ph.D., professor of psychology at the university and the study's author. This study is a first step in understanding a complex issue, he says. Whether stress has an actual impact on colds is still unknown. Still, using stress management on a daily basis can't hurt, and it may help defend you against a season of sniffles.

Cold Sores

If you're over age 60, you stand a better chance of seeing a blizzard in Phoenix than of getting a cold sore, dentists say. "As you get older, cold sores tend to burn themselves out," says Michael Siegel, D.D.S., associate professor of oral medicine and diagnostic sci-

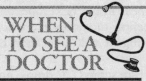

WHEN TO SEE A DOCTOR

Most cold sores heal within 10 days with or without treatment. If a mouth sore persists beyond this time, see your doctor or dentist, urges Brad Rodu, D.D.S., professor in the department of pathology at the University of Alabama School of Medicine in Birmingham. He can determine if an underlying infection is causing the problem and can prescribe medication to solve the problem.

ences at the University of Maryland School of Dentistry in Baltimore.

Why cold sores, which appear on the outsides of your lips and are also known as fever blisters, subside as you age is a mystery. But some researchers suspect that the body, in a process that can take decades, gradually becomes more resistant to herpes simplex, the virus that causes cold sores, Dr. Siegel says.

If you are among the few older Americans who continue to get cold sores, you probably have years of experience in dealing with them and know a number of ways to ease an outbreak. But here are a few reminders.

Drop a tannic bomb. Over-the-counter (OTC) drops (such as Zilactin-L) that contain tannic acid can, if applied soon enough, prevent a cold sore from forming or, at the very least, help to reduce its size, says Brad Rodu, D.D.S., professor in the department of pathology at the University of Alabama School of Medicine in Birmingham.

The key is to start using the drops as soon as your lip begins tingling. That's an early warning sign that a cold sore may appear in the next four to 12 hours, Dr. Rodu says. Reapply the drops every hour while you feel the tingling. It will help keep the sore small.

Have a tea party. Like some OTC drops, non-herbal tea contains tannic acid, too. The OTC medications are more effective, but you may want to try putting a wet tea bag on the sore for a few minutes every hour to provide temporary relief until you can get to the drugstore, Dr. Rodu says.

Give it a frosty reception. If your lip starts tingling, put ice on it to slow the growth of the virus that causes cold sores. That should lessen the severity of an outbreak, Dr. Rodu says. Wrap an ice cube in a towel and apply it to the affected spot for five to 10 minutes, repeating about once an hour.

Lube up. Moisturizing ointments such as petroleum jelly can soothe the pain and prevent cracking and bleeding skin, Dr. Rodu says. Apply them as needed.

Play it safe in the sun. Sun exposure can trigger a cold sore outbreak. To prevent it, be sure to wear a lip balm that contains a sun protection factor of at least 15, Dr. Rodu suggests. Reapply it every hour, as necessary.

Bundle up on blustery days. Cold, windy weather is a well-known trigger for cold sores. Always wear a ski mask or cover your mouth with a scarf when the wind kicks up and temperatures tumble, Dr. Rodu advises.

Colitis

If you have been diagnosed with chronic colitis, you are already familiar with some of its unpleasant symptoms—diarrhea, abdominal pain, and rectal bleeding.

Colitis is one of a group of conditions known collectively as inflammatory bowel disease. Ulcerative colitis causes open sores in the large intestine and almost always results in bloody, watery stools. Plain colitis, which is less severe, doesn't involve ulcers and tends to be confined to the upper part of the large intestine.

Although having a chronic inflammatory condition like colitis is no picnic, there is encouraging light on your health horizon. With good care, proper diet, and a less stressful approach to life, you may be able to ease some of the discomfort of colitis and keep it under control. But flare-ups do happen. And when the symptoms start up again, the first thing you'll be looking for is some fast-track roads to relief.

Here are some routes top doctors recommend—and some detours around future problems.

Supernourish yourself. "During colitis flare-ups, you may feel too rotten to eat well, so it's important to eat a high-quality diet the rest of the time," says Joel Mason, M.D., a nutritionist and gastroenterologist with the USDA Human Nutrition Research Center on Aging at Tufts University in Boston. "You want to build an adequate store of nutrients in your body."

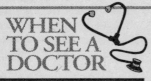

WHEN TO SEE A DOCTOR

The fact is, colitis can get out of control. That's why you need to see your doctor during an acute flare-up, says Joel Mason, M.D., a nutritionist and gastroenterologist with the U.S. Department of Agriculture Human Nutrition Research Center on Aging at Tufts University in Boston. "Self-medicating is not a good idea. The antidiarrheal medications Imodium and Lomotil can be very harmful if used inappropriately," he says.

Dr. Mason also recommends a regular screening for colon cancer if you've had chronic ulcerative colitis for more than seven years, because the disease does increase your risk. "If a cancer is detected very early, it increases the likelihood that you can be adequately treated and even cured," he says.

Be your own diet detective. Since each individual case of colitis is so different, you need to be on the lookout for specific foods that your body may not tolerate well, says Stephen McClave, M.D., a gastroenterologist and associate professor of medicine at the University of Louisville School of Medicine in Louisville, Kentucky. If a specific food causes trouble on multiple occasions, avoid it. But if it happens only once, retest. If you find that cabbage makes your symptoms worse, for example, don't avoid all leafy vegetables.

Tell it to Dear Diary. Recording your foods, moods, and flare-ups can help, says James Scala, Ph.D., a nutritional biochemist and lecturer at Georgetown University School of Medicine in Washington, D.C. "Keep track not just of what you ate or drank but also where, when, why, and how you felt at the time. If you can relate the onset of a flare-up to a food or an emotional experience, you'll be able to manage your illness more effectively in the future."

Try pectin protection. Fiber may be an important dietary help for colitis sufferers, says Danny Jacobs, M.D., a surgeon at Brigham and Women's Hospital and assistant professor of surgery at Harvard Medical School, both in Boston. And pectin, the soluble fiber found in apples and other fruits and vegetables, is particularly pleasing to the colon. "Apples are a marvelous source of pectin," he says, "and as long as you don't eat the seeds (or peels), there's no limit to how many you can consume."

But phase out fiber during flare-ups. "If you're having a flare-up, use a very low-fiber diet," says Dr. Mason. "You want to pass as little undigested residue through the bowel as possible. But as soon as the flare-up is over, return to a normal or high-fiber diet."

Fix friendly fruits. Dr. Scala offers these suggestions for taking the trouble out of fruit by reducing the amount of fiber. Be sure to peel all fruits (even grapes!), he advises. And if you're eating a citrus fruit, cut it into sections, removing all white, fibrous material. Dr. Scala also recommends eating canned fruit that's preserved in juice rather than sugar syrup. And be sure to avoid dried fruit.

Supplement your strategy. Since colitis can attack your nutritional status, multivitamin/mineral supplements are important, says Dr. Scala. "Take a multivitamin/mineral supplement that provides twice the Recommended Dietary Allowance of key nutrients," he recommends. "For about seven cents a day, it's worth it."

Fuel yourself with folate. People with ulcerative colitis should consider taking a daily multivitamin/mineral supplement that contains at least 400 micrograms of folate, recommends Dr. Mason. This is particularly true for those individuals who use sulfasalazine (Azulfidine), the most commonly prescribed drug for controlling colitis. The drug tends to inhibit your body's ability to use this B vitamin, he says. If more than 400 micrograms of folate is taken per day, however, it should be done under the supervision of a physician.

De-stress for less distress. After food intolerance, emotional stress is the biggest challenge for colitis sufferers, says Dr. Scala. To reduce stress, he calls for "a regular exercise program. Exercise will dissipate the effects of stress better than anything." In addition, Dr. Scala recommends stress counseling.

Lighten up on lactose. Inability to digest lactose, the sugar in milk, can be a factor in colitis, says Dr. McClave. "A lot of us teeter on the edge of milk intolerance, and a bowel disease like colitis can tip the balance." By avoiding all milk products, you may be able to reduce your symptoms.

Avoid crunchy veggies. You need to take the crunch out of carrots, asparagus, zucchini, squash, and other popular vegetables, says Dr. Scala. The best way is to cook them until they are very tender, he says. Pressure cooking is especially effective.

Check your medicine chest. Ulcerative colitis patients need to be cautious about using nonsteroidal anti-inflammatory drugs, warns Gary R. Gibson, M.D., assistant professor of medicine at Northeastern Ohio University College of Medicine in Warren. Over-the-counter ibuprofen (Advil), aspirin, and a dozen prescription drugs (including Naprosyn, Voltaren, and

Feldene) can erode the lining of the small intestine and colon. Be sure to check with your doctor before taking any of these medications.

Constipation

Do you take *War and Peace* into the bathroom instead of *Reader's Digest*? If so, you're probably constipated.

Constipation actually has two forms. Some people have to strain to move their bowels every time they want to go. But others just feel the urge too seldom.

How often is often enough? Routines vary. But if you have to go fewer than three times per week and each time it's a strain, there's a mighty good chance you're constipated. Here's how to get things moving again.

Lotion the motion with fiber. "Go on a high-fiber diet," says Edward P. Donatelle, M.D., professor emeritus of the department of family practice and community medicine at the University of Kansas School of Medicine in Wichita. Soluble fiber, found in grains, legumes, and fruits, is particularly effective. Oatmeal, rice, wheat germ, corn bran, prunes, raisins, apricots, figs, and an apple a day are all good sources, Dr. Donatelle says.

Try a natural laxative. For a concentrated constipation buster, go for a fiber supplement that will budge that balky bowel. One of the best is psyllium, which is sold in health food stores. Marvin M. Schuster, M.D., chief of the department of digestive diseases at Francis Scott Key Medical Center in Baltimore, recommends one teaspoon of psyllium with meals. Add the teaspoonful to a glass of water or juice and stir thoroughly before drinking. (You can also make a "paste" of one teaspoon of psyllium moistened with water, but be sure to drink at least a full glass of juice or water afterward.) Another alternative: Metamucil, a bowel regulator that contains psyllium and is sold in most drugstores and some supermarkets.

Use fluids to fuel the fiber. "Drink plenty of fluids," suggests John Sutherland, M.D., clinical professor of family practice at the University of Iowa College of Medicine in Iowa City and director of the Waterloo Family Practice Residency Program in Waterloo. Fluid expands and softens the fiber you're eating, allowing it to form bulk in the colon. That bulking action in turn triggers the urge to move your bowels. "Ordinarily you need to drink about a gallon of fluid a day—the more, the better," Dr. Sutherland says.

Avoid milk and cheese. If you have a problem with constipation, try avoiding milk products temporarily, says Dr. Donatelle. Both milk and cheese contain casein, an insoluble protein that tends to plug up the intestinal tract.

Get your body moving and your bowels will, too. "Exercise can help that lazy bowel to function better," according to gastroenterologist Nicholas Talley, M.D., Ph.D., associate professor of medicine at the Mayo Clinic in Rochester, Minnesota. "Aerobic exercise such as walking, running, and swimming is best." If you're a walker, for instance, go for a brisk 20- to 30-minute arm-swinging stroll every day.

Be Selective about Laxatives

Many over-the-counter products are sold as laxatives, but not all laxatives are recommended by doctors. In fact, heavy use of some laxatives can be counterproductive and even risky, according to Ronald L. Hoffman, M.D., director of the Hoffman Center for Holistic Medicine in New York City.

Heavy use of some laxatives can give you diarrhea, according to Dr. Hoffman. And many are habit-forming. If you always rely on a laxative to prompt bowel movements, your body may begin to need it to trigger the action. Laxatives containing castor oil can damage your intestinal lining, and those that have mineral oil can interfere with your ability to absorb certain vitamins and minerals, according to Dr. Hoffman.

Safest are the natural or vegetable laxative products, high-fiber bulking agents such as Metamucil, Citrucel, or Perdiem that are sold in most drugstores. "If you can't tolerate a high-fiber diet, these bulking agents are very safe, helpful supplements," according to gastroenterologist Nicholas Talley, M.D., Ph.D., associate professor of medicine at the Mayo Clinic in Rochester, Minnesota.

Dr. Talley recommends taking the cautious approach with bulking agents. Follow the directions on the package, increasing the dosage slowly if needed.

Listen when your body talks. "Sometimes people who are constipated ignore 'the urge' and wait until later. This can aggravate the problem," says Dr. Sutherland. When your body tells you it's time to go, head for the bathroom as soon as possible.

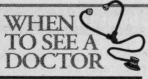

WHEN TO SEE A DOCTOR

Although constipation is usually not a serious problem, there are times when you should seek a doctor's advice. If you've had symptoms for more than three weeks and home remedies don't help—even with lots of fluid, fiber, and exercise—be sure to see your doctor.

You should also consult your doctor if there is blood in your stool. Although rare, constipation can sometimes signal a serious intestinal disease or disorder, including cancer, according to gastroenterologist Nicholas Talley, M.D., Ph.D., associate professor of medicine at the Mayo Clinic in Rochester, Minnesota.

Get into training. You can actually train your bowels to get on a regular schedule, says Vera Loening-Baucke, M.D., a pediatrician at the University of Iowa Hospitals and Clinics in Iowa City. Her advice: Sit on the toilet for about ten minutes after the same meal every day. The key is to stay relaxed. Eventually, says Dr. Loening-Baucke, your body will catch on.

Reach for the rhubarb. "When it's in season in early summer, fresh rhubarb is a delicious and powerful antidote to constipation," says Ronald L. Hoffman, M.D., director of the Hoffman Center for Holistic Medicine in New York City. It contains a good amount of fiber, which helps keep things moving. For a rhubarb juice refresher that will get your tract on track, try this cooling recipe. Chop three stalks of rhubarb (remove the leaves, which are toxic) and mix with 1 cup of apple juice, one-quarter of a peeled lemon, and 1 teaspoon of honey. Put all the ingredients in a blender or food processor and puree until smooth. Some advice: Try a small amount of rhubarb juice at first and see how your body responds. It can be as powerful and quick-acting as prune juice. Also, depending on how you like the taste, you might want to mix it with other juices. Caution: Rhubarb should be avoided by people with a history of calcium kidney stones.

Watch out for water robbers. Coffee, tea, and alcohol are all diuretics that can leave you somewhat dehydrated, says Dr. Hoffman. Since you need fluids in your system to aid bowel movements, you're more likely to have constipation if you drink these beverages. When you do have them, go for moderation and help compensate by drinking plenty of water, Dr. Hoffman suggests.

Give a high-fiber cookie to the kid in you. When you need a break from bran cereals, don't give up on fiber. Instead, try a fiber cookie supplement like Fiberall or Fibermed wafers, says Arnold Wald, M.D., head of the gastroenterology division at Montefiore University Hospital in Pittsburgh. "Be sure to take them with plenty of fluids—at least a six- to eight-ounce glass with each," he suggests.

Renew your Rx. Medicines that can contribute to constipation include prescription antidepressants and painkillers as well as some over-the-counter remedies such as iron supplements and aluminum-containing antacids. Dr. Hoffman recommends that you check with your doctor if you suspect your medication is causing your constipation.

Corns and
Calluses

The average Joe or Josephine takes as many as 10,000 steps a day, most of them on hard surfaces. Multiply that by 365 days a year and then multiply that by 75 or so years, and you've taken enough footsteps to walk around the world—several times over.

The only problem is that most of this traveling is done in shoes designed for fashion rather than function. The very same footwear that protects your feet from the hard realities of glass-littered streets and pebble-pocked lawns is an Achilles' heel to your toes. The friction shoes cause, as you may be uncomfortably aware, can leave you with corns and calluses.

These ugly bumps and lumps of thickened and hardened dead skin cells produce discomfort that can range from minor to extreme. So here are some treatments for the next time corns or calluses crop up.

Support your arches. "People with high arches are particularly susceptible to corns," says dermatologist Joseph Bark, M.D., past chairman of the department of dermatology at St. Joseph's Hospital in Lexington, Kentucky. How do you find out whether the shape of your arches is a contributing factor? "Check for corns on three pressure points on your feet that carry your weight: on the ball of the foot, right below

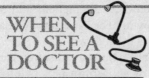

WHEN TO SEE A DOCTOR

Corns and calluses may require the attention of a doctor if they are very painful. And you should also consult a doctor if you have numbness or reduced sensation in your feet.

"Should pumice stones, moleskin, and pads fail to eliminate pain, medical attention is recommended," says Robert Diamond, D.P.M., a Pennsylvania podiatrist affiliated with Muhlenberg Hospital Center in Bethlehem and Allentown Osteopathic Hospital. For some people, surgery may be necessary, according to Dr. Diamond.

If you have reduced feeling in your feet, however, you may have a medical problem such as diabetes or possibly poor circulation. If you have a serious cut or injury on your foot, you might not feel it—and you could wind up with a dangerous infection.

If you have diabetes or poor circulation in your feet, Dr. Diamond recommends that you see a doctor any time you have corns or calluses. Those with diabetes, he notes, should not try any home remedies.

the smallest toe, and on your heel," Dr. Bark suggests. If this is your problem, try store-bought arch supports.

Be a beachcomber. "Walking barefoot on the beach can get rid of your calluses," says Robert Diamond, D.P.M., a Pennsylvania podiatrist affiliated with

Muhlenberg Hospital Center in Bethlehem and St. Luke's Hospital of Allentown. "The sand acts as a natural pumice stone and files them down."

Bag 'em with aspirin. One way to soften hard calluses is to crush five or six aspirin tablets into a powder, then add ½ teaspoon each of lemon juice and water. Apply this paste to all hard-skin areas. Wrap your entire foot with a warm towel, then cover with a plastic bag, suggests Suzanne M. Levine, D.P.M., adjunct clinical instructor at New York College of Podiatric Medicine and clinical assistant podiatrist at Wycoff Heights Medical Center, both in New York City. After sitting still for at least 10 minutes, remove the coverings and file the callus with a pumice stone. *Caution*: Don't try this remedy if you are allergic or sensitive to aspirin.

Soak your feet in Epsom salts. To relieve pain, Dr. Levine recommends soaking your feet in Epsom

Avoid "Medicated" Corn Pads

One of the most popular store-bought remedies for corns is among the worst, says podiatrist Robert Diamond, D.P.M., a Pennsylvania podiatrist affiliated with Muhlenberg Hospital Center in Bethlehem and St. Luke's Hospital of Allentown.

"Medicated corn pads cause more problems than they're worth," says Dr. Diamond. "The 'medication' is salicylic acid, which turns the corn white and blister-free, so it can peel off. But what happens frequently is that the acid is so strong it goes through the corn and eats at the toe, causing an ulcer in the toe."

salts and warm water. Soaking twice a day, for 10 minutes each time, should provide some relief.

For footwear, think round. "Many women who wear pointy-toed shoes get corns on the fourth or smallest toe," says Dr. Bark. "Even if you don't get corns there, you're much better off with round-toed shoes or any style shoes with a large toe box." If corns are a recurring problem, he recommends getting a pair of open-toed shoes or sandals and wearing them as often as possible. With no friction on the toes, there's less discomfort—and you're less likely to develop *new* corns.

Lay on the low-cost lotion. There are many products that can help soften corns and calluses. Lotions and bath oils that contain lanolin, glycerin, or urea start at around $2 in most drugstores. "Fruit acid moisturizers such as LactiCare are also very effective when you apply them heavily," says Dr. Bark.

Pump up the padding. Place "horseshoe" moleskin or foam pads around a corn if it continues to hurt when you walk. Be cautious with these pads, though, as they can pressure the surrounding area too much when you're walking. "And if you wear nylons, which can be very irritating, even putting a bandage over the corn helps reduce the friction," says Dr. Diamond.

Go for the insole. "Wearing a Spenco insole to give you more padding is a good idea," says Dr. Diamond. The insole helps protect against calluses on the sole of the foot.

Cracked Skin

Dry, itchy skin is bad enough, but when eczema gets an attitude or psoriasis gets super serious, you may make the transition from considerable discomfort to full-fledged torture. Your skin can crack, leaving painful slits that bring agony with even the most basic body movements, such as stretching.

Doctors call these cracks skin fissures. You will probably call them something a little more colorful. Hands and feet are the most likely spots for cracked skin, but there are other vulnerable places, too.

"Sometimes the feet are so dry that they crack, particularly on the heel and between the toes—and these cracks are like little portholes for infection," says Houston podiatrist William Van Pelt, D.P.M., former president of the American Academy of Podiatric Sports Medicine. "Women who wear open-backed heels and slides are particularly prone."

Here's how to take the fire out of painful fissures.

Give yourself a good soak. "The best way to beat very dry skin is to hydrate it every night," says Dr. Van Pelt. "Each skin cell is like a little sponge, so each night before going to bed, I recommend soaking your feet or whatever part of your body is especially dry in warm water for about 20 minutes. During this soak, the skin cells will absorb water. Then pat yourself dry."

Seal up with a lube job. After soaking, seal in the moisture by applying a coating of a petroleum jelly product such as Vaseline, adds Dr. Van Pelt. "It works

Cracked Lips?
Maybe It's Your Toothpaste

Brushing twice daily with a tartar control toothpaste may be a good way to fight plaque, but that tooth-paste apparently doesn't do much good for your lips. Regular use of these toothpastes can leave skin cracked and cause an itchy rash around the mouth, according to research conducted by Bruce E. Beacham, M.D., associate professor of dermatology at the University of Maryland School of Medicine in Baltimore.

The reason: Tartar control toothpastes contain compounds that can irritate mucous membranes and other tissues, especially if you have atopic dermatitis or sensitive skin. In Dr. Beacham's research, however, he found that cracked lips and the accompanying rash *don't* occur when tartar control brands are used less often than once a day. So if you use the tooth-paste every other day or so, you'll help prevent your lips from cracking.

much better than commercially sold moisturizers, which don't have the same 'sealing' effect," he says. For foot care, he suggests, "after you apply Vaseline, put on a pair of socks and go to bed." If it's your hands that need attention, put on light cotton gloves at night after you give them the Vaseline treatment.

"Glue" the cracks. Although it doesn't cure skin fissures, you can lessen the pain by applying Super Glue to the slits, says Rodney Basler, M.D., a dermatol-ogist and assistant professor of internal medicine at the University of Nebraska Medical Center in Omaha. "A little dab of Super Glue takes the air away from the nerve endings and seals the slits." He says this procedure is perfectly safe on slits and minor paper cuts but shouldn't be tried on deep wounds.

Cuts and Scrapes

The rough-and-tumble years may be behind you, but somehow you never fully outgrow your vulnerability to cuts and scrapes. In fact, the chances of minor wounds can increase once you're over 60, because your skin isn't as protective as it once was.

"Ultraviolet rays make the skin more fragile and thin, especially as you grow older," says Frederic Haberman, M.D., assistant clinical professor of medicine (dermatology) at Albert Einstein College of Medicine in New York City and director of the Haberman Dermatology Institute in Ridgewood, New Jersey. "Fragile skin is much more vulnerable to cuts and scrapes if you bump up against a hard surface."

If you have a minor wound or scrape, you can use the advice here to deal effectively with it. And once you have your cut under control, you may want to consider the tips on reducing your chances of injury.

Stop the bleeding. Use gauze, a bandage, a clean cloth such as a towel or washcloth, or your hand to stop the bleeding, says Wyatt Decker, M.D., consultant and trauma coordinator in the department of emergency

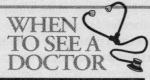

WHEN TO SEE A DOCTOR

If your cut is bleeding bright red and the blood is spurting, get to a doctor quickly. You may have punctured an artery, says Wyatt Decker, M.D., consultant and trauma coordinator in the department of emergency medicine at the Mayo Clinic in Rochester, Minnesota.

Also see a doctor if you experience these symptoms, which indicate a budding infection.

■ The wound is slow to heal and there is increased pain, redness, swelling, or heat.

■ The cut oozes pus or thick greenish fluid.

■ Red streaks run from the site of the wound toward your torso.

■ You have a fever.

medicine at the Mayo Clinic in Rochester, Minnesota. Apply pressure directly to the wound. If the wound is on your arm or hand and it is bleeding profusely, raise your arm above the level of your heart and continue to apply pressure to the wound until the bleeding stops, he says.

Clean the cut. Once the bleeding has stopped, clean the injured area thoroughly with ordinary soap and water, says Larry Millikan, M.D., chairman of the department of dermatology at Tulane University School of Medicine in New Orleans. Keep the wound clean by soaping and rinsing it three times a day.

Keep it moist. Apply an antibiotic ointment or ordinary petroleum jelly, says Dr. Millikan. Moist wounds heal quicker and are less susceptible to scarring.

Put on a second skin. Try using a colloidal dressing, a new over-the-counter product that can cut healing time in half, according to Wilma Bergfeld, M.D., head of clinical research in the department of dermatology at the Cleveland Clinic Foundation in Ohio. Like a second skin, a colloidal dressing is a membranous, jellylike material that breathes, allowing air, but not water, to pass over your wound. This locks moisture in, which helps you to heal quickly.

Wear protective clothing. Older people who have diabetes or who are taking steroids for arthritis must be especially careful when working outdoors, says Dr. Decker. "They have skin that is prone to tearing easily," he says. "I would advise wearing gloves for any kind of manual labor outside the house." Also, when doing yard work, wear trousers, long sleeves, and gloves.

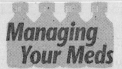

Managing Your Meds

If you've just cut yourself and you want to take something for the pain, make sure you reach for acetaminophen rather than aspirin or nonsteroidal anti-inflammatory drugs (NSAIDs) such as ibuprofen, naproxen, or ketoprofen. Aspirin and, to a lesser degree, NSAIDs can inhibit blood clotting, says W. Steven Pray, Ph.D., R.Ph., professor of nonprescription drug products at Southwestern Oklahoma State University in Weatherford.

The anticoagulant drug warfarin (Coumadin) can also slow clotting time because it thins the blood, says Dr. Pray.

Moisturize your skin. Cover your skin with a good moisturizer, even if the skin itself will be covered by long sleeves or pants. "Skin that is dried out is subject to more cuts, scrapes, and fissures than moist skin," Dr. Haberman says.

Know the problem spots in your home. Be careful on stairs and never move quickly on hardwood stairs in stocking feet, Dr. Haberman advises. Hardwood stairs are slippery, and you can fall easily and scrape or cut yourself. "Also, be careful getting in and out of the shower, which is where many older people injure themselves each year. Often, there's a counter that we bump into over and over again or some object in the house that causes us trouble. That's the kind of thing that we have to change to prevent injury."

Block those rays. Use plenty of sunscreen with a sun protection factor of at least 15 to protect any exposed area of your body from the sun, especially your face, hands, and neck, Dr. Haberman says. This will reduce the ultraviolet damage that makes your skin fragile.

Cysts and Sties

If you have something that looks like a pimple on or underneath your eyelid, you've turned to the right chapter. Never mind that you can't quite decide what to call that pimplelike annoyance—neither can doctors. Eye doctors frequently use both names interchangeably—cyst or sty—or even fancier terms like chalazia or hordeolum. Naming this bump can be as tricky as getting rid of it.

In plain English, here's what's going on. You have 33 oil glands per eyelid. When all is running well, these glands secrete oil to prevent your tears from evaporating. But sometimes a gland gets clogged. The oil can't get out. So it backs up and begins to swell and redden, becoming inflamed and sometimes painful. "It's like a blind pimple that won't come to the surface and pop," says Joseph Kubacki, M.D., professor and chairman of the ophthalmology department and assistant dean for medical affairs at Temple University School of Medicine in Philadelphia.

Sties slowly come and go on their own. If they become big enough or painful enough to inhibit your daily routine, then you should see your doctor, who may be able to drain the sty. Regardless of why you have this bump, here are some ways to get rid of it and prevent future occurrences.

Bathe it in hot compresses. Sties can sometimes stick around for weeks. But you can shorten that time with some moist heat, which stimulates blood flow, hastens the healing process, and encourages the cyst to drain, says James Gigantelli, M.D., director of ophthalmic plastic and reconstructive surgery at the University of Missouri in Columbia.

Fill your sink with the hottest water you can stand. Immerse two washcloths in the basin. Wring out one washcloth and hold it across your closed eyelid. When it cools, place it back in the basin and swap it for the other, says Dr. Gigantelli. Do this for 5 to 10 minutes four to six times a day. "If you do it any less than that, you won't do any good," he says. You

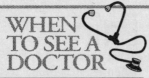

WHEN TO SEE A DOCTOR

If a sty keeps popping up in the exact same spot, if your eyeball is red or your vision blurry, or if you notice a discharge from the sty, see a doctor. These symptoms may signal an uncommon form of cancer (sebaceous carcinoma) that can affect people older than 60. If it doesn't spread to the lymph nodes, this type of cancer is curable.

should notice a difference within two to three weeks. Normally, sties could last for months.

Clean your lids regularly. To keep your glands from getting clogged, first close your eyes and place a warm washcloth over your eyelids for a minute or two. Next, cleanse your eyelids with a cotton swab dipped in "no tears" baby shampoo and gently run it back and forth along your lids, says Howard Barneby, M.D., spokesperson for the Better Vision Institute and ophthalmologist in Seattle. Then rinse with a warm washcloth.

Keep your eyes lubricated. When you have a sty, using artificial tears that are available at the drugstore can make you more comfortable. Use one drop four to six times a day if you have dry eyes to prevent future sties, says Dr. Gigantelli.

Throw away old makeup. Discard mascara brushes and other cosmetic items that come in contact with a sty. They could carry germs that might cause you to reinfect yourself. Also, don't share makeup with others, says Dr. Barneby.

Denture Pain

It's a well-worn legend that George Washington had wooden dentures. But that story, historians say, is just a load of mahogany. In reality, the Father of Our Country, who began losing his teeth at age 22, endured dentures made from an odd assortment of elephant, hippopotamus, and walrus tusks, which he called his "sea horse teeth."

He probably had a lot worse names for them.

But even modern dentures aren't perfect. Over time, your dentures may not fit as well as they once did, says Kenneth Shay, D.D.S., chief of dental services at the Veterans Affairs Medical Center in Ann Arbor, Michigan. No matter what your age, your gums continue to change over time, and as they do, dentures that once fit like a glove may begin to feel like hippo teeth. In these cases, your dentures will need to be adjusted or replaced. If you are getting dentures for the first time or having an old pair replaced, expect some discomfort. Denture pain is particularly common in the first few days after you get a new set. Here are a few suggestions that can help you adapt to new dentures.

Stick with what is comfortable. When you first get your dentures, continue eating what you have been eating until you get accustomed to them.

"Many of my patients think, 'Boy, the first thing I'm going to do after I get my dentures is go out and eat a big, juicy steak.' That simply isn't a good idea," Dr. Shay explains. "Your mouth needs time to adjust to

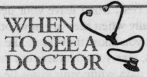

having two pieces of plastic inside of it. So continue eating what you were eating before you received your dentures, until you feel comfortable and confident that you can chew your food well."

Let a lozenge lounge around. Dentures can cause excess saliva in your mouth for a couple of weeks after you begin using them, Dr. Shay says. That's because your mouth thinks your dentures are food and produces saliva to begin digesting them. Eventually, your mouth will adapt to your dentures, and saliva production will return to normal.

In the meantime, suck on sugarless candies or lozenges frequently, Dr. Shay suggests. It will help you swallow more often and get rid of some of the excess saliva.

Give your gums a rest. Don't leave your dentures in too long, especially when they are new, otherwise your gums will let you know they don't like it. If you develop sore gums, take your dentures out and set them aside for a few days while your gums heal. Then try using the dentures again, suggests Flora Parsa Stay, D.D.S., dentist in Oxnard, California, and author of *The Complete Book of Dental Remedies*.

Take your dentures out for at least six hours a day, either while you're sleeping or when you're at home doing household chores, Dr. Shay says.

Clean 'em right. Take your dentures out of your mouth before bed, brush them thoroughly with a denture cleanser, then place them in a glass of water overnight. Avoid using regular toothpastes, because they are too abrasive for most dentures, according to Dr. Shay. These pastes can damage your dentures to the point that they don't fit properly, which will cause sore gums.

Douse the ache. Take out your dentures, then rinse your mouth three times a day with a rinse made with goldenseal, a potent herbal remedy, to help soothe denture pain, Dr. Stay says. To prepare the rinse, add ½ tablespoon of dried goldenseal and ½ teaspoon of baking soda to ½ cup of warm water. Cool and strain before using.

Seek an herbal solution. Dab a bit of aloe vera gel or eucalyptus oil on a cotton-tipped swab and apply it directly to your gums where the dentures are causing pain, Dr. Stay suggests. These products soothe and heal sore gums. You can use the gel or oil as needed, but for best results, avoid eating for at least one hour after applying these products.

Rule out allergies. Some people are allergic to denture cleansers and adhesives, Dr. Stay says. A few

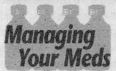

Managing Your Meds

Any drug that dries out the mouth can contribute to denture pain, says Gretchen Gibson, D.D.S., director of the geriatric dentistry program at the Veterans Administration Medical Center in Dallas. Without enough saliva, your dentures will rub against your gums and cause discomfort.

Medications that are used to control high blood pressure, like prazosin (Minipress), and antidepressants like amitriptyline (Elavil) are among the common drugs prescribed to seniors that can dry out your mouth and lead to denture discomfort, Dr. Gibson says. Denture pain also may be a side effect of:

✦ Diuretics such as chlorothiazide (Diuril) or furosemide (Lasix)

✦ Nitroglycerin (Nitrostat) and other drugs used to control angina

✦ Oxybutynin (Ditropan) and other drugs used to control urinary incontinence

✦ Oral steroids used for asthma, like beclomethasone (Beclovent)

are even allergic to materials in the dentures themselves. In addition to a burning sensation in the mouth, these allergies can irritate the gums and cause mouth ulcers.

If you suspect that you have an allergy, ask your dentist about substitutes for the cleansers and adhesives you're using. Then try out the alternative products one by one and see whether the irritation subsides. If no change occurs after this elimination process, leave your dentures out and see what happens. If your dentures are causing the problem, you may need new dentures that are made with different materials, Dr. Stay says.

Diarrhea

As they say in football, the best offense is a good defense. And diarrhea is your body's best *offensive* defense. Whether its much-ballyhooed revenge can be blamed on Montezuma, the blue plate special, a disagreeable antibiotic, a sneaky viral infection, or even stress, diarrhea is the body's painful way of saying "No, thanks!"

Sure, diarrhea lacks a certain something in elegance, but it sure makes up for it in effectiveness. A couple of trips to the toilet (okay, so maybe more than just a couple) and you're usually back on your feet.

Although it typically takes nature anywhere from two to four days to run this course, here's how to help take the kick out of the "runs."

Be clear on your diet. Most folks know that liquids are the suggested nourishment for the first 24 hours when diarrhea hits. But don't assume that any old liquid will do. "You should take only clear

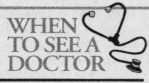

WHEN TO SEE A DOCTOR

See your doctor if your diarrhea symptoms include any of the following:

■ A sustained fever of over 101°F

■ Abdominal pain more severe than the "churning stomach" sensation normally associated with diarrhea

■ No progress or a worsened condition after three or four days

■ Blood, pus, or mucus in your stool

■ Inability to keep liquids down, lasting for more than 24 hours—or other signs of dehydration such as constant extreme thirst, tongue dryness, sunken eyeballs, and cracked or dry lips

Although these may be symptoms of minor ailments, all require a doctor's attention for diagnosis.

liquids: If you *can't* see through it, stay away from it," says William B. Ruderman, M.D., chairman of the department of gastroenterology at the Cleveland Clinic–Florida in Fort Lauderdale and an expert on diarrhea. "That means you *should* consume soda, tea, bouillon, and apple juice. Sports drinks like Gatorade are especially good, because they replace sugars and electrolytes (potassium and sodium). But *avoid* acidic citrus juices, such as orange and grapefruit, and *especially* tomato juice." Exceptions? Beer doesn't qualify, even though you can see through it. Nor do wine, clear alcohol, and mixed drinks. In fact, too much beer, wine, or any other kind of alcohol can cause diarrhea.

Food-wise, the best choices after the initial 24 hours include "translucent" foods like chicken broth and Jell-O. Whatever you choose to eat at this time should be bland and easily digested.

Get cultured with yogurt. One of the few exceptions to the clear cuisine rule is yogurt, whose active cultures contain "good" bacteria your bowel loses to the "bad" bacteria that prompted the diarrhea. "Yogurt is especially effective when the diarrhea is caused by food poisoning (like traveler's diarrhea)," says Manfred Kroger, Ph.D., professor of food science at Pennsylvania State University in University Park. "And it's also effective when diarrhea is the result of stress or antibiotic or radiation treatment. Basically, yogurt's active cultures help Mother Nature speed up the process of replacing the beneficial benign bacteria, and you feel a lot better faster." If yogurt isn't your thing, any acidophilus or fermented dairy product will do. Check the supermarket's dairy case.

Exercise your sweet tooth. A spoonful of sugar helps your body hold on to whatever you're drinking. "Glucose aids the absorption of water by the gut, so if you have sugar in whatever you're taking, you can absorb it more easily," says Dr. Ruderman. "If you're drinking tea or apple juice, add a teaspoonful of sugar to aid in absorption. If you're drinking soda, stick with regular sugared types and stay away from 'diet' varieties." (If you do drink soda, he adds, open the cap and let the soda go flat before you imbibe.)

Forget about high fiber—for now. Now's not the time for oat bran and other high-fiber foods or

Avoiding Traveler's Diarrhea

Sure, you want to "experience" a foreign country—but only to a point. So here's how travelers can stay one step ahead of the "runs" while abroad, according to William B. Ruderman, M.D., chairman of the department of gastroenterology at the Cleveland Clinic–Florida in Fort Lauderdale and an expert on diarrhea.

■ "When traveling abroad, drink *only* bottled or canned beverages—including water. Just because you're staying in a fancy hotel, don't assume the water is safe. The hotel gets its water from the same city water supply as everyone else."

■ Don't use ice in your drinks. "People think they're safe drinking bottled sodas, but then they use ice, get diarrhea, and wonder what happened. It may not be as refreshing, but you're better off with a warm soda."

■ Don't eat any food that is unpeeled or raw. If you're having any local fruit, peel it—even if it's an apple or a pear. And make sure everything you eat is cooked thoroughly."

■ Don't assume you're A-OK when traveling in the U.S.A. "I would be suspicious of the water supply in every camping area in the country that's in a backwoods, mountainous area. Take your own water supply."

complex carbohydrates. "It's unwise to stress your system with a lot of nonabsorbable fiber," adds Dr. Ruderman. "When you have diarrhea, the blander, the better." That means choose white toast, not wheat. And go for light foods such as cooked carrots, applesauce, baked chicken (without the skin), and other things that don't cause gas. Avoid pasta, corn, oats, and most fruits, particularly prunes, pears, and apples. Also, have some bananas: Diarrhea can cause potassium depletion, and bananas are high in potassium.

Be anti-antacid. Yesterday's heartburn often becomes today's diarrhea, especially when you treat it with over-the-counter medications. "Antacids are the most common cause of drug-related diarrhea," says Harris Clearfield, M.D., professor of medicine and director of the division of gastroenterology at Hahnemann University Hospital in Philadelphia. "Maalox and Mylanta both have magnesium hydroxide in them, which acts exactly like milk of magnesia, making these antacids a common cause of diarrhea." Meanwhile, antacids with aluminum hydroxide, such as Riopan and Amphojel, can cause constipation. (True, this is the opposite effect, but it's just as unwanted.)

Keep drinking. "The more you drink, the better you'll be," says Dr. Ruderman. "Even if you're not thirsty, it's important to take in a lot of fluids, because diarrhea can cause dehydration." His advice? At least six to eight ounces every two hours. "You should drink between two and three liters a day," Dr. Ruderman adds. That's the equivalent of 1½ 32-ounce bottles of soda.

Note: Drink even more if you haven't urinated in the past six hours, feel thirsty, or experience sunken eyeballs. And drink a lot if your tongue feels very dry or your lips become dry and start to crack.

Don't assume you'll be in the pink with the pink stuff. If you think diarrhea is the result of something you ate and you also have a fever, don't take Pepto-Bismol. "Antidiarrheals such as Pepto-Bismol can prolong salmonella (food poisoning)," says Dr. Ruderman. The medication slows down "gut motility"— that is, the speed at which the food moves through your system—so the bad stuff stays in your body longer. (However, if you have familiar traveler's diarrhea, *without* fever, Pepto-Bismol may help.)

Diverticulosis

D iverticulosis is a classic good-news–bad-news condition. On the one hand, it's a disease with virtually no symptoms, and it may never cause problems. On the other, diverticulosis can progress and become a related, though more serious, problem known as diverticulitis. Together, the two ailments are known as diverticular disease.

No question, you're at greater risk of getting diverticular disease as you get older. Diverticulosis, especially, is a common problem in America, reports Peter McNally, D.O, chief of gastroenterology at Evans Army Hospital in Colorado Springs, Colorado, and

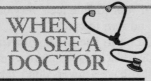

WHEN TO SEE A DOCTOR

Most people never know they have diverticuli (small multiple pouches that generally develop on the colon) until one of the sacs becomes inflamed. By then, the disease may have progressed into diverticulitis, a more serious complication.

Talk to your doctor if you feel unexplained pain in the lower left part of your abdomen, says Peter McNally, D.O., chief of gastroenterology at Evans Army Hospital in Colorado Springs, Colorado, and spokesperson for the American College of Gastroenterology. The pain may be accompanied by a fever and sweating, especially during bowel movements. If you have these symptoms or if you notice bloody stool, "see your doctor that day," says Dr. McNally.

spokesperson for the American College of Gastroenterology.

After you cross the treacherous waters of middle age, there's a very good chance that you'll get diverticulosis. According to the National Digestive Disorders Clearinghouse, about half of all Americans between 60 and 80 have diverticulosis, and almost everyone over 80 does.

Some definitions: A diverticulum is a grape-size pouch or sac that protrudes from the wall of the colon (large intestine). Sacs occur in other places along the gastrointestinal tract as well, but rarely. The pouches are thought to arise from excess pressure buildup in the colon, usually due to a lack of fiber in the diet. Doctors often compare the condition to an inner tube poking through weak spots on a tire.

Typically with diverticulosis, diverticuli (small multiple pouches) appear. Once established on the colon, they're permanent. Most people never know they have the condition, says Michael Epstein, M.D., founder of Digestive Disorders Associates in Annapolis, Maryland.

Diverticulitis occurs, however, when the diverticuli trap bits of stool or undigested food and become inflamed. This inflammation causes abdominal pain, usually around the left side of the lower abdomen. If the diverticuli become infected, the pain is accompanied by fever, nausea, vomiting, chills, and cramping. At this point, people often see their doctor, who diagnoses the disease. Because diverticulosis usually "flies below radar," people can miss opportunities to stop its transformation, says Dr. Epstein.

Fortunately, that transition from diverticulosis to diverticulitis may not occur—the statistical likelihood is 10 to 25 percent—and you can do things to improve your odds of never developing either affliction.

Viva variety. In countries where dietary fiber is high, such as Africa and China, diverticular disease is virtually nonexistent. Although there's no conclusive evidence, that's a strong case for increasing your intake of fiber as part of a regular healthy diet, says Dr. McNally. "Try to get from 25 to 40 grams of fiber in your diet a day," he says. That's combined soluble and

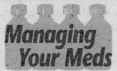

Managing Your Meds

Sometimes, taking medicine is a catch-22. That's especially true if you have diverticulitis, because taking a pain medication may make your situation worse. Sure, the pain may go away for a time, but the pain medication may make your already sluggish colon move even slower and make your diverticulitis worse, says W. Steven Pray, Ph.D., R.Ph., professor of nonprescription drug products at Southwestern Oklahoma State University in Weatherford. Beware of constipation-causing pain medications, especially narcotics like codeine, which is found in products such as Tylenol with codeine, and morphine (Duramorph).

Before taking corticosteroids, for example, fludrocortisone (Florinef), cortisone (Cortone Acetate), and dexamethasone (Decadron), be sure to tell your doctor that you have diverticulitis. These drugs can mask symptoms of diverticulitis and ulcers, says Dr. Pray.

Several drugs may even cause diverticulitis, warns Dr. Pray. Before taking donepezil (Aricept), which is used to

insoluble fiber because both can help. Soluble fiber, which dissolves easily in water, takes on a soft texture in the intestines that helps prevent dry, hard stools. Insoluble fiber passes almost unchanged through the intestines and adds bulk to the stool. Dr. McNally recommends incorporating high-fiber foods such as beans, whole grains like buckwheat, bran cereals such as Kellogg's All-Bran, fresh fruits like avocados, and vegetables such as artichokes into a daily regimen. Add

treat Alzheimer's disease; risperidone (Risperdal), which is prescribed for psychotic disorders like schizophrenia; or sertraline (Zoloft), which is used to treat depression, alert your doctor if you have diverticulosis or are at risk for it.

If you already have diverticulitis, your doctor may have prescribed an antispasmodic such as hyoscyamine (Gastrosed). This powerful medication may interact with certain other medications. Be sure to tell your doctor if you are also taking any of the following:

✦ Over-the-counter diarrhea medicine containing kaolin and pectin (Kapectolin) or attapulgite (Kaopectate)

✦ Antifungals such as ketoconazole (Nizoral) that are used to treat serious fungus infections

✦ Tricyclic antidepressants such as amitriptyline (Elavil)

✦ Over-the-counter and prescription potassium supplements, which may be used to treat high blood pressure, such as potassium chloride (Kay Ciel)

fiber to your diet slowly. Too much, too soon may lead to gassiness, bloating, and diarrhea. Each week, increase your daily intake by no more than five grams, the amount of fiber in one cup of cooked carrots, says Dr. McNally.

Raise your glass. Dr. Epstein says that increasing water and fiber at the same time is a good idea. Lacking sufficient fiber, the bowel has to work harder to push the stool out. He advises drinking plenty of fluids, six to eight glasses daily, which just means a tall glass every couple of hours. Not sure you're getting enough water? Test yourself by examining your urine. "It should look light, not dark," says Dr. Epstein.

Build a base at breakfast. Another good idea: Mix a tablespoon of powdered fiber with a glass of orange juice in the morning. "It's a real simple, healthy way to start the day," says Dr. McNally. Check your pharmacy shelves for powdered fiber that comes in different flavors, consistencies, and sizes, like Metamucil and Citrucel.

Investigate veggies. "In the best of all possible worlds," says Joanne Curran-Celentano, Ph.D., R.D., associate professor of nutritional sciences at the University of New Hampshire in Durham, "you want to get a lot of fiber from vegetables" and not only because of their fiber content. Vegetables contain other desirable nutrients that are good for the body, such as cancer-fighting beta-carotene. Her favorites include kale and squash.

Subtract seeds. Doctors are currently debating the effects of seeds on diverticulosis. Some experts say that seeds of all types can aggravate the condition and lead to diverticulitis. Dr. Epstein, for instance, tells people to at least cut back on seeds as well as corn, nuts, and popcorn.

Stay active. As you age, physical activity falls off, notes Bryant Stamford, Ph.D., director of the Health Promotion and Wellness Center at the University of Louisville in Kentucky. Without the benefits of exercise, the gastrointestinal tract slows down, which can make diverticular disease worse. So try to get a little bit of exercise—even if it's just a walk around the block—every day, he suggests.

Dizziness

Scientists are discovering that the topsy-turvy sensations astronauts endure following prolonged space flights are similar to the dizzy feelings that many Americans experience as they age, says William H. Paloski, Ph.D., director of NASA's life sciences research laboratories at the Johnson Space Center in Houston.

For astronauts, the answer is simple—the body's balance system needs gravity to work properly. In the weightless environment of space, the balance system essentially shuts down, and astronauts must adapt to living in a world where up and down are meaningless. Once astronauts land, it takes time to get used to relying on their balance mechanisms again. So they may feel dizzy and disoriented for a few days, Dr. Paloski says.

On earth, particularly for older adults, dizziness also is a sign that the body's balance mechanisms are out of whack. Fatigue, stress, anemia, anxiety, inner-ear infections, and other common ailments can cause dizziness at any age. But many chronic conditions associated with aging, such as diabetes, heart disease, high blood pressure, and arteriosclerosis (hardening of the arteries), also can affect your balance, says Brian W. Blakley, M.D., chief of otolaryngology at the University of Manitoba Faculty of Medicine in Winnipeg and author of *Feeling Dizzy*. Here are a few ways to stop feeling topsy-turvy.

Get down. For mild dizziness, the best thing you can do is lie down, relax, and wait for the dizziness to go away, Dr. Blakley suggests. Often, the sensation will

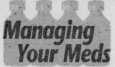

Managing Your Meds

Almost any drug can cause dizziness, particularly when taken in conjunction with another medication made with the same active ingredient, says W. Steven Pray, Ph.D., R.Ph., a professor of nonprescription drug products at Southwestern Oklahoma State University in Weatherford. Sleeping pills like Nytol and allergy medications like Benadryl, for instance, both contain the antihistamine diphenhydramine. If you take these two over-the-counter (OTC) products together, it may cause an overdose of antihistamines and greatly increase your risk of developing dizziness and other side effects. Always ask your doctor or pharmacist about drug interactions before taking any combination of medications, he suggests. In addition, be aware that the following drugs also can turn your world upside down.

✦ High blood pressure medications including terazosin (Hytrin) and prazosin (Minipress)

✦ Anticonvulsants that contain phenytoin (Dilantin)

✦ Antibiotics such as cephalosporins (cephalexin)

✦ OTC and prescription pain medications including aspirin, ibuprofen (Advil), and codeine as found in many pain medications, such as Tylenol with codeine

disappear within a few minutes. Even if you're at some social occasion, excuse yourself, take a break, and lie down on a couch or stretch out in a lounge chair with your feet as high as possible, at least higher than your heart. You want to elevate your legs to stimulate blood flow to your brain. If there's no place to lie down, just retire for a minute—even go to the john if you have to—sit down, and lower your head between your legs until the dizziness subsides, he suggests.

Eat three squares a day. Skipping meals can result in low blood sugar, a common cause of dizziness, Dr. Blakley explains. Similarly, eating unusual fare like an all-liquid diet can create a mineral imbalance in your body that could cause wooziness. Eat at least three well-balanced meals a day consisting of three to five servings of fruits and vegetables; six to 11 servings of breads, cereal, and other foods made with grains; two to three servings of dairy products like milk and cheese; and two to three servings of meat and fish.

Shake the salt habit. Too much salt in the diet causes the body to retain fluid, which can disrupt the workings of the inner ear, according to Dr. Blakley. Avoid cheese, bacon, and salty snacks like potato chips, popcorn, and french fries. Read package labels carefully and reach for foods that are advertised as having no salt added or being low in sodium or reduced-sodium. Use herbs, spices, and fruit juices to season foods, he says. And be sure to rinse canned foods like tuna to remove salty juices.

Move like a snail. Rapid changes in head positions, particularly when you shift from lying down to standing up, can cause dizziness, Dr. Blakley explains. Move in stages. If you're getting out of bed, for instance, sit on the edge of the mattress for at least 30 seconds before standing.

Jump into the deep end. Practicing the very movements that cause dizziness can help your brain learn to compensate for the problem. As a starting

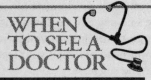

WHEN TO SEE A DOCTOR

Seek immediate medical attention if any of the following are true:

■ Your dizziness is unexplained, severe, recurrent, or persistent.

■ You also have difficulty speaking or swallowing.

■ You also develop sudden weakness, numbness, or tingling on one side of your body.

■ You also have a severe headache.

■ Your vision suddenly gets worse or you develop double vision.

■ You also have ringing in your ears or sudden loss of hearing in one ear.

■ You feel dizzy after a fall or after a head injury.

point, Dr. Blakley suggests doing three repetitions of the following exercises, three or four times a day. These exercises are designed to stimulate the balance sensors in your inner ear. They are supposed to make you dizzy and should be done while sitting in a chair or other safe place so that you will not fall if you become dizzy. Keep your eyes open.

First, try some horizontal head rotations.

1. Start in a sitting position looking straight ahead.

2. Turn your head all the way to the right, keeping your chin parallel to the floor and moving it toward your right shoulder. Then turn all the way to the left, going back and forth, slowly increasing the speed of rotation of your head as much as you can in 20 seconds.

3. Rest a few seconds.

You can also try some vertical head rotations.

1. Start in the sitting position with your head turned a little, as if you are looking at an object to your right, and your chin parallel to the floor.

2. Move your head so that your left ear moves toward your left knee. Your ear will not touch your knee in this exercise. You will have to bend your neck. Move in this direction until your head is horizontal, usually about a foot above your knee.

3. Alternate between these two positions as quickly as you can for 20 seconds.

4. Rest a few seconds.

5. Do steps 1 and 2 in the opposite direction, turning your head to the left and then moving your right ear toward your right knee. Alternate between these positions as quickly as you can for 20 seconds.

Dry Eyes

Every time you blink, a film of tears spreads over your eyes. For the wet-eyed crowd, that film can turn to an eye bath when you're watching a classic weeper like, say, *Old Yeller*. But if you suffer from dry eyes, even the tear-jerkingest flick can leave your hanky dry.

But another thing happens when you have dry eyes: They actually ache. Lacking the ability to cover or coat the cornea (the clear front surface of the eye) with a thin, protective coating of tears, your eyes start burning and stinging. At worst, it may feel as though a grain of sand is permanently embedded in your parched peepers. And because of this ongoing problem, your vision may be mildly blurred, or your eyes may become sensitive to light.

There are many causes: Medicines such as decongestants, tranquilizers, and antihistamines, as well as drugs for high blood pressure, may all cause dry eyes. You can also get dry eyes if you have an allergy to contact lens products. Winter winds, air-conditioning, and indoor heating are all potential culprits as well. Chronic cases often result from menopause, rheumatoid arthritis, or Sjögren's syndrome, a gland condition that also causes dry mouth and vaginal dryness. Sometimes dry eyes occur for no apparent reason. But whatever the cause, here are some ways to get your peepers dewy again—and to give you a chance to shed a tear the next time you hear a sob story.

Oil your eyes with a washcloth compress.
Place a warm washcloth on your closed eyelids for five to 10 minutes several times a day to help open the clogged oil glands in the eyelids," says Eric Donnenfeld, M.D., associate professor of ophthalmology at North Shore University Hospital/Cornell Medical College in Manhasset, New York.

Here's why it works. Tears are made up of three components: water, oil, and mucus. Artificial tears, the kind sold in eyedropper form in drugstores, can replace the water component of your tears. But those drops don't replace the oil. Only your own eyes can do that. So the warm compress helps your eyes do the work they're supposed to, according to Dr. Donnenfeld.

Using a compress is *especially* helpful if you have "crusty" eyes when you wake up or at other times of the day, says Dr. Donnenfeld. (About 50 percent of dry-eye sufferers get this crusty condition—called blepharitis—in the morning or during the day.)

Choose the right artificial tears. Over-the-counter artificial tears are a mixture of saline and some type of film-forming substance, such as polyvinyl alcohol or synthetic cellulose. This solution can be used several times a day, because it mimics real tears and provides a soothing balm whenever your eyes feel dry.

When choosing a brand, keep in mind that thicker formulas remain in the eyes longer, so you'll need to use them less frequently. But the thicker kind can blur vision and leave a gooey residue on your eyelashes. Thinner drops, on the other hand, need to be used more frequently. "You'll need to experiment to see what drops work for your condition," says Paul

Nighttime Is the Right Time for Treatment

Even when your lids are closed, eyes can dry out, which is why your doctor will probably suggest that you use either a combination tear-replacement/moisture-sealing ointment or a "moisture chamber" at night.

These over-the-counter superthick ointments, which contain petroleum and mineral oil, last longer than drops, says Paul Amber, M.D., assistant clinical professor of ophthalmology at Harvard University in Cambridge, Massachusetts. To insert, pull the lower lid down, look up, and squeeze a dab of ointment in the trough between your lid and eye. Blink to spread the ointment around. Keep in mind that ointments can blur your vision for a while, so be sure you don't use them before driving.

Your eye doctor can supply you with ready-made moisture chamber glasses to wear during sleep, but a pair of ordinary watertight swim goggles will also do fine. In a pinch, says Mitchell H. Friedlaender, M.D., director of the Cornea Service at the Scripps Clinic and Research Foundation in La Jolla, California, you can even make your own chamber by taking a piece of plastic food wrap and securing it with petroleum jelly around your eyes. As tears evaporate, the air inside the chamber becomes slightly more humid, preventing further tear evaporation and creating a comfortable, moist atmosphere. To boost the moisture content, use ocular ointments along with your moisture chamber.

Michelson, M.D., senior staff ophthalmologist at the Mericos Eye Institute in La Jolla, California.

"But use only commercially prepared, preservative-free products," warns Donald Doughman, M.D., professor of ophthalmology at the University of Minnesota in Minneapolis. "If it doesn't say 'nonpreserved' or 'preservative-free' on the label or box, don't buy it. Preservatives can damage your eyes."

Turn heating and cooling vents away. A blast of heat or air-conditioning may be what your body craves, but it's no good for your eyes. "When you're driving, keep air vents pointed down, away from your face," according to Dr. Donnenfeld. "And when you're home, do the same: Point heating and cooling ducts away from areas where you spend a lot of time. This is really important if your home has forced hot-air heating, because that can dry out your eyes very quickly."

Dress for the slopes. The Great Outdoors can deliver a one-two punch to dry eyes. The sun's brightness makes them supersensitive, and the wind and low humidity dry them out. That's why many experts suggest that you wear eye-protecting sunglasses or goggles for any outdoor activity. "Wraparound sunglasses are very helpful because they protect the sides of the eyes, which are vulnerable to the wind," says Dr. Donnenfeld. "But if you have *very* dry eyes, the best thing you can do is wear ski goggles when you're outside. They create a moist chamber for the eyes."

Take a blink break. Doing close work—typing at a video display terminal, driving, sewing, even watching television—can exacerbate even mild cases of eye dryness, says Dr. Michelson. "People doing tasks that require concentration tend to stare and not blink as much." And when you don't blink very often, eye moisture evaporates rapidly. So if you're doing concentrated work and notice dry eyes, look away and take a blink break whenever possible. Blinking helps restore the tear film over your eyes.

Humidify your surroundings. Moisturizing the air can keep mucous membranes from drying out during sleep, especially in the winter, doctors suggest. "When moisture is low, your eyes dry up fast," says Dr. Donnenfeld. "If you can, get a humidifier for your bedroom or other places where you spend a lot of time." And when you're using a hair dryer, don't run it any longer than necessary.

Moisten up and fly right. If you know you'll be in the arid environment of an airplane cabin, be extra vigilant in using artificial tears. And be sure the overhead air vents are pointed away from your eyes, says Dr. Donnenfeld.

Dry Mouth

Ever notice how drooling seems to come naturally to the very young? From the mouths of innocent babes comes enough saliva to turn a bib to a bath mat. But as we grow up, we tend to dry up. The addition of years seems to translate to a loss of saliva.

Aging alone, however, isn't the only cause of xerostomia, or dry mouth. More often, we can blame it on all the 24-karat hassles that we live with in the golden age of our lives: Most cases of dry mouth can be blamed on some 400 medicines used to treat nearly everything from arthritis to ulcers. Even caffeine and over-the-counter pain relievers such as ibuprofen (Advil) can contribute to dry mouth.

Besides making your mouth feel like it's plugged with cotton, dry mouth can make swallowing, eating, and even talking difficult. Worst case: Mouth tissue becomes cracked and irritated, and you begin to suffer related problems such as bad breath, lost fillings, gum infections, and tooth decay. But here's how to permanently wet your whistle if you're among the one in three Americans with dry mouth.

Take a hard line against soft drinks. Drinking more is the obvious solution to dry mouth—as long as you're *not* slurping soda, orange juice, or other beverages that contain either citric or phosphoric acid.

"Soft drinks are very acidic, and people with dry mouth lack the saliva necessary to neutralize these acids that can harm the teeth," says James Sciubba, D.M.D., Ph.D., chairman of the department of dental medicine at Long Island Jewish Medical Center in New Hyde Park, New York, and founding chairman of the Sjögren's Syndrome Foundation.

Instead, Dr. Sciubba says carrying a flask of water and taking frequent sips is the best way to get your mouth moist again. "The key is how frequently you drink, not necessarily how much you drink," he says.

Suck on fruit pits. Pits from peaches, nectarines, and cherries help increase saliva flow without adding any calories. Just be careful not to swallow them.

Eat mushy foods. Eating any food will stimulate saliva. But the best choices are soft foods and those moistened with sauces or gravies that go down the hatch easily, says Nelson Rhodus, D.M.D., associate

Brush Frequently to Beat Bad Breath

Brushing your teeth is even more important than usual when you suffer from dry mouth. Since saliva usually washes away trapped food morsels, when you're short on saliva, food hangs around longer—and that creates bad breath.

Since dry mouth almost guarantees bad breath, Nelson Rhodus, D.M.D., associate professor of oral medicine at the University of Minnesota in Minneapolis, suggests that you dip your toothbrush in baking soda moistened with water and scrub your teeth and tongue twice daily to help neutralize odor and bacteria. That's also good for your teeth, since anyone with dry mouth is at greater risk for cavities and other dental problems.

professor of oral medicine at the University of Minnesota in Minneapolis.

Go sugarless. "Use of sugar by a patient with a dry mouth will produce tooth decay within six months," warns Dr. Sciubba. "One of the best ways to keep saliva flowing is to suck on hard candies or to chew gum, but the gum and candy must be sugarless." In fact, sucking on sorbitol-containing sugarless candies, mints, and gum has been found to increase saliva tenfold in some people.

Rinse your mouth with some fluoride. When saliva production is low, your risk of cavities and gum disease is high. Swishing with a fluoride mouth rinse at bedtime helps remineralize teeth and can help protect you against cavities and gum disease.

There are also artificial saliva products that help. "In our studies, we found that over-the-counter products such as MouthKote provide a nice, moist coating over mucous membranes," says Dr. Rhodus. Other products include Xero-Lube, Salivart, and Evian mineral water spray.

Moisturize the air. Using a cool-air vaporizer in your home is a good way to add much-needed extra humidity to the air—especially if you're a mouth breather, says Dr. Sciubba. But make an effort to always breathe through your nose to prevent saliva from evaporating.

Use lemon sparingly. While full-fledged lemonade should be avoided, tasting some lemon juice diluted in water or rinsing with a bit of lemon juice and glycerin is a good way to stimulate the flow of saliva, says Dr. Rhodus. But here's the drawback: If your mucous membranes are so dry that you have developed sores, the citric acid could further irritate your mouth. (If you do have these sores, go light on lemon as well as spicy foods and anything else that can irritate your mouth.)

Dry Skin

Life can be hard on your skin. So many showers, baths, and swimming pools. So many hours in the sun, wind, and rain. Like the natural forces that can erode mountains, these everyday experiences have the unfortunate power to erode the skin's protective layer of lipids, or oils.

By the time you've seen the passage of 22,000 days or so, your skin has been through a lot. Whatever it shows on the surface, just underneath it's wearing a bit thin—and where skin cells are skimpy, your body has a harder time holding moisture. The diminished lipid layer no longer holds moisture very well, says Norman Levine, M.D., professor and chief of dermatology at the University of Arizona Health Sciences Center in Tucson. And when you have only a skinny layer for moisture storage, you tend to get dry, sensitive skin.

But you don't have to give in to the forces of nature. You can even counteract the wear-away work of the elements that are against you. As it happens, there are a number of ways you can recapture your lost moisture. Here's how you can literally save your skin.

Rebuild your barriers. The best answer to dry skin, say Dr. Levine and other experts, is to rebuild your skin's protective barrier with a good moisturizer. Apply it all over at least twice a day. The moisturizer can replace some of the missing elements that used to allow your skin to retain fluids and keep itself moist.

Almost any moisturizer is fine, says Guy F. Webster, M.D., Ph.D., associate professor of dermatology at Thomas Jefferson University in Philadelphia. "Even petroleum jelly is a good moisturizer because it seals the skin and prevents moisture from being exposed to air and then evaporating." Dr. Webster also notes that when purchasing a moisturizer, you should look for the ingredient urea acid or lactic acid. The better moisturizers will contain one of those.

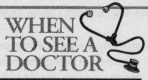

Go for a lipid cleanser. Most soaps contain detergents that break down and wash away the skin's natural oils, which is precisely what you don't want to happen. When you wash, use a gentle soap substitute that is designed to cleanse your skin without removing the oil. Look for body washes that contain lipids. (Lipid cleansers will have an oil such as mineral, linseed, castor, or soybean oil listed as part of the ingredients.) These products are gentle on the skin and are excellent moisturizers, says Mary Ruth Buchness, M.D., chief of dermatology at St. Vincent's Hospital and Medical Center in New York City and associate professor of dermatology and medicine at the New York Medical College in Valhalla. Cleansers that contain lipids include Nivea Visage Gentle Cleansing Lotion, Noxzema

Plus Cleansing Cream, and Ponds Cold Cream Deep Cleanser.

Lather up with moisturizing soaps. There are many moisturizing soaps available. Among the most widely recommended by dermatologists are Basis for Dry Skin and Neutrogena Dry Skin. Other good soap substitutes include Cetaphil and pHisoderm.

Or go the water route. The fact is, you don't have to use a soap or soap substitute all over your body. Just wash your face, hands, and odor-producing areas of your body such as your armpits and groin. Just rinse off the rest, suggests Dr. Levine.

Ration your bathing. It seems ironic, but one of the greatest threats to a skin's ability to stay moist

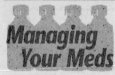

Managing Your Meds

Many medications can dry out your skin, says W. Steven Pray, Ph.D., R.Ph., professor of nonprescription drug products at Southwestern Oklahoma State University in Weatherford. Drugs prescribed for edema (water retention) are meant to dry out the body. These include loop diuretics such as furosemide (Lasix) and potassium-sparing ones like triamterene (Dyrenium). And many high blood pressure medications such as chlorothiazide (Diuril) have a similar diuretic effect. If you are currently taking medication and are concerned about dry skin, ask your doctor about the side effects of your medications. But be sure you don't stop any medication, especially for high blood pressure, unless your doctor is informed and gives consent.

is water itself, especially when it's piping hot. Hot water is especially destructive to the skin's natural oils, says Dr. Levine. Bathe as infrequently as possible, he advises, especially in winter when the air is dry. Once every two, three, or even four days might be enough for you. And when you do take a bath or shower, use lukewarm water and avoid lingering too long.

Leave a little water behind. After your shower or bath, pat yourself dry, leaving a little moisture on your skin, advises Dr. Buchness. Then apply your moisturizer. By applying your moisturizer on top of your slightly wet skin, you are sealing in the moisture and thus preventing it from escaping.

Hydrate with alpha hydroxy. Doctors may argue over the value of alpha hydroxy acids (AHAs) for eliminating wrinkles. But AHAs can remove dry, dead, and scaly skin and then moisturize the new tissue below. AHA moisturizers, which are made from milk, fruit, and sugarcane, trap water and hold it within your skin. By eliminating dead cells and plumping up the new ones, these moisturizers help keep your skin moist and youthful, says Dr. Buchness.

Give your skin a vacation. Before you go on your next vacation, consider what the climate will be like. "Very often, people who suffer from dry skin don't think about where they go on vacation and then find that their skin is even drier and more irritated when they go," explains Dr. Buchness. If you're in a humid place like New Orleans, your dry skin condition may ease a little. But what if you head for Arizona, where the temperatures are high and the humidity is down in the single-digit figures? That's just the kind of place where your skin could be most miserable. Instead, plan a trip to a place where your skin will get relief, too.

Earache

If you've been spending a lot of time with a box of tissues and a bag of throat lozenges and now you're lying awake with an aching ear, you already know two things about earaches: They often accompany bad colds and sore throats, and they're always nastier at night.

A typical earache begins when a congested eustachian tube—which runs from the back of the throat to the eardrum—can't regulate pressure or fluids in the ear. Pain starts when mucus or pus builds up behind the eardrum. The more the fluid builds, the greater the pressure and pain.

While antibiotic treatment can resolve the infection that's causing the pain, there are some things you can do for yourself to get temporary relief.

Warm up to relief. "The greatest pain reliever is warm, moist heat around the ear," says Stephen P. Cass, M.D., assistant professor of otolaryngology at the Eye and Ear Institute of Pittsburgh. A warm compress—such as a towel rung out in hot water and pressed against the ear—brings the most immediate relief, he says. Resoak the towel as it cools and use it as often as

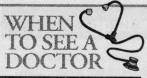

WHEN TO SEE A DOCTOR

If your ear hurts when you chew, it may be a tip-off that you have trouble in the jaw joint, says Clough Shelton, M.D., an otolaryngologist with the House Ear Clinic in Los Angeles. You might be a nighttime jaw clencher or have an inflamed or misaligned jaw caused by temporomandibular joint disorder—which can be diagnosed by a doctor.

Also, sudden or severe pain in your ear without an accompanying cold or sore throat is not typical. See your doctor if you notice blood or pus in the ear, redness or swelling around the ear, dizziness, or hearing loss. These could be signs of a severe infection that needs immediate attention.

you need to, even while you are being treated for an underlying infection, he suggests.

Try a liquid pillow. A hot water bottle wrapped in a towel also makes a comforting pillow for an aching ear, says Dr. Cass. If you get a lot of earaches and need something more portable, you can invest in a mini hot water bottle that's made to fit directly over the ear, he says.

Press on a gel pack. Another ear-warming alternative: Use a dual-purpose first-aid gel pack that you can warm up in hot water or the microwave, suggests Anthony J. Yonkers, M.D., chairman of the department of otolaryngology/head and neck surgery at the University of Nebraska Medical Center in Omaha. "Make

Don't Be Bugged

Tiny insects that find their way into ears usually find their way out pretty quickly—but not always. Some get stuck inside.

What should you do if you're bugged by a bug in your ear? Using an eardropper full of alcohol, flood the ear to kill the bug, suggests Stephen P. Cass, M.D., assistant professor of otolaryngology at the Eye and Ear Institute of Pittsburgh. Then gently irrigate the ear with water from an ear syringe.

"*Do not* try to fish for it with a tweezers, pencil, fingernail, or Q-Tip," he warns. You'll just push it in farther or damage your ear.

sure the gel pack is not too hot, then press it right on your ear, and it will make you feel better," he says.

Put your ear to the plate. Some people swear by old-time heat treatments like this: Warm up an oven-safe plate, wrap it in a towel, and rest your aching ear right on it. The plate should be warm and comforting, not hot, cautions Dr. Cass.

Find relief in your medicine cabinet. An adult with a cold or fever who develops ear pain can take aspirin, ibuprofen (Advil), acetaminophen (Tylenol), or another nonprescription painkiller, says Jerome C. Goldstein, M.D., executive vice president of the American Academy of Otolaryngology/Head and Neck Surgery in Alexandria, Virginia. Children with earaches should never be given aspirin, and other pain relievers should get a doctor's go-ahead. Your doctor may recommend children's Tylenol.

Get the drop on pain. A couple of drops of warm mineral oil may soothe a sore ear, says Clough Shelton, M.D., an otolaryngologist with the House Ear Clinic in Los Angeles. Warm the oil by putting it in hot water. Test it on your wrist as you would a baby's bottle. It should feel barely warm. Use an eyedropper to drip the oil in and gently pull the outside of the ear to make sure it goes down, he says. One caution: You can't use this method if the doctor says you have a perforated eardrum.

Decongest your head. If you're really congested, Sudafed or other decongestants can shrink your eustachian tube and bring ear pain down to size, says Dr. Goldstein. Ask your doctor what might be best for you.

Stay away from wind. If wind bothers your aching ears, wear a scarf when you're outside or put cotton in the opening of the ear, suggests Dr. Cass. But don't push the cotton down where you can't retrieve it with your fingers.

Soar above ear pain in airplanes. If your ears hurt when the pressure changes during an airplane flight, chew gum or suck on candy, especially during descent and landing, which is the most troublesome time of changing pressure. The chewing or sucking will activate the muscles that send air to your inner ears, says Dr. Shelton. When you hear your ears "pop," you'll feel better, because pressure in the ear is balanced.

If chewing doesn't work, close your mouth, relax your cheek muscles, hold your nose, and blow gently until you feel relief, Dr. Shelton says.

Take a dose before and after. Experienced flyers who expect painful flights can take Sudafed or use a nasal decongestant at the recommended dose for a day *before* they fly, says Dr. Yonkers. And if the pain is unresolved *after* you land, use decongestants for a day after your flight, too, adds Dr. Shelton.

Eczema

Eczema is a term doctors use to describe all kinds of red, blistering, oozing, scaly, brownish, thickened, and itchy skin conditions. Outbreaks can occur on the face and neck, in the folds of elbows and knees, on the hands, or, in extreme cases, over the entire body. While no one knows the cause, doctors say that allergies, sensitivity to environmental conditions like dry furnace air and scratchy clothes, and possibly stress can trigger eczema flare-ups.

Although many people outgrow eczema when they reach adulthood, others have outbreaks their whole lives. Eczema can be especially irritating for seniors because their oil-producing glands are not as active as they used to be, says John F. Romano, M.D., clinical assistant professor of dermatology at New York Hospital–Cornell Medical Center in New York City. This can lead to dry skin and greater irritation. And sometimes older skin heals more slowly, especially in the lower legs, because of reduced circulation, Dr. Romano adds.

There are several types of eczema, and some of them require very different treatments. Since many types appear alike, it might be tricky to get a correct diagnosis. But that's what you need, says Dr. Romano.

Once you know what you're dealing with, you can manage eczema a number of ways, all of which begin with an effective skin-care routine.

Maintain moisture. To prevent the dry skin that is at the root of eczema, you need to trap some moisture. Apply a soothing skin cream right after you finish bathing, says K. William Kitzmiller, M.D., dermatologist in private practice in Cincinnati. The best of the heavy creams or lotions, called emollients, are oily but unscented. Nivea cream, petroleum jelly, and even solid vegetable shortening are excellent for people with eczema, says Dr. Kitzmiller.

Emollients are safe to use as often as needed. "When you step out of the bath or shower, liberally apply your emollient and then blot your skin dry," suggests Dr. Kitzmiller. Since water gets into your skin when you bathe, the emollient helps trap the moisture and hold it there, he says.

Have some hydrocortisone cream. Most eczema flare-ups can be relieved by nonprescription 1-percent hydrocortisone cream such as Cortaid, according to Dr. Romano. Don't apply it every day, however, because it can cause spider veins and stretch marks. Intermittent use, no more than three times a week, should keep irritation in check, he says.

Time your baths. Doctors used to tell people with eczema to take quick baths—no longer than 10 minutes—to avoid having their skin dry out. Ignore that old thinking, says Kristin Leiferman, M.D., professor of dermatology at the Mayo Medical School in Rochester, Minnesota. Instead, take a leisurely bath for 10 to 20 minutes per day. Your skin cells will absorb water through their membranes and become hydrated. "You'll know that you've been in long enough when

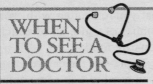

WHEN TO SEE A DOCTOR

Eczema can have many different causes, so if you develop an outbreak, it's smart to see a doctor to determine what's causing the itching, says John F. Romano, M.D., clinical assistant professor of dermatology at New York Hospital–Cornell Medical Center in New York City. Definitely get checked out if you have patches of skin that are:

■ Painful

■ Hot to the touch

■ Oozing a puslike discharge

your skin starts to pucker and crinkle," notes Dr. Leiferman.

Turn down the temp. When you take that bath, though, use lukewarm water. Hot bath water *can* dry out the skin. And hot water can also irritate skin that's already tender, explains Dr. Kitzmiller.

Eliminate scented products. Added fragrances are a chief cause of skin allergies and irritant reactions, according to Dr. Kitzmiller. If you have eczema, try to avoid any skin-care products that have fragrances.

Dr. Leiferman recommends nonirritating soaps and cleansers, like Dove or Aveeno, that don't have a lot of fragrance, color, or additives.

Milk it for all it's worth. Whole milk compresses are a low-cost way to soothe eczema flare-ups and reduce itchiness, says Dr. Kitzmiller. Saturate a gauze pad or cotton cloth with equal parts cold milk and ice water and apply it to the skin for about three minutes, he says. Resoak the cloth and reapply it at least two more times for three-minute soaks. You can repeat this treatment several times a day, he suggests, but be sure to rinse your skin with cool water after each application. Otherwise, you'll start to smell like sour milk.

Ice the itch. Another way to control the itch of eczema is to hold a plastic bag of ice on the affected area, says Dr. Kitzmiller. Wrap the ice pack in a towel and hold it on the inflamed zone as long as necessary.

Choose nonitchy clothing. Anything you can do to reduce itchiness is going to minimize damage to your skin caused by scratching, says Karen K. Deasey, M.D., chief of dermatology at Bryn Mawr Hospital in Pennsylvania. Choose cotton clothing and cotton bedding whenever possible. When your body is in contact with cotton, your skin stays cool and can breathe. Synthetic fabrics can be irritating and so can wool.

Turn to mild detergents. You can further reduce the itchiness of clothes by using mild laundry detergents such as Tide and Ivory and by rinsing garments twice to clear away all traces of detergent, says Dr. Deasey.

Shun the softeners. Avoid fabric softeners, advises Dr. Deasey, because they contain fragrances that can make your skin itch. She also suggests staying away from the newer blue liquid detergents because they leave residues on clothes, and if your skin reacts to those residues, you'll itch.

Humidify your surroundings. Anything you do to add moisture to the air is going to help relieve the dry skin and itch of eczema, says Dr. Kitzmiller. Ideal humidification, he says, is about 50 percent, "just

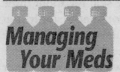

Managing Your Meds

If your eczema is normally under control but you have a flare-up, your doctor may prescribe a topical steroid cream such as fluocinonide (Lidex). Although many people express concerns about the side effects of topical steroids, side effects are rare as long as the medication is used appropriately, says John F. Romano, M.D., clinical assistant professor of dermatology at New York Hospital–Cornell Medical Center in New York City. Just be sure to use topical steroids as directed by your doctor.

Also, be on the alert for prescription drugs that can dry out skin and aggravate an eczema condition, says Dr. Romano. Among those known to cause problems are:

✦ Diuretics used to treat heart disease and high blood pressure, such as hydrochlorothiazide (Esidrix), that reduce fluid levels in the body and can dry the skin

✦ Some neurological and psychiatric medications, such as lithium (Eskalith), which can also irritate sensitive skin

Be careful with niacin, advises Dr. Romano. Too much can cause flushing, a trigger for at least one kind of dermatitis. If you are taking a prescription for niacin, be sure to take your recommended daily dose and no more. And alert your doctor if you have dermatitis symptoms accompanied by oily skin or seeping in the itchy area.

short of making the windows sweat." You can add moisture to the air in your home with a cold-air humidifier or by placing shallow pans of water near radiators, Dr. Kitzmiller says.

Protect your hands. Hand rashes are an extremely common form of eczema. Many household items could be causing these rashes, including soaps and detergents, solvents, cleaning agents, chemicals, and the ingredients in skin and personal care products. And once your hands become dry and chapped, they're even more vulnerable to household agents that could make them itch. Even innocuous-looking substances like water and baby products can make an outbreak worse when your hands are super-dry.

If you have eczema on your hands, doctors recommend wearing a pair of vinyl gloves with cotton liners to protect you from irritants whenever you do dishes or housework. Have four or five pairs and keep them in the kitchen, bathroom, and laundry areas. Be sure to dry out your gloves between cleaning jobs, he says. And always replace gloves that develop holes.

Relax for your rash. "Stress is a definite contributing factor in eczema as well as in other skin conditions," notes Dr. Kitzmiller. "Skin disorders have multiple causes, and a person's emotional state can play a large part. If you are feeling stressed-out or are particularly worried about something, it will only aggravate your condition."

Stress causes your body to release histamines, which make you itch, Dr. Kitzmiller explains. When you start to feel stressed, take 10 deep breaths, meditate, or go for a walk, he says. "Do whatever it takes to calm down and relax."

Reduce dust mites. Many doctors think that people with certain types of eczema may be affected by allergens produced by dust mites in the house. Take measures to ban the mites from contact, and your skin condition might improve, says Dr. Kitzmiller.

Bedding, mattresses, curtains, and carpets are all prime real estate for these mites. Regular vacuuming, damp dusting, and routine washing and airing of bedding are the most effective ways to reduce their population, he says.

Eyestrain

Eyestrain can happen to anyone. In fact, it usually happens to everyone, especially if you're over age 40. You're likely to have eyestrain at least occasionally if you use a computer, watch TV, drive a car, or live in a smoggy city.

You know you've got eyestrain when normally clear images (such as words on the computer screen or print on the page) begin to appear blurry. Your eyes start to ache so much that you just want to close them for a while. Well, that's *one* thing you can do. But here are some other ways you can put a lid on eyestrain.

Try time-outs from close work. "When you're using a computer or doing any other type of close work that strains your eyes, stop every hour for about two minutes and give your eyes a rest," suggests Eric

Donnenfeld, M.D., associate professor of ophthalmology at North Shore University Hospital/Cornell Medical College in Manhasset, New York. "Just close your eyes and do nothing for a couple of minutes."

Stop reading—and refocus. "When you're reading, stop every 30 minutes or so and focus on something far away for a few seconds," adds Merrill M. Knopf, M.D., an ophthalmologist in Long Beach, California, and an officer of the California Association of Ophthalmology. There's a muscle in your eye that contracts when you're doing close-up work, Dr. Knopf explains. By refocusing, you relieve the spasms in that eye muscle. If you want something to look at, hang a sheet of newspaper on a far wall and try to read the larger print.

Take a tea break. Warm eyebright tea is a gentle balm for eyes that are strained. "Take a towel and soak it in brewed eyebright tea," says Meir Schneider, director of the Center for Self Healing in San Francisco and author of *Self Healing: My Life and Vision*. "Lie down, place the warm towel over your closed eyes, and leave it there for 10 to 15 minutes. It will make your eyestrain go away."

Be very careful not to let the towel drip tea into your eyes, though—and be sure the tea has cooled down enough before you soak the towel in it.

Note: Eyebright tea is not a real tea but a mixture of herbal ingredients, sold in loose tea form at most health food stores, specifically for eyestrain.

Put your eyes "on the blink." Your eyes have their own personal masseuse—the eyelids. "Make it a point to consciously blink your eyes frequently and not squint," says Schneider. "Each blink cleanses your eyes and gives them a tiny little massage."

Fine-Tune Your Workstation

If you're a frequent computer user, you have probably discovered how important it is to reduce the glare on your computer screen in order to minimize eyestrain. "It's not so much the intensity of the surrounding light that's important; rather, it's the positioning," says Merrill M. Knopf, M.D., an ophthalmologist in Long Beach, California, and officer of the California Association of Ophthalmology. "The light source should be positioned close enough to you that it's comfortable but far enough away that it doesn't shine on your screen or into your eyes." Of course, placing a special antiglare shield on the screen also helps.

But here are some lesser-known tips to help prevent video-screen eyestrain, from R. Anthony Hutchinson, O.D., an optometrist in Encinitas California, and author of *Computer Eye Stress: How to Avoid It, How to Alleviate It.*

■ Adjust your computer monitor so that the letters on the screen are at least five times brighter than the background.

■ Screen size isn't significant, but letter size is: Capital letters should be at least ⅛ inch high.

■ Avoid overhead fluorescent lighting when using your computer, because its flickering can interact with the flicker on your screen, causing eyestrain. (Even though you can't see the fluctuation in light, a fluorescent tube actually flickers about 60 times a second.)

Get glasses. Most eyestrain is the result of vanity, says Dr. Donnenfeld. "Obviously, you're going to strain your eyes if your vision is off, so get a pair of glasses if you need them." If you have good distance vision and just have trouble seeing up close, reading glasses, sold in most drugstores, are sometimes enough to cure eyestrain.

Exercise your eyes. Standing about five feet from a blank wall, have someone toss a tennis ball at the wall while you try to catch it each time it bounces off. Or hold your thumb out at arm's length. Move it in circles and Xs, bringing the thumb closer, then farther away, as you follow it with your eyes. Both exercises help offset damage caused by eyestrain and improve the brain-muscle connection of your vision, says Don Teig, O.D., an optometrist and sports vision specialist in Ridgefield, Connecticut.

Fatigue

Everyone suffers from fatigue now and then—usually as the result of being under too much physical or mental strain. The usual Rx is some R and R. But if you're all caught up on your rest and relaxation and you still feel pooped, it's time to wonder why.

Of course, anyone who feels totally drained most of the time should pay a visit to the doctor. But for the usual, run-of-the-mill worn-out feeling, here are some ways to perk up your get-go.

Add some stress to your life. It's no surprise that too much stress can knock you out. But if there's not *enough* stress in your life, you can feel fatigued because of boredom and lack of motivation. "It's sort of like the tension or stress on a violin string," says Paul J. Rosch, M.D., clinical professor of medicine and psychiatry at New York Medical College in Valhalla and president of the American Institute of Stress in Yonkers. "If you have too much, the string will snap. If you have too little, you'll get a dull, raspy sound. But just the right amount creates a beautiful tone. Similarly, we need to find the right amount of stress that allows us to make beautiful music in our lives."

The key is to add the kind of stress that will make you feel challenged, not beaten. "I suggest becoming a volunteer," says consumer health expert John Renner, M.D., clinical professor of family medicine at the University of Missouri at Kansas City. The only additional stress is your commitment to show up on time and do the job, but you have the challenge of working with people and producing results.

But avoid stress carriers. "Some people are Typhoid Marys of stress, and just being around them can fatigue you," says Maria Simonson, Ph.D., Sc.D., professor emeritus and director of the Health, Weight, and Stress Program at Johns Hopkins Medical Institutions in Baltimore. "They tend to be the people who are insensitive, complainers, and blamers. The best thing you can do is try to stay clear of them."

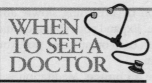

WHEN TO SEE A DOCTOR

When that tired, worn-out, run-down feeling just won't go away no matter what you do, it's a good idea to see the doctor.

Fatigue can be a warning sign of serious illness, including diabetes, lung disease, and anemia, according to Rick Ricer, M.D., associate professor of clinical medicine at Ohio State University College of Medicine in Columbus.

In some cases, fatigue can be a symptom of hepatitis, mononucleosis, thyroid disease, or cancer, according to doctors. And a pattern of extreme fatigue could be one sign of chronic fatigue syndrome, which is more debilitating than normal fatigue and requires a doctor's diagnosis and treatment.

So be sure to see a doctor if you can't shake off that pooped-out feeling.

Close your mouth for better breathing. One often overlooked cause of fatigue is poor breathing. People who breathe shallowly and rapidly get fatigued easily because the body gets less oxygen. The problem is often due to mouth breathing, says Robert Fried, Ph.D., director of the Biofeedback Clinic at the Institute for Rational Emotive Therapy in New York City and author of *The Psychology and Physiology of Breathing in Behavioral Medicine*.

Remedy the situation by breathing slowly and steadily through your nose. Expand your abdomen and keep your chest down with each breath; that way, you use your whole diaphragm.

Give (inner) peace a chance. Meditation is a great way to offset fatigue, and anyone can do it. Start by turning on some soft music, lying back on the sofa, and telling yourself that you're feeling relaxed, says Dr. Simonson. "Concentrate on the softness of the music and breathe deeply. With each exhalation, repeat a word, phrase, or prayer that brings feelings of peace. (Many people say the word *peace*.) While doing this, imagine yourself on a beach; imagine the breeze, the waves, and the seagulls." If your doctor has found no reasonable cause for fatigue, Dr. Simonson recommends meditating for 20 minutes twice a day.

Color your world. "If you live in a dark, dark house, you're going to feel fatigued," says Rick Ricer, M.D., associate professor of clinical medicine at Ohio State University College of Medicine in Columbus. Add some color and more light to your life, he suggests. Studies show that wearing red or being in red surroundings energizes. The color green has been found to evoke peacefulness and serenity, while brown helps induce feelings of warmness and camaraderie.

Use your head to exercise your body. Studies show that as you exercise, no matter what kind of daily exercise you choose to do, your body becomes better at handling the everyday emotional and physical stressors, says Ralph Wharton, M.D., clinical professor of psychiatry at Columbia University in New York City. "Just be sure you exercise a minimum of three times a week for 30 minutes each time."

If exercise causes pain, of course, you should see your doctor first. And whatever you do—walking, running, aerobics—ease into it slowly. If you are a regular exerciser, stick with lighter-than-usual workouts until you begin to feel more energetic.

Don't be a sundown sprinter. Beware of late-night activity, whether it's a light workout or intense training. Most experts agree that exercising after 7:00 P.M. can cause a disruption of regular sleeping habits, which can translate into fatigue the following morning.

Stomp out cigarettes. Smoking is an oxygen robber that can cause fatigue. But doctors say you shouldn't expect an immediate energy boost upon quitting. Nicotine is a stimulant, and withdrawal from smoking can cause temporary tiredness.

Lose weight . . . but not too quickly. It's true, lugging around extra weight can tire you out faster, but don't try to lose too much too soon. Crash diets can send your energy into a nosedive. (Because ultra-low-calorie diets usually concentrate on one type of food, such as grapefruit, they don't give you all the nutrients you need for sufficient energy.)

When your calorie intake is restricted too much, it's very stressful for the body, according to Manfred Kroger, Ph.D., professor of food science at Pennsylvania State University in University Park. "And one of the many symptoms of this type of stress is fatigue."

For responsible dieting, men should consume at least 1,500 calories a day, and women should have 1,200 calories or more.

Turn off the tube. Sure, television helps you unwind after a hard day of hassles—but maybe you're unwinding too much. TV is notorious for lulling folks into a state of lethargy. Instead of watching the tube, try something a little more mentally stimulating, like reading, says Dr. Ricer. "That will be more energizing."

Fever

When your forehead feels hot enough to fry an egg, your body is shaking like Jell-O, and your teeth are chattering, it's hard to believe that fever is your friend.

But it is.

A fever isn't a disease. It's a *symptom* of an infection, typically caused by a cold or the flu. When you have a cold, for instance, your immune system signals to your brain that it needs more body heat in order to attack infectious cells, and your body temperature rises.

There are some tried-and-true procedures that can help bring down the fever and make you more comfortable.

If it's mild, hands off. Some doctors believe a mild fever (under 100°F in adults) should not be treated.

"Taking antipyretics such as aspirin or acetaminophen (Tylenol) brings down the fever, but there's also some evidence that immune activity is suppressed," says Donna McCarthy, Ph.D., assistant professor of nursing at the University of Wisconsin-Madison.

Don't be stoic—pop a pill. On the other

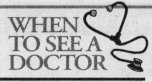

WHEN TO SEE A DOCTOR

For adults over the age of 60, fever can be more taxing on the heart and thus more risky than for younger people. With that in mind, contact the doctor immediately for:

- Fever above 103°F in an adult
- Fever of 101°F if you're over age 60
- Any fever if you have a chronic illness such as diabetes, heart disease, or lung disease
- Fever that lingers more than three days
- Fever accompanied by a rash, severe headache, stiff neck, confusion, back pain, or painful urination

hand, there's no good proof that not treating fever helps your recovery, says Thomas Rosenthal, M.D., associate professor of family medicine at the State University of New York at Buffalo. "Let your comfort be your guide," says Dr. Rosenthal. "If you have headache or muscle aches, by all means take an aspirin or acetaminophen. Both are equally effective, and you should feel effects in a half-hour." (Children should be given only child-size doses of acetaminophen. Aspirin is not advised by pediatricians because of its link to Reye's syndrome, a potentially fatal neurological disease.)

Have a massage. If you go the nondrug route, having a massage and listening to soothing music help boost comfort, says Dr. McCarthy.

Tools for Temperature Taking

Here's a rundown of the old and the new.

■ The "standard" glass thermometer filled with silver mercury or red alcohol is still recommended for temperature taking. Place the thermometer in the deep pocket alongside the tongue, not under the tongue. The pocket ensures an accurate reading, because it's closer to the artery where the heat originates. For the record, the proper way to use one is to shake it until the mercury is below 96°F, place it in the mouth, and leave it for three minutes.

■ Temperature "strips" turn colors as your temperature rises. While forehead strips are not supersensitive, you can distinguish between a temperature of 100°F and 102°F by looking at the colors. The mouth strips are more reliable but must remain in the mouth a full two minutes.

■ Digital thermometers are affordable, plastic, paddle-shaped probes containing a tiny computer chip that receives an electric signal. Within a minute, the beep alerts you to the temperature displayed in the window. You don't have to shake them, but you must wash the tip and keep a battery on hand. They are available at most pharmacies.

A warm bath is best. "The advice to immerse a fevered person in cold water is outdated," says Dr. Rosenthal. "A cold bath makes the body temperature drop too quickly. You'll shiver—which raises your temperature even more, because the rapid muscle movement generates body heat." For the same reason, he adds, you should avoid alcohol rubs, which also cool the skin too quickly.

Fill 'er up. With fever, your system is pumped up, and you lose double or triple your normal water loss without even knowing it, says Dr. Rosenthal. Drinking lots of liquid makes it easier to sweat and get rid of the heat.

Back off from heavy exercise. Both fever and exercise boost your body's heat production, making your heart work harder. Also, if you can't lose the extra heat fast enough, heat exhaustion could result. "The 'work' of fever is enough of a workout to skip exercise for a day," says Herbert Keating, M.D., chief of medicine at the Veterans Administration Medical Center in Des Moines, Iowa.

Flu

Do you feel the onset of a brain-mashing headache—along with major muscle aches, bone-tiring fatigue, vomiting, and a fever that makes you sweat and shiver? These are all clues that the flu has its hold on you.

Anyone who's had the flu before will probably be tempted to get a flu shot before the season begins—and a shot can prevent the flu or lessen its severity. But if it strikes, most of the recovery action is on the home front. Here are some things you can do to make your flu flee.

By all means, feed your flu. You need vitamins and minerals to mount an effective defense against the flu bug, says Herbert Patrick, M.D., assistant professor of medicine and medical director of the respiratory care department at Jefferson Medical College of Thomas Jefferson University in Philadelphia. Aim for well-balanced meals or at least try some bland fruit such as mashed bananas or applesauce.

Sip your nutrition. "Drinking your nutrients is a good idea when you have the flu, especially if you're not up for eating solid foods," says Frederick Ruben, M.D., professor of medicine at the University of Pittsburgh and spokesperson for the American Lung Association. Wash down your meals with a vitamin-rich juice such as vegetable juice or have a bowl or two of soup. The more fluid you drink, says Dr. Ruben, the more your tissues are hydrated and the more mucus flows.

Beware of fluid flu remedies. Combination cold/flu liquid remedies can contain as much as 80-proof alcohol. "That's equal to the amount in a shot of liquor," says Dr. Ruben. Alcohol can depress your immune system and also dry out your mucous membranes, so you should avoid it when you have the flu, he says.

Toss your old toothbrush. The virus continues to linger on wet toothbrush bristles, and you can reinfect yourself day after day, says Dr. Patrick. To prevent this, throw away your toothbrush three days after the onset of the flu and use a new one.

Steer clear of crowds. There *is* a season when you're more likely to be hit by this viral bully, according to Dr. Patrick. "Spending time in offices, malls, theaters, or other crowded environments between December and February increases your chances of ending up flat on your back with the flu, especially if your resistance is low," he says.

Consider postponing that flight. Some years ago, researchers from the Alaskan division of the Centers for Disease Control and Prevention (CDC) in Atlanta traced an outbreak of flu to a single infected passenger in an airplane. Due to a faulty ventilation system, the air inside the cabin recirculated the flu virus as the plane sat waiting for takeoff. Later, 38 of the 54 people on the flight came down with the flu. There have not been follow-up studies, "but an airplane has cramped quarters and air blowing all around, which may create a high-risk situation for exposure to airborne infectious diseases," says Nancy Arden, chief of the influenza epidemiology division of the CDC. If you have any kind of chronic condition (such as diabetes or heart or lung disease), a bout with the flu could be serious. You may want to reduce risk of exposure by avoiding long trips in peak flu season, from December through February.

Develop the hand-washing habit. "Ordinary soap kills the flu virus, but in order to reduce your chance of infection, you've got to remember to wash your hands throughout the day, not just before meals or after going to the bathroom," says Carole Heilman, Ph.D., chief of the respiratory diseases branch at the National Institute of Allergy and Infectious Diseases in Bethesda, Maryland. When a family member is sick, you can use a disinfectant spray on the sink and countertops. Use hot, soapy water to wash towels, telephones, and dishes.

Go for the tiny droplets. Humidifying a room can help lick the flu, according to Dr. Patrick. The vapor emitted by a room humidifier moistens the mu-

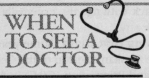

WHEN TO SEE A DOCTOR

If you are over age 65 or have certain chronic conditions such as heart disease or lung disease, doctors recommend getting a flu shot *before* flu season begins. Residents of nursing homes and most medical personnel are also advised to have flu shots, which can usually prevent the flu entirely or lessen its severity.

If you do get the flu, you should see a doctor immediately if you have any of the following symptoms.

- Hoarseness
- Pains in the chest
- Difficulty breathing

Also, be sure to consult a doctor if you have vomiting that continues for more than a day or severe abdominal pain. Prolonged vomiting can leave you dehydrated, which is especially risky for young children and elderly people. And abdominal pain can be a sign of another problem, such as appendicitis.

cous membranes in your nose and throat, so germs are more easily trapped and expelled.

If you use an ultrasonic room humidifier, be sure to rinse it out daily to prevent mold and fungus growth in the water reservoir, says Dr. Patrick. (And you should run a hot-water-and-bleach mixture through the machine at least once a week, following directions on the humidifier.) Better yet, use a hot steam humidifier that moisturizes *and* kills any microbial growth in the water.

Breathe deeply . . . and meditate. Relaxation techniques may protect you from influenza and other infections, according to the results of a study at the University of Pittsburgh School of Medicine that involved the use of self-hypnosis for relaxation. But you don't have to do self-hypnosis to get the benefits of relaxation therapy. Other ways to relax include deep breathing and stretching, meditation, and yoga.

Don't exercise. Once you have been hit by the flu, get in bed and cancel your daily run. "There is some evidence that pushing yourself when you have the flu can depress your immune system and slow your recovery," says David Nieman, Ph.D., a health researcher at Appalachian State University in Boone, North Carolina.

After your symptoms clear—which usually takes about a week—wait another two weeks before returning to your regular exercise schedule.

Foot Pain

When you really think about it, it's amazing that our feet last as long as they do. The 26 bones, 33 joints, 107 ligaments, and 19 muscles and tendons in your feet take 8,000 to 10,000 steps a day, covering more than four times the circumference of the globe in a lifetime. An average day of walking puts several hundred tons of pressure on your feet, which is partly why your feet are easier to injure than any other part of your body.

And when your feet have a problem, they'll let you know it. First, they send you signals like calluses, black toenails, and bunions. If you deal only with the signals or the symptoms but don't solve the underlying problem, your feet will eventually send you another message that's impossible to overlook—pain.

Usually, the problem in question is that your shoes don't fit right or that you were born with certain foot problems that need to be corrected by a doctor, says Neil Scheffler, D.P.M., podiatrist and president of health care and education for the Mid-Atlantic Region of the American Association of Diabetes in Baltimore. Other factors, however, also come into play. For instance, putting on extra weight as you age can add a tremendous amount of pressure to your feet. Here are some other age-related causes of foot pain.

Plantar fasciitis (fas-ee-EYE-tis). The most common cause of heel pain, plantar fasciitis becomes more prevalent as you get older. That's probably because your plantar fascia (a strong, elastic band of fibrous tissue that runs from your heel to your forefoot) gets less flexible over time. As the fascia inflames under the constant strain of walking or standing, it pulls at your heel, sometimes creating a bony prominence called a spur. Though the spur sounds painful, it's really the tight pull against your heel that causes the pain, says Tzvi Bar-David, D.P.M., podiatrist with Columbia-Presbyterian Medical Center in New York City.

"Think of the plantar fascia as a bowed string

that creates the arch of your foot. When you step on this bow, you flatten it and tighten it," says Dr. Bar-David.

The telltale sign that you have plantar fasciitis is that you feel pain on the inner part of your heel. This usually occurs when you first get out of bed or stand up after sitting for some time.

Fat-pad loss. When you were born, you had nice cushy fat pads under your heels and your forefeet. But as you walked and walked over the years, these pads eventually got flattened out and slowly shrank away. This is a natural process but can be a painful one since now you have little there to cushion your feet and absorb shock. You'll feel pain from fat-pad loss under your heel and the ball of your foot.

Arthritis. Use any joint often and rigorously enough and eventually you'll wear away the cartilage that cushions it. In most cases, an injury fails to heal correctly. Then inflammation causes your protective cartilage to rub away, and walking becomes painful. The feet tend to suffer mightily from arthritis because there are so many joints to damage. Arthritis manifests itself with pain, swelling, and lumps, most often in the top of your midfoot or in your toes.

Regardless of why your feet hurt, here are some strategies to nip pain in the bud.

Stomp on pain. Nonsteroidal anti-inflammatory drugs (NSAIDs) such as ibuprofen (Advil) can relieve the pain and swelling of most types of foot pain. Follow package directions. This is a temporary fix, however. You don't want to stay on over-the-counter painkillers for more than a few weeks, advises Dr. Bar-David. So make sure to try other strategies to relieve your specific foot problem.

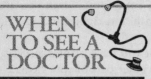

WHEN TO SEE A DOCTOR

Usually, simple remedies are all you need to banish pain. But if home remedies don't help, see your regular doctor or podiatrist, advises Tzvi Bar-David, D.P.M., podiatrist with Columbia-Presbyterian Medical Center in New York City.

Persistent heel or other types of foot pain may signal more serious problems such as a stress fracture or adult flatfoot syndrome when the tendon that holds your arches up gets torn. Such conditions may require surgery or immobilization. Also, your heel pain may result from another cause such as a disc problem or arthritis in your spine.

Bend some toes to stretch a tendon. Much of the pain from plantar fasciitis stems from a tight Achilles tendon (the band that runs down through your heel and connects with your plantar fascia). When it's tight, your plantar fascia gets less flexible. "Often, if you stretch the Achilles tendon, you'll end up relieving the plantar fasciitis," says Dr. Bar-David.

To stretch your Achilles tendon, get in a relaxed position—sitting or lying down—and bend your leg until your toes are within reach. Using both hands, pull your toes toward your shin and hold for 20 seconds.

Or lean in for tendon relief. Another Achilles tendon stretch can be done standing up in front of a wall. Place your hands against the wall and lean forward with your feet firmly planted flat on the ground behind you. Keep your back and feet flat and your knees locked. You will feel your calf stretching if you do this properly, notes Dr. Bar-David. Repeat this 10 times, holding each stretch for 30 seconds.

Vary your stretch times. The Achilles tendon stretches can help alleviate heel pain when it strikes, but you should also do them routinely. Be sure to stretch before and after exercising. Also, stretch before going to sleep and before getting out of bed in the morning. Though you might think your legs and feet are relaxed at night, most people sleep with their feet pointed, keeping the plantar fascia and the Achilles tight all night long, Dr. Bar-David says. So plantar fasciitis is often worse during the first few steps in the morning. By stretching before you rise, you can get your feet off to a good start.

Cushion that heel. Shop around for heel cups or ask a podiatrist about some cushioning that will make your heel feel better. With extra cushioning, your heels aren't jarred so much by everyday walking or running. And with the slight heel lift, your Achilles tendon has a chance to relax, which eases the pull on your plantar fascia, explains Dr. Bar-David.

Switch to running or walking shoes. If your foot's natural padding has eroded over time, wear sneakers. They have extra cushioning in the heel, which helps make up for your somewhat-reduced natural fat pads, says James Michelson, M.D., associate professor of orthopedic surgery at Johns Hopkins School of Medicine in Baltimore. Lace-up shoes also will put less stress on the front of your foot if you have pain there.

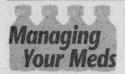 **Managing Your Meds**

Over-the-counter nonsteroidal anti-inflammatory drugs (NSAIDs) such as ibuprofen (Advil) and naproxen (Aleve) can zap pain, but they may also cause side effects in some people. They include:

✦ Confusion

✦ Swelling of the face, feet, or lower legs

✦ Sudden decrease in urine output

✦ Stomach upset

If you suffer from any of these symptoms, talk with your doctor or pharmacist about a pain-relieving alternative that doesn't produce these kinds of side effects, advises W. Steven Pray, Ph.D., R.Ph., professor of nonprescription drug products at Southwestern Oklahoma State University in Weatherford.

Lose weight. If you've gained weight over the years, common sense tells you the extra pounds are putting extra pressure on your feet. This can create heel or forefoot pain, warns Dr. Bar-David. The lighter your body, the less your foot pain.

Get cushioned inserts. You can buy inserts to put in the sole of your shoe to absorb more shock. "Usually, it's all that's needed," adds Dr. Michelson.

Go for depth. If inserts and running shoes don't do the trick, go to a specialty orthopedic shoe store and ask for shoes that provide extra depth. These will allow you to stick even more cushioned inserts into your shoe to absorb even more shock, according to Dr. Michelson.

Avoid high heels. If you're a woman, wearing high heels could contribute to arthritis and other foot pain. High heels also push all of the force of walking into the front of your foot, where things are tight and immovable. Switch to flats, says Dr. Michelson.

Get your feet measured. Shoes that are too tight will make your feet hurt even more. Most women wear their shoes two sizes too small, notes Dr. Michelson, and many haven't had their feet measured in at least five years. Since your feet grow as you age, the shoe that fit when you were 40 may be too small now. Have a clerk or a friend measure your feet for you while you are standing. And do this every time you buy a new pair of shoes, advises Dr. Michelson. Some other ways to make sure you get the right fit:

♦ Shop at the end of the day. Your feet swell over the course of the day, and you'll want shoes that fit when your feet are at their largest.

♦ Keep in mind that one foot might be larger than the other. When you're shoe shopping, always fit shoes to your larger foot. (Use cushioning, if necessary, to fill in the gaps in the shoe for your smaller foot.)

♦ Make sure there's at least a half-inch between your longest toe and the end of the shoe.

Make ginger a habit. Fresh ginger is a great remedy for arthritis and other pain related to swelling, because it's a natural anti-inflammatory, says Neal Barnard, M.D., author of *Foods That Fight Pain* and president of the Physicians Committee for Responsible

Medicine in Washington, D.C. Though you don't have to use a lot of it to get significant relief, you do have to take it regularly, he says.

Buy fresh ginger at the supermarket. Mince up ½ to one teaspoon per day. Either put it in your food as a flavoring or mix it into some water and swallow it like a pill. Cloves, garlic, and turmeric, though less studied, have shown similar effects in some people, according to Dr. Barnard.

Rub hot peppers on them. Over-the-counter creams made from capsaicin, the active ingredient in hot peppers, can relieve arthritis and other foot pain, says Dr. Barnard. The lotion may at first cause a burning sensation, which goes away the more you use the stuff. Rub just enough to lightly cover the affected area on your feet whenever you feel pain. Wash your hands thoroughly after each application and keep the cream away from your eyes and other mucous membranes. It can really burn.

Modify your exercise. If your feet hurt because you give them a regular pounding every time you take a brisk walk, change your routine, says Donna Astion, M.D., associate chief of foot and ankle service for the Hospital for Joint Diseases, Orthopaedic Institute in New York City. For instance, try taking every other day off, alternating between weight-bearing activities such as running and nonweight-bearing activities such as cycling. If you run, alternate between hard tar roads and softer surfaces like trails.

Soak them. Treat your feet to a soak in Epsom salts and warm water. The soak can drain swollen tissues and help relieve pressure. Follow the directions on the package, which usually recommend one tablespoon of Epsom salts dissolved in each quart of water.

Forgetfulness

Hmmmm, now what were we going to discuss next? Oh, yeah, how to cure those blasted bouts of forgetfulness. You know, when a name or date is on the tip of your tongue . . . or you can't seem to remember where you parked your car . . . or left your keys.

Frustrating as it is, a memory slip doesn't mean you're edging toward Alzheimer's disease. (Alzheimer's is marked by things such as not knowing the year or forgetting the names of immediate family members.) Everyone has occasional episodes of forgetfulness, so even if you've forgotten the last time it happened to you, here's how to build a better memory.

Get in shape. Scientific research confirms that a healthy body indeed helps breed a healthy mind— memory-wise, at least. Several studies show that people over age 40 who exercise aerobically at least three times a week have 20 percent better memory skills than people who don't exercise. So if you're not a regular exerciser, change those sedentary ways.

"Regular exercise improves blood flow to the brain," explains Richard Gordin, Ph.D., professor of physical education at Utah State University in Logan. "And improved blood flow often means improved thinking and memory."

Tune in talk shows. "The most troublesome tasks for everyone are remembering names and faces and remembering dates and appointments. I recommend you watch TV shows that will help improve those skills," says Douglas Herrmann, Ph.D., a research scientist at the National Center for Health Statistics in Hyattsville, Maryland, and author of *Super Memory*. "Since meeting new people challenges memory, watch talk and game shows and try to recall each guest's name as the show goes on. A show like 'Wheel of Fortune' is good for improving your vocabulary and recalling word definitions."

Write it down. Putting information in writing also puts it into your memory, says Dr. Herrmann. So try writing down important information in order to remember it more easily later on. Many memory experts suggest you "make lists."

Think in rhymes. Want to *know it*? Become a *poet*. "Make a rhyme for uninteresting things or hard-to-recall facts or when the information is complicated or highly detailed," says Dr. Herrmann. "Rhymes give us a structure that helps us remember things."

Remember your beta-carotene. Consuming at least one serving daily of foods rich in beta-carotene can improve some aspects of your memory and word fluency or recall, particularly if you're over age 60, according to James G. Penland, Ph.D., research psychologist at the U.S. Department of Agriculture Human Nutrition Research Center in Grand Forks, North Dakota. Dark green vegetables and orange fruits and vegetables are abundant in beta-carotene.

Observe rather than see. Seeing something allows for a momentary experience, which may or may not give you the opportunity to soak up details. But observing means paying attention to detail. For instance, you've seen a $20 bill countless times, but can you remember who's pictured on the front of it? Unless you know it's Andrew Jackson, you're not an observer.

"By noticing special properties or features of commonplace items, you will have a better chance to commit them to memory," says psychologist Robin West, Ph.D., of the University of Florida in Gainesville, author of *Memory Fitness over Forty*.

Play mental games. Playing cards or board games like Scrabble is a good way to practice improving your memory, advises Forrest R. Scogin, Ph.D., associate professor of psychology at the University of Alabama in Tuscaloosa. "But choose the games you like, because it can be very frustrating for someone having memory problems to say, 'If I just start playing Scrabble, my memory will improve.'" The process is like building up your strength with exercise. Don't expect too much too soon.

Fragile Skin

Yes, you're familiar with the crow's-feet around your eyes and the subtle skin folds along your neck, but what are these cracks, these flakes, these spots and growths?

They're all signs that, like the rest of your physical body, your skin is getting a little more fragile as you age. In fact, your skin is likely to become more fragile in several ways. It becomes drier and more wrinkled and also tends to heal more slowly than it did when you were younger. The good news is there are several things you can do to protect your skin. But first, here's a look at what causes fragile skin.

"One of the major reasons skin becomes fragile is because it becomes thinner the older you get," says Arthur K. Balin, M.D., medical director of the Sally Balin Medical Center for Dermatology and Cosmetic Surgery in Media, Pennsylvania, and co-author of *The Life of the Skin*. The top two layers of the skin, the epidermis and dermis, become thinner and contain fewer blood vessels, he says. With the decline in the number of blood vessels and overall quantity of blood flowing to cells, the tissues shrink.

A big contributor to this form of skin aging is the sun. "The sun breaks down capillaries, which reduces the amount of blood getting to tissues," says Frederic Haberman, M.D., assistant clinical professor of medicine (dermatology) at Albert Einstein College of Medicine in New York City and director of the Haberman Dermatology Institute in Ridgewood, New Jersey. "It also dries out the skin and breaks down the underlying layer. The result is that the sun makes the skin thinner, drier, and more fragile."

Doctors advise that your best line of defense for protecting and soothing fragile skin is to prevent overexposure to sunlight and, as much as possible, to keep your skin moisturized. It's also a good idea to support your skin with antioxidants, those immune-boosting and cancer-fighting nutrients in food that prevent the decay of cells and tissues, experts say.

Go soak yourself. Once your outer layer of skin becomes thin, it can no longer hold moisture as well as it did during its youth, says Hillard Pearlstein, M.D., assistant clinical professor of dermatology at Mount Sinai School of Medicine in New York City. So you

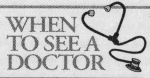

need to take steps to replenish the moisture. The best way, says Dr. Pearlstein, is to soak in a lukewarm bath for 15 minutes. But don't overdo it.

Many doctors recommend that people with fragile skin bathe only two or three times per week and use only the mildest soaps. Also, they say, you should avoid hot showers or baths because hot water is more drying than cool water. And you should use soap only on odor-producing areas such as the armpits, genitals, and feet; rinse the rest of your body with cool water.

Moisturize twice a day. You should moisturize your skin every morning and evening whether or not you've bathed that day. If you apply moisturizer after you've bathed, it will help hold the water in. "The moisturizer will not rebuild skin," Dr. Pearlstein says, "but it will make the skin feel better and offer some protection against further moisture loss."

Use a moisturizer that contains petroleum jelly or lanolin, advises the American Academy of Dermatology. These are among the best and least irritating of moisturizing ingredients. If your moisturizer irri-

Managing Your Meds

If you find that your skin is becoming more fragile, it may be because of a prescription you're taking. The category of drugs known as adrenal corticosteroids, which includes such prescription medications as cortisone (Cortone), prednisone (Deltasone), and dexamethasone (Decadron) used to treat adrenal problems, arthritis, and skin diseases, may in some cases thin your skin and make it more susceptible to injury, says W. Steven Pray, Ph.D., R.Ph., professor of nonprescription products at Southwestern Oklahoma State University in Weatherford.

tates your skin, consult a dermatologist for recommendations.

Try an antioxidant. Many people see an improvement in their skin after daily application of a skin lotion that contains the antioxidant vitamins C and E, says Dr. Haberman. (One brand containing both vitamins is Neutrogena New Hands.) Those who benefit from these topical lotions say the lotions make their skin feel stronger and that they appear to delay some of the damage done by overexposure to sunlight.

Create a daily shield. The sun's rays attack your skin like piercing arrows. "You have to stay out of harm's way to protect fragile skin," advises Dr. Pearlstein. "That protection starts with applying an adequate sunscreen each day of at least a sun protection factor of 15."

Cover up, especially in summer. You should never deliberately sunbathe. And always wear a wide-brimmed hat to shade your face and neck, Dr. Pearlstein recommends. Also, wear long sleeves and light trousers. Finally, be sure to put on gloves when you're gardening to protect the backs of your hands.

Walk on the shady side of the street. "I tell my patients to walk before 10:00 A.M. and after 4:00 P.M., when the sun's rays will do less damage to the skin," Dr. Pearlstein says. "I also tell them to walk on the shady side of the street to avoid the direct rays of the sun."

Try some acid on your skin. Alpha hydroxy acids (AHAs) are showing promising signs in the skin's fight against aging and sun damage, according to the American Academy of Dermatology. Some studies suggest that AHAs may reduce wrinkles and improve the skin's overall appearance. AHAs, which are found in milk, fruit, and sugarcane, are present in many moisturizing creams and lotions. You may see them listed as glycolic acid or lactic acid. You can safely use AHAs at home, notes Dr. Pearlstein. Look for over-the-counter skin preparations containing AHAs. Follow the package directions for usage.

Gallstones

Like a good friend, the gallbladder quietly serves us well until we mistreat it and it demands our attention. Located on the right side of the body under the liver, the gallbladder is a small pear-shaped organ that aids in digestion. Its main function is to store bile from the liver until the bile is needed to break down fats during digestion.

If too much cholesterol or calcium is in the bile, gallstones can form, but that in itself is not always a problem. Most people with gallstones never even know that they have these deposits, which can range in size from a grain of sand to a golf ball. Sometimes, when gallstones pass through a duct, they can get stuck, and that can cause a gallbladder attack. You'd know if you had one: You'd experience pain in your upper-middle or right abdomen, moving around to your back; nausea; and vomiting. These are all signs of gallstone problems, says Robert Charm, M.D., gastroenterologist in Walnut Creek, California, and professor of gastroenterology and internal medicine at the University of California, Davis. At that point, surgery is sometimes the best option.

If others in your family have had the problem or if you're overweight, you could be more prone to gallstones. Women who have had several children or who are on estrogen replacement therapy also tend to have a higher risk of developing gallstones, says Roger Gebhard, M.D., gastroenterologist at the Veterans Affairs Medical Center and professor of medicine in the division of gastroenterology at the University of Minnesota, both in Minneapolis. While many older people have gallstones, age doesn't put you at risk for them. But once you have gallstones, they don't go away on their own, explains Dr. Gebhard.

Even if sex and heredity are ganging up to raise your risk, that doesn't mean you're destined to get gallstones. Here are some things you can do to discourage the stones from getting started.

Eat light. Since being overweight is a common

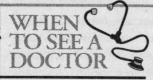

WHEN TO SEE A DOCTOR

In most cases, when you have gallstone pain, you'll need to see a doctor to confirm the diagnosis and determine the best way of dealing with the problem, says Martin Brotman, M.D., gastroenterologist at the California Pacific Medical Center in San Francisco. If your doctor decides to remove your gallbladder, your worries about gallstone pain are over. And don't fret; your digestive system will function just fine without that extra internal appendage.

But if your doctor doesn't operate, be alert to any recurrence of symptoms. If the pain returns, you'll need to return to your doctor.

risk factor for gallstones, do what you can to keep the weight off. Especially steer clear of large fatty meals, says Mike Cantwell, M.D., clinician and coordinator for clinical research at the Institute for Health and Healing at the California Pacific Medical Center in San Francisco. "Fat makes the gallbladder work harder, increasing the likelihood of gallstones."

Lose a little at a time. While it's important to avoid being overweight, don't embark on a crash diet to get there. Losing weight fast can actually increase your risk of developing gallstones, explains Dr. Cantwell. Yo-yo dieting (a cycle of quick weight loss followed by weight gain) is especially hard on the gallbladder. It creates a situation where the gallbladder sits

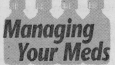

Managing Your Meds

Thankfully, hardly any drugs can cause gallstones to develop or worsen. But gemfibrozil (Lopid), a drug prescribed to reduce triglyceride blood levels and raise high-density lipoprotein (HDL) cholesterol, has been linked to gallstone formation, says W. Steven Pray, Ph.D., R.Ph., a professor of nonprescription drug products at Southwestern Oklahoma State University in Weatherford. If you've been using this drug, talk to your doctor about this side effect. He may wish to prescribe an alternative.

unused for a time, then suddenly gets overused. This stop-start activity only increases the likelihood of gallstone formation. A slow, steady weight-loss program that includes regular meals of low-fat foods and plenty of exercise is the way to go.

Put on your walking shoes. If you don't exercise regularly, you could be risking gallstones. Regular exercise steps up metabolism (the pace of energy-burning), notes Dr. Charm. "When metabolism is slow, small gallstones can develop. Even simple activities like stretching or walking help gallbladder health."

Pump up the fiber. Yet another reason for eating meals high in fiber is that it'll reduce gallstone risk, says Dr. Charm. "Fiber helps lower cholesterol produced by the liver." And cholesterol, remember, is one of the building blocks of gallstones.

Glaucoma

Political opponents were fond of saying that President George Bush lacked "vision" for America's future. They were almost right.

In April 1990, White House doctors discovered that the 65-year-old president had a budding case of glaucoma in his left eye. Although he had not lost any vision, he immediately began using eyedrops twice a day to prevent future loss of sight.

"I haven't felt a thing," Bush told the press at the time.

Like Bush, many people afflicted with this insidious disease aren't aware that they have it. In fact, glaucoma is often called the silent thief of sight because it usually strikes slowly, painlessly, and without warning. Yet it afflicts more than three million Americans—most of them over age 60. Each year, it affects another 50,000 people worldwide and causes blindness in more than 1,000.

"Most people don't realize that they have had vision losses from glaucoma until the losses are very advanced. Your vision may be 20/20 right up to the end—and then it's snuffed out. And unfortunately, those losses are irreversible," says Anne Sumers, M.D., ophthalmologist in Ridgewood, New Jersey, and a spokesperson for the American Academy of Ophthalmology.

But if glaucoma is detected and treated early, the progress of the disease can be halted and most of your vision can be saved with a simple regimen of eyedrops once or twice a day, Dr. Sumers says.

To understand how glaucoma robs vision, imagine that your eye is like a small sink, says Robert Ritch, M.D., medical director of the Glaucoma Foundation in New York City. The faucet is a tiny gland behind the iris that is constantly producing fluid that bathes the eye. The drain is a $\frac{1}{50}$-inch-wide opening called the trabecular meshwork. As you age, this drain tends to clog, and the fluid meets more resistance in flowing out of the eye. Since the eye is a closed compartment, fluid buildup results in raised pressure, or intraocular pressure (IOP), inside the eye, putting excessive pressure on the optic nerve. As the IOP increases, the nerve slowly begins to die, and your peripheral (side) vision fades. Untreated, it eventually leads to almost total blindness. Once it is detected, the first line of treatment is to lower IOP. You'll need to regularly take medication to control it.

If you've been diagnosed with low-pressure glaucoma, in addition to taking medication, there are several things you can do to help keep it under control.

Go for ginkgo. In addition to any prescription medications, ask your doctor about using ginkgo biloba, an over-the-counter herbal remedy that Dr. Ritch believes helps preserve vision. "Ginkgo appears to increase blood flow to the eye and prevent the death of cells in the optic nerve," he says.

Look for ginkgo extracts containing 6 to 7 percent terpenes, a component of the herb that Dr. Ritch suspects plays a key role in stopping optic nerve damage. He suggests taking 120 milligrams of the herbal remedy twice a day for two months, then cutting back to 60 milligrams twice a day. Doses of ginkgo

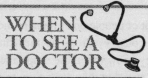

WHEN TO SEE A DOCTOR

Because it has no symptoms, glaucoma will sneak up on you. That's why it's important for everyone over age 60 to have an annual eye exam that includes a glaucoma check, says Anne Sumers, M.D., ophthalmologist in Ridgewood, New Jersey, and a spokesperson for the American Academy of Ophthalmology.

In between exams, see an optometrist or ophthalmologist if you experience any of the following symptoms:

■ Morning headaches

■ Recurrent blurry vision

■ Seeing rainbow-hued halos around lights at night

■ Decreases in your peripheral (side) vision

■ Pain around your eyes after watching television or leaving a dark theater

biloba higher than 240 milligrams of concentrated extract can cause skin rash, diarrhea, and vomiting. Don't use ginkgo if you're taking monoamine oxidase (MAO) inhibitor drugs like phenelzine sulfate (Nardil) or tranylcypromine (Parnate), aspirin or nonsteroidal anti-inflammatory medications, or blood-thinning medications like warfarin (Coumadin).

Set your sights on antioxidants. Studies strongly suggest that antioxidant vitamins C and E can

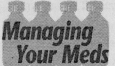

Managing Your Meds

A lot of people don't think of their glaucoma eyedrops as medicine. They know that these drops affect the eyes, but they don't seem to realize that the drugs in eyedrops can get into the bloodstream and cause side effects in the entire body, says Anne Sumers, M.D., ophthalmologist in Ridgewood, New Jersey, and a spokesperson for the American Academy of Ophthalmology. "So whenever you are being treated for glaucoma, it is extremely important to let all of your doctors know what medications you are taking."

Medications known as beta-blockers (Timoptic, Betoptic, Betagan) that are often used to treat glaucoma can cause asthma attacks, dizziness, impotence, fatigue, depression, memory loss, and other symptoms that your physician

relieve low eye pressure and slow the development of glaucoma, Dr. Ritch says. He recommends taking 2,000 milligrams of vitamin C and 800 international units (IU) of vitamin E daily. (Vitamin C in amounts above 1,200 milligrams may cause diarrhea in some people. Also, although vitamin E is generally sold in doses of 400 IU, one small study showed risk of stroke in dosages higher than 200 IU. Consult with your doctor if you are at high risk for stroke.)

Walk away from it. Regular aerobic exercise like walking can help lower pressure in the eye, increase blood flow to the optic nerve, and slow the progression of the disease, Dr. Ritch says.

In fact, research conducted at Oregon Health Sci-

wouldn't necessarily associate with glaucoma unless he knew you were being treated with these drugs, Dr. Sumers says.

Ask your ophthalmologist or pharmacist about side effects before taking any glaucoma medications, including:

✦ Pilocarpine (Isopto Carpine, Pilocar) and other miotics; can cause headaches and blurred vision

✦ Methazolamide (Neptazane, MZM) and other carbonic anhydrase inhibitors; can cause depression and kidney stones

✦ Brimonidine tartrate (Alphagan); can cause headaches and fatigue

✦ Latanoprost (Xalatan); can cause a pigmentation of the iris, which may turn the patient's blue eyes to brown

ences University in Portland on a group of sedentary people who began a program of brisk walking for 40 minutes three times a week found that those with glaucoma reduced their eye pressure by 20 percent. And those people who did not have glaucoma saw a 9 percent reduction in eye pressure.

Stick to your schedule. Timing is critical when using glaucoma medications, Dr. Sumers says. To get 24-hour coverage from your medication, you have to properly space out your doses. "Some people think that three doses a day means at breakfast, lunch, and supper. That's not going to work, because the last dose of medication is going to wear off before you get another one the next day," she says. "So if you're supposed to use eyedrops three times a day, allow a full eight hours between treatments."

Don't skimp. If you don't think you got enough medication into your eye, try again, Dr. Sumers suggests. "You can't overdose on eyedrops. It's better to use an extra drop than to not get enough in."

Try the squeeze play. After you insert your eyedrops, press a finger against the tear duct in the inner corner of your eye for about one minute, Dr. Ritch says. It will help keep medication in your eye, where it is needed, rather than allowing it to run down your face. Keep your eyes shut while doing this, so the drug can be properly absorbed, he suggests. It is particularly important to leave about 10 minutes between medications if you're using two different eyedrop medications. If you don't wait long enough, the second drop will wash the first drop out of the eye before it has chance to do its job.

Gout

O nce known as the "kings' disease" because it almost always afflicted the well-heeled, this form of arthritis is an equal opportunity deployer: It delivers a *royal* pain to the toe, knee, and other joints.

You'll qualify for gout if your kidneys lose some of their ability to flush away excess amounts of a by-product called uric acid. When uric acid crystallizes, it lodges in the joints, causing more than a crystal's worth of pain. "Think of what happens when you put too much sugar in a glass of iced tea," says Jeffrey R. Lisse, M.D., director of the division of rheumatology at the University of Texas Medical Branch at Galveston. "The sugar will dissolve up to a point, and the remaining crystals pile up at the bottom."

When that occurs, the joint can get hot, swollen, and tender. Sometimes the pain is so bad that it can actually wake you from a sound sleep. "Gout occurs sporadically, but it hits like gangbusters, often in the middle of the night," says Paul Caldron, D.O., a clinical rheumatologist and researcher at the Arthritis Center in Phoenix. "We're talking about pain so intense that the weight of the sheet feels excruciating."

This megagrief can last for hours or days, but a gout bout can vanish almost as swiftly as it comes, leaving you totally pain-free until the next episode. If you've had that experience, here's how to avoid a future round with the crystal attackers.

Lose weight, but not too quickly. The majority of gout patients are overweight—usually 15 to 30 percent over their ideal weights. The greater your girth, the higher your uric acid level. And the more uric acid, the more frequent and more intense the gout attacks. But lose weight gradually: A crash diet can actually raise uric acid levels.

Control your blood pressure. Gout patients with hypertension have twice as much to worry about. That's because some blood pressure medications boost uric acid levels, says Branton Lachman, Pharm.D., clinical assistant professor at the University of Southern California School of Pharmacy in Los Angeles. His ad-

Foods to Avoid

The best way gout patients can avoid a purine-packed flare-up is to avoid foods high in purine. Among the most loaded, containing from 100 to 1,000 milligrams per 3½-ounce serving:

Anchovies	Meat extracts
Brains	Mincemeat
Consommé	Mussels
Gravy	Pork roast
Heart	Poultry
Herring	Roast beef
Kidney	Sardines
Liver	Sweetbreads

The following foods should be limited to no more than one serving daily, because they contain nine to 100 milligrams per 3½-ounce serving.

Asparagus	Mushrooms
Beans (dry)	Oatmeal
Lentils	Peas (dry)
Luncheon meats	Spinach

vice: Try to control your blood pressure naturally by decreasing sodium intake, exercising regularly, reducing excess weight, and controlling stress.

Live without liver. Foods high in a substance called purine contribute to higher levels of uric acid. "You can't get away from purine, because it's in most foods," says Dr. Caldron. "But it's useful to avoid red meat, especially organ meats, some types of fish, and even some dark green leafy vegetables such as spinach."

Eschew the brew. Alcohol is a double whammy for those with gout, because it boosts the production of uric acid, says rheumatologist John G. Fort, M.D., clinical associate professor of medicine at Thomas Jefferson University Hospital in Philadelphia. Beer is particularly bad, because it has an even higher purine content than wine or other spirits.

But drink lots of water. You can help your kidneys flush excess uric acid from your system by going heavy on H_2O. (Besides, dehydration can trigger an attack.) "Brisk urinary output certainly may help," says Dr. Caldron. To accelerate "urinary output," Robert H. Davis, Ph.D., professor of physiology at the Pennsylvania College of Podiatric Medicine in Philadelphia, recommends no fewer than five glasses of water each day.

Give your sex life a kick. Urinating isn't the only way to get rid of uric acid. One study showed that among men, frequent sexual activity reduces uric acid levels. The study suggests that more sex means less gout—for men, anyway.

Be sweet to your feet. Injure a big toe and you increase gout risk, say researchers. So wear shoes around the house to protect your feet from everyday accidents.

Gum Pain

They say that pain is nature's way of ringing us up to tell us something's wrong. But when it comes to our gums, nature doesn't always use the hotline. More often, the message of gum pain seems to come via the old-time pony express. By the time we get the news, the situation at the point of origin is likely to have gone from bad to worse. So if your gums are hinting that something unusual is going on, it may be an understatement.

But why do gums hurt? "The causes could be either serious infections caused by bacteria or a situation where the skin on the gums has something wrong with it," says Kenneth Kornman, D.D.S., Ph.D., clinical professor and former chairman of the department of periodontics at the University of Texas Health Science Center at San Antonio. There are many infectious conditions that can cause pain. And every now and then, gum surfaces can be plagued with a maddening host of abrasions, burns, growths, and lesions.

But all these problems have one thing in common: If they persist, they can really gum up your life, so don't take any chances when pain makes a rare cameo appearance. Head for the dentist's chair as soon as possible. And meanwhile, take these steps to find some relief.

Brush away gum pain. Removing bacteria with regular tooth care not only prevents gum disease but can also provide some short-term pain relief, says Dr. Kornman. Proceed with gentle brushing (with a soft brush), flossing, and warm-water rinsing. In addition, an over-the-counter rinse like Listerine, diluted or at full strength, may diminish some of the bacteria and ease some pain. (For some people, though, the alcohol content of a rinse may make pain worse. Discontinue using it if that happens.)

Don't rub. Massaging your gums may only cause further irritation, according to Dr. Kornman.

Try a warm saltwater rinse. "Take a few swigs of warm saltwater and swish it between your teeth and gums," advises Leslie Salkin, D.D.S., director of postgraduate periodontics and professor of periodontology at the Temple University School of Dentistry in Philadelphia. "It has a general soothing effect. If you have an abscess, the salts will help draw it out and drain it." He recommends one teaspoon of salt in a glass of lukewarm water. (Saltwater is also your first line of defense for any gum burn, cut, abrasion, or wound.)

Suppress the pain with an analgesic. Any over-the-counter medicine that reduces pain and inflammation could do wonders for your sore gums. It can also help reduce a fever if your pain is caused by an infection. "We're finding that in most cases of dental disease, it is inflammation that causes discomfort," says Samuel Low, D.D.S., associate professor and director of graduate periodontology at the University of Florida College of Dentistry in Gainesville. "Consequently, we are recommending anti-inflammatory products such as ibuprofen (Advil)." Or you can take aspirin if you don't have adverse reactions to it (but children should avoid aspirin because of the risk of Reye's syndrome).

Don't put aspirin on your gum. "For some reason, many people have the idea that applying aspirin directly to the affected gum area is beneficial," says Kenneth H. Burrell, D.D.S., director of the American Dental Association's Council on Dental Therapeutics in Chicago. That couldn't be farther from the truth, he notes. "Unfortunately, the only thing that happens is that you create a chemical burn in the gum tissue. Don't ever try it."

Ice it down. For an all-natural anti-inflammatory effect, Dr. Low recommends using ice. "It really works on swelling," he says, "and also serves as a local anesthetic to dull nerve endings." Apply an ice pack wrapped in a towel to your cheek or lip near the area of pain.

Moisten your mouth. Dr. Salkin recommends sucking on ice chips or a lemon drop if you are suffering from gum irritation due to dry mouth. That should be enough to replenish any missing saliva.

Use peroxide power. Many of the bacteria that cause gum pain cannot survive in oxygen, so some dentists recommend the use of everyday hydrogen peroxide, which you can pick up at any pharmacy and dilute. Dr. Low advises using a rinse of half water, half hydrogen peroxide.

Dab with baking soda. Another way to discourage bacteria is with household baking soda. Just make a paste of baking soda mixed with water and apply it gently on the gums, suggests Dr. Low. But be careful. Overzealous use can abrade gum tissue.

Numb that gum. If you have a burn, a cut, an ulceration, or any problem on the skin of the gum, Dr. Kornman says the best thing you can do is apply one of the many over-the-counter gels or ointments that contain benzocaine. Its numbing action delivers instant relief. It also knocks out much of the pain associated with serious gum infections.

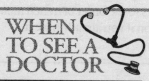

WHEN TO SEE A DOCTOR

If you think that a twinge of pain is only the first sign of gum disease, you may be sorely mistaken (no pun intended). Gum disease could already be in the advanced stages by the time you experience pain. So be sure to see a doctor even if the pain seems to go away.

Also, you should visit your dentist when gums are red, tender, discolored, or bleeding, *whether or not you feel pain.*

"See your general dentist first before going to a periodontist (a gum specialist)," says Samuel Low, D.D.S., associate professor and director of graduate periodontology at the University of Florida College of Dentistry in Gainesville. "A dentist is equipped to handle many of these problems and then can direct you to a periodontist if needed."

Anyone for tea? Some doctors suggest holding a wet tea bag against a gum abrasion or canker sore. Tea leaves contain tannic acid, an astringent that also has some pain-relieving power.

Say no to tobacco. "We see greater gum destruction in smokers," warns Dr. Salkin. He points out that smoking contributes to gum problems and can exacerbate any infectious or ulcerative conditions. Chewing tobacco is another gum irritant and can lead to a variety of gum cancers, according to Dr. Salkin. In addition, smoking often contributes to the onset of trench mouth and worsens the condition if you already have it.

Heartburn

What can you do when that burning sensation right under your rib cage won't go away? You belch. But there's no Ladder Company Number 9 to put out this fire. This is the inferno of that after-dinner bother—heartburn.

The cause of this post-dining fire storm is actually the hardworking sphincter in your lower esophagus. This muscle relaxes to let food pass into your stomach, then quickly closes. But when it doesn't close properly, the contents of your stomach can back up—a condition known as esophageal reflux—creating burning or irritation under your rib cage. Hello, heartburn.

In everyone over age 40, the esophageal sphincter is likely to weaken a bit. Not much you can do about that. But the main causes of heartburn are usually obesity, stress, and the wrong diet. And those things (unlike age) you *can* do something about.

There's other good news. Your esophagus can heal from the burning caused by stomach acid within seven weeks with proper care, decreasing your chances of recurring episodes. So here's some body-plumbing help that will give your pipes a soothing rest.

Watch out for repeat offenders. Coffee, alcohol,

spicy foods, and citrus fruits often bring on a five-alarm blaze, according to John Sutherland, M.D., clinical professor of family practice at the University of Iowa College of Medicine in Iowa City and director of the Waterloo Family Practice Residency Program in Waterloo. And watch out for fried and fatty foods as well as tomatoes and chocolate. Any of these can "irritate your esophageal lining or relax your sphincter muscle, triggering reflux," says Ronald L. Hoffman, M.D., director of the Hoffman Center for Holistic Medicine in New York City.

Obliterate that onion. Do you suffer after spicy meals with onions? The onions, not the spices, may be the cause, says Melvin L. Allen, Ph.D., a gastroenterology researcher at the Presbyterian Medical Center of Philadelphia. It helps to refrigerate raw onions before you slice them. That reduces their potency. Better yet, cook them!

Or opt for a different onion. "There are three types of onions that don't cause heartburn," says Stephen Brunton, M.D., director of family medicine at Long Beach Memorial Medical Center in Long Beach, California. "Try the Texas sweet onion, the Maui, and the Walla Walla varieties." (You may not find these in your grocery store unless it has a large and diverse produce section, but be persistent and check your local farmer's market or food co-op.)

Try less on the plate. "Eat small meals to avoid heartburn," advises William J. Ravich, M.D., associate professor of medicine in the division of gastroenterology at Johns Hopkins University School of Medicine in Baltimore. It's best to eat more frequent meals of small portions, instead of three "normal" meals a day. And try to have your last meal of the day at least three hours before bedtime, since you're more likely to get heartburn when you're lying down.

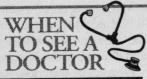

WHEN TO SEE A DOCTOR

If you have heartburn daily or even several times a week, see your doctor, says William J. Ravich, M.D., associate professor of medicine in the division of gastroenterology at Johns Hopkins University School of Medicine in Baltimore. Frequent or repeated symptoms *could* be an indication of esophagitis, or inflammation of the esophagus.

Other warning signs may indicate an ulcer. According to *Seven Weeks to a Settled Stomach*, by Ronald L. Hoffman, M.D., director of the Hoffman Center for Holistic Medicine in New York City, sometimes the first indication of an ulcer is a lot of belching and bloating, which might lead you to think you have severe gas pains. The pain may be worse between meals when your stomach is empty, and you may feel better after you eat something. If these symptoms sound like yours, consider the possibility of an ulcer and see a doctor.

Drink water with your meals. Drinking water will wash stomach acids from the surface of the esophagus back into your stomach, says Dr. Hoffman. The saliva you swallow with the water will help neutralize the acid.

Four after-dinner no-no's. Your after-dinner habits may be causing your heartburn. For greater comfort, avoid drinking, smoking, napping, and strenuous lifting. After-dinner drinks tend to bring on night-

If you are experiencing what you think may be heartburn accompanied by any of the following symptoms, you should be checked out by a physician *fast*.

- Difficulty or pain when swallowing
- Vomiting
- Bloody or black stool
- Shortness of breath
- Dizziness or light-headedness
- Chest pain or pain radiating into the neck and shoulder

According to Samuel Klein, M.D., associate professor of medicine in the division of gastroenterology and the division of human nutrition at the University of Texas Medical School at Galveston, these symptoms indicate problems far more complex than heartburn, ranging from obstruction of the esophagus to a heart attack.

time reflux, Dr. Hoffman says, and "smoking may weaken your lower esophageal sphincter." Avoid lying down after dinner, because gravity helps food stay in your stomach where it belongs. ("Try to resist the after-dinner nap, especially after eating a heavy meal," says Dr. Sutherland.) And as for taking out the garbage after dinner, lifting heavy things after eating can also bring on heartburn, Dr. Ravich says.

Sleep on a slope. "Place the head of your bed on

six-inch blocks," advises Dr. Hoffman. "This seems to reduce heartburn by minimizing the flow of reflux from your stomach into your esophagus at night." Also, if you're in the habit of lying on your right side, try sleeping on your left side instead, suggests William B. Ruderman, M.D., chairman of the department of gastroenterology at the Cleveland Clinic–Florida in Fort Lauderdale. "The stomach is lower when you're lying

Hiatal Hernia Isn't the Problem: Heartburn Is

Nearly one in every three people has a hiatal hernia, a condition where the upper portion of the stomach protrudes upward through an opening in the diaphragm into the chest. This usually occurs as a result of weakening of the tissue around the diaphragm.

Although hiatal hernia causes no pain and produces no symptoms, it's often confused with heartburn, says William B. Ruderman, M.D., chairman of the department of gastroenterology at the Cleveland Clinic–Florida in Fort Lauderdale. That's because people who have reflux heartburn often have a hiatal hernia as well.

But if you're *not* prone to heartburn, having a hiatal hernia usually means little, says Dr. Ruderman. In fact, many people are completely unaware they have a hiatal hernia—even though it affects half of all people over age 50. "The bottom line is that it isn't necessary to do anything about a hiatal hernia," says Dr. Ruderman. "But it is necessary to take care of heartburn if you're feeling pain."

Don't Forget Antacids

You can reach for relief with antacids, but timing is important, says Dennis Decktor, Ph.D., scientific director of the Oklahoma Foundation for Digestive Research in Oklahoma City. Use antacids after you eat but before heartburn occurs. Food and drink wash them away.

It appears to be the coating action rather than the acid-neutralizing action of antacids that matters, according to Dr. Decktor. For this reason, he advises, "don't drink water with an antacid or you may wash the coating away."

Tablets, pills, or liquid? Take a chewable, Dr. Decktor recommends. When you chew, you create saliva, which helps neutralize some of the "burning" acid.

on your left side," observes Dr. Ruderman. In that position, stomach acid is less likely to make its way up into your esophagus.

Run not, burn not. Although exercise is a great habit, running can cause "runner's reflux," says Dr. Hoffman. If that's a problem, try other forms of exercise that don't jostle the body as much—such as bicycling or working out with weights. (But avoid doing any form of exercise except a relaxed stroll right after a meal.)

Review your Rx. Some medications lead to heartburn. For example, "make sure your stomach doctor knows what your heart doctor has prescribed," says John Horn, Pharm.D., associate professor at the University of Washington School of Pharmacy in Seattle. "Certain medications for high blood pressure, particularly calcium channel blockers, can cause reflux."

Try the vomit nut. It's unappealingly named, but the so-called vomit nut, or nux vomica, is a homeopathic remedy that relieves heartburn, says Dr. Hoffman. Check your local health food store for availability and follow the directions on the bottle.

Heart Palpitations

There's nothing like an off-beat ticker to scare the daylights out of you. Some irregularities in heartbeat are considered harmless and self-correcting. You may sense that your heart has skipped a beat, a condition known as ectopic (from the Greek *ektopos*, "misplaced") atrial heartbeat. Or your heart may suddenly speed up, a condition called tachycardia. Sometimes this kind of arrhythmia passes quickly, with no serious effects.

But—and this is a big but—only a doctor can say with certainty that your heart palpitations are nothing to worry about. "If you have any question about what you are experiencing, the safest thing is to have it checked out," says Jeremy Rushkin, M.D., director of the Cardiac Arrhythmia Service at Massachusetts General Hospital and associate professor of medicine at Harvard Medical School, both in Boston. That advice holds true whether you're young or old. (And even if other heart problems are ruled out during an exam, the doctor may want to prescribe medication specifically for arrhythmia.)

You may think of your heart simply as a muscular pump, but the fact is, this organ is very sensitive to many things going on in the body. A near accident, cigarette smoke, drugs (both prescription and nonprescription), emotional upsets, and overindulgence in food, alcohol, or caffeine can all upset the carefully orchestrated pattern of electrical charges that leads to a normal heartbeat.

"People are often unaware of how they are setting themselves up for an arrhythmia problem," says Stephen Sinatra, M.D., chief of cardiology and director of medical education at Manchester Memorial Hospital in Manchester, Connecticut, and assistant clinical professor of medicine at the University of Connecticut School of Medicine in Farmington. "They need to address a number of things that could be contributing to their problem."

Here are some steps to consider.

If you smoke, stop. "Smoking is an extremely dangerous activity if you have cardiac arrhythmia," Dr. Rushkin says. "It can undo even the best of medical care."

Warm up and cool down. If you exercise, add at least 10 minutes to the beginning and end of your routine to give your heart time to change pace gradually. And no 50-yard dashes to the bus stop or sudden sprints up the stairs, unless you've warmed up first with a few passes around the block.

"Sudden exercise is a very common trigger in people prone to arrhythmia," Dr. Rushkin says. Cooling down is equally important, especially if you've been running, cycling, or doing other exercises that involve your legs, Dr. Rushkin says.

Save skydiving for another lifetime. If you've never had arrhythmia, chances are you won't develop it pursuing even the most daring of avocations. "But if you're prone to arrhythmia, we suggest you not put yourself into such stressful circumstances," Dr. Rushkin says. That goes for occupational stress, too. A firefighter or police officer may need to switch to a less hair-raising job.

Stick with noncompetitive sports. "I have the opportunity to take care of a number of competitive athletes with heart arrhythmias, and they tend to have problems only when they are in a competitive situation," says Dr. Rushkin.

"The combination of competition and physical stress is a much more powerful trigger of arrhythmias than is either one alone, and that's not surprising."

Restrain yourself at all-you-can-eat buffets. Stuffing yourself to the gills—what doctors politely call metabolic overload—can bring on heart palpitations in those prone to them, Dr. Rushkin says. So eat lightly.

Go easy on alcohol. "Some people with arrhythmias are extremely sensitive to alcohol, and they usually know it—they sometimes get palpitations after just one drink," Dr. Rushkin says. "We advise them to be very cautious and moderate in their drinking. I prefer that they not drink at all."

Say no to joe. Coffee, tea, chocolate, and certain drugs that contain caffeine, such as diet pills, can exacerbate arrhythmia problems in some people. "I recommend that people who have a history of arrhythmias should avoid caffeine as much as possible," says Dr. Rushkin.

Give your medicine chest the twice-over. Quite a few drugs can cause heartbeat problems, including those sometimes prescribed to correct ar-

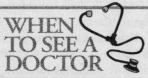

WHEN TO SEE A DOCTOR

A single skipped heartbeat or an extra beat that you sense occasionally throughout the day usually is no cause for concern, according to Jeremy Rushkin, M.D., director of the Cardiac Arrhythmia Service at Massachusetts General Hospital and associate professor of medicine at Harvard Medical School, both in Boston. "Almost everyone experiences these, especially as we get older."

But if you feel more than that, such as a string of skipped beats, or if your heart seems to race without provocation, you should see a doctor right away. You should also see the doctor if you have additional symptoms of dizziness or faintness.

rhythmia. Culprits include digitalis, beta blockers, calcium channel blockers, all anti-arrhythmic drugs, tricyclic antidepressants, and cimetidine (Tagamet), a popular ulcer drug.

"A doctor can sometimes tell early on that a drug is going to cause problems, and that's why many of these drugs are started in the hospital," Dr. Rushkin says. "But some effects may occur later and may occur unexpectedly." Contact your doctor immediately if you think you're having a problem.

And be especially wary of decongestants. Even popular over-the-counter drugs can cause problems, says Dennis Miura, M.D., Ph.D., director of cardiac arrhythmias and electrophysiology at Albert

Einstein College of Medicine of Yeshiva University in New York City. "Decongestants and asthma sprays that contain ephedrine or pseudoephedrine are the most common offenders," he says. They can cause a faster and somewhat more forceful heart rate and, in some circumstances, can cause or exacerbate serious arrhythmias. If you're already prone to arrhythmia problems, don't use these drugs without your doctor's okay.

Breathe calmly and fully. If you tend to hold your breath, as some people do when they're frightened, tense, or straining in some physical activity, or if your breathing is shallow and rapid, you can upset your heart's natural rhythm, says Robert Fried, Ph.D., director of the Biofeedback Clinic at the Institute for Rational Emotive Therapy in New York City and author of *The Psychology and Physiology of Breathing in Behavioral Medicine*. So pay attention to your breathing. Allow yourself to exhale fully, then relax your belly and give your lungs time to fill before you exhale again.

Roll with the punches. "I am convinced that stress can be a powerful factor in enhancing or increasing susceptibility to arrhythmia," Dr. Rushkin says. "I would certainly endorse any program or activity that reduces stress. People simply need to find what works best for them." Meditation, biofeedback, yoga, prayer, music—all can ease tension.

Fill up on fish. Preliminary studies from researchers in Australia suggest that omega-3 fatty acids from fish such as salmon and mackerel may help reduce arrhythmias. The researchers think these fats may alter the composition of heart muscle cells, making them less prone to rhythmic disturbances.

Hemorrhoids

It's easy enough to see a bulging varicose vein in your leg. But when a vein bulges where the sun doesn't shine, you're more likely to *feel* it than see it. A hemorrhoid is exactly that: a varicose vein in the anus or rectum that can cause considerable discomfort—itching, burning, and, occasionally, throbbing pain.

Hemorrhoids can bleed when they are scraped by a hard bowel movement. Your first symptom may be an alarming streak of bright red blood on the feces or drops of blood on the toilet paper. (The bleeding usually stops by itself in a few minutes.)

If the doctor says you have hemorrhoids, you probably know what causes them, too. Hemorrhoids are most often caused by constipation, or "straining at stool." Just as the veins in your temples pop out when you're trying to lift something heavy, the veins in your anus can pop out when you try too hard, for too long, to have a bowel movement.

It's true that hemorrhoids do tend to shrink when the pressure's off, but daily straining can make them continually protrude (or prolapse), bleed, and hurt. But here are some ways to ease the discomfort and help heal the hidden annoyance.

Clean with care. While it's important to keep your bottom clean, vigorous wiping will only aggravate your hemorrhoids, says Max M. Ali, M.D., director and president of Hemorrhoid Clinics of America in Oak Park, Michigan. Wipe first with moistened toilet paper, or use a premoistened wipe. Then pat with dry toilet paper. Or try using a plastic squeeze bottle of water to gently "shower" your bottom, then pat dry with toilet paper. Avoid using scented or colored toilet paper containing chemicals that irritate tender tushies. If you must use soap to clean, use an unscented, hard-milled bar such as Ivory.

Dab on petroleum jelly or zinc oxide paste. In studies, both of these low-priced drugstore items worked just as well as more expensive creams. You can try either, or both, to reduce the pain and swelling of hemorrhoids. After wiping, dab a small amount of the cream or paste on a cotton ball and apply to the anal area.

Sit in a sitz. "Of all the things you can do when your hemorrhoids are sore, sitz baths are the best, in my opinion," says Lester Rosen, M.D., chairman of the National Standards Task Force of the American Society of Colon and Rectal Surgeons and associate clinical professor of surgery at Hahnemann University School of Medicine in Philadelphia.

"Warm water relaxes the anal sphincter muscle," Dr. Rosen explains. A relaxed anal sphincter muscle takes the squeeze off tender protrusions.

Fill your bath with three to four inches of warm (not hot) water. Don't add anything to the water—not Epsom salts, bubble bath, or bath oil, Dr. Rosen says. Sit in the tub for 15 minutes or so.

Pay heed when nature calls. "Try to tune in to the stomach/bowel reflex that should occur twice a day, within 20 minutes after breakfast and dinner," says Sidney E. Wanderman, M.D., author of *The Hemorrhoid Book* and former senior clinical instructor in surgery at Mount Sinai School of Medicine in New

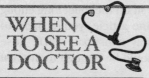

WHEN TO SEE A DOCTOR

It's best not to assume that bleeding during a bowel movement is caused by hemorrhoids until a doctor verifies that's the case. Intestinal polyps, anal fissures, even colon cancer can also cause rectal bleeding.

"Everyone, even people with diagnosed hemorrhoids, should get regular examinations for bowel cancer and should see a doctor if there is a change in bowel habits," says Max M. Ali, M.D., director and president of Hemorrhoid Clinics of America in Oak Park, Michigan.

York City. The reflex is a signal that feces have moved into your colon and are ready to come out. Schedule your day to give yourself time to go when the urge strikes, Dr. Wanderman suggests. "You'll have less straining if you work with nature on this one."

Get up and moving. "It really works," Dr. Rosen says. Exercises such as walking, running, biking, and swimming make food move through your bowel faster. That helps prevent constipation and hemorrhoids. "Good overall muscle tone and a firm tummy also let you respond decisively to nature's call," Dr. Wanderman says.

Go or get off the pot. If you want to go, should you sit and wait? Some people believe that having good reading material handy makes for a leisurely, relaxing (even enjoyable) excretory experience. "I personally believe that if you sit on the toilet long enough to read an entire magazine article, you're there too long, and you are probably constipated," Dr. Rosen says. "Several minutes should be enough to evacuate your bowels."

Eat foods that fight hemorrhoids. Include in your diet high-fiber foods that naturally produce softer stools that move easily past tender spots. Try oats, oat bran, or barley, suggests dietitian Patricia H. Harper, R.D., of North Huntingdon, Pennsylvania. Aim for several servings a day of fruits and vegetables. In addition, if you can eat a cup or so of beans, chances are your hemorrhoids will shrink to a mere memory.

If chewing is a problem for you, get your fiber by eating applesauce mixed with oat bran; hot oat or rice cereals; mashed carrots or sweet potatoes; and creamy vegetable or bean soups, Harper suggests.

Drink up. It's equally important to get plenty of fluids. Try to get a minimum of six to eight glasses of water or other fluids a day, Harper suggests. Since some kinds of fiber absorb fluids, the more you drink, the more you'll help keep stools soft.

Hot Flashes

As a woman reaches menopause—usually around age 50—hormone levels fall rapidly as the ovaries halt production of the hormone estrogen. Sensing this, the body's internal thermostat tends to react quite strongly. Blood vessels on the skin's surface open up like a radiator, enveloping you in intense heat and flushing your face. About 80 percent of all women experience these hot flashes as they go through menopause.

Your doctor may prescribe estrogen tablets if your hot flashes are severe. But many women find they can deal with milder symptoms with home treatments.

Track those flashes. Hot flashes may occur more predictably and less randomly than you think, studies show. To prove it, take note of the date, time, intensity, and duration of the hot flash, suggests Linda Gannon, Ph.D., professor of psychology at Southern Illinois University at Carbondale. Also record the circumstances preceding it—what you ate or drank, how you felt emotionally.

"Some women find that hot flashes worsen when they drink alcohol or coffee, smoke cigarettes, or encounter stressful situations that elicit strong emotions," says Dr. Gannon. Your hot flash diary can show you what triggers you need to avoid to keep cool.

Lower the temp. Keeping cool is important for menopausal women, since many of the precipitating factors in hot flashes are related to heat, says Sadja Greenwood, M.D., assistant clinical professor of gynecology at the University of California, San Francisco, Medical Center. She suggests sipping cool drinks and wearing natural fabrics that "breathe." And one study at Columbia University in New York City showed that menopausal women had fewer and milder hot flashes in cool rooms than in hot rooms. So turn on the fan or the air conditioner to keep the temperature down. And when you're going out, carry a fold-up fan with you, Dr. Greenwood advises.

Keep a cool head—meditate. Some brain research has shown that hot flashes are stimulated by a brain chemical (neurotransmitter) known as norepinephrine, which influences the temperature-regulating center in the brain, says Dr. Greenwood. "This may explain why daily stress-reduction practices such as meditation, deep breathing, and yoga, which result in lower levels of norepinephrine, help some women reduce their hot flashes," she says.

In one study, menopausal women with frequent hot flashes were trained to slowly breathe in and out six to eight times for two minutes. These women had fewer hot flashes than women trained to use either muscle relaxation or biofeedback.

Douse it with vitamin E. "This nutrient often does a commendable job of relieving the severity and frequency of flashes. Lots of my patients have good luck with it," says Lila E. Nachtigall, M.D., associate professor of obstetrics and gynecology at New York University School of Medicine in New York City. She recommends starting with 400 international units (IU) twice a day (a total of 800 IU).

But check with your physician before beginning vitamin E supplementation. While the vitamin is generally considered safe, it can have a blood-thinning effect. Meanwhile, try to include more vitamin E–rich foods in your diet: wheat germ, wheat germ oil, safflower oil, whole-grain breads and cereals, peanuts, walnuts, filberts, and almonds.

Sip some sarsaparilla. For centuries, herbalists have used special "women's herbs" that have a weak regulating effect on estrogen and may help control hot flashes, according to Susan Lark, M.D., medical director of the PMS and Menopause Self-Help Center in Los Altos, California. The herbs include sarsaparilla, dong quai, black cohosh, false unicorn root, fennel, and anise.

These herbs are available combined in ready-made formulas, or they can be used alone, says Dr. Lark. To make a tea, empty one herb capsule into a cup of boiling water and let it steep for a few minutes. Don't drink more than two cups of herbal tea (along with meals) daily. Discontinue the herbs if you notice nausea or other symptoms, says Dr. Lark. And talk to your doctor before taking these herbs if you're at risk for cancer or other conditions that rule out estrogen replacement therapy.

Get up and go. In one Swedish study, severe hot flashes and night sweats were only half as common among physically active postmenopausal women as among bench warmers. "Possibly, exercise elevates the level of endorphins, the feel-good hormones that drop when there is an estrogen deficiency," says Timothy Yeko, M.D., assistant professor in the department of obstetrics and gynecology, division of reproductive endocrinology, at the University of South Florida in Tampa. The endorphins affect the thermoregulatory center—your thermostat, says Dr. Yeko. Regular physical activity may increase endorphin activity and therefore diminish the frequency of hot flashes.

Don't aim to be a skinny-mini. "Estrogen is actually manufactured in body fat from other hormones after menopause," says Dr. Greenwood. "A very thin woman will have less natural estrogen in her system, which may give her more problems with hot flashes."

Impotence

Cary Grant fathered a daughter at age 62. Clint Eastwood had a baby girl at 67. Charlie Chaplin had a son at 73. Tony Randall sired a daughter when he was 77. And Anthony Quinn had his 13th child at age 81.

"Men shouldn't lose potency as a result of getting older. There are age-related diseases that men develop that can lead to difficulty in getting erections. But if men are healthy, they should be able to function all of their lives," explains Drogo K. Montague, M.D., director of the Center for Sexual Function at the Cleveland Clinic Foundation.

Normally, an erection occurs when there is increased blood flow into the penis and penile veins are compressed to make sure that the blood is sealed there, causing stiffness. Nerves in the penis provide pleasurable sensations and help retain the erection until ejaculation, Dr. Montague says.

A man, however, is not a machine. Almost every

man fails to achieve an erection rigid enough for intercourse at some point during his adult life, notes Dr. Montague. And for up to 30 million American men, getting and maintaining an erection is a persistent problem. Though it's commonly known as impotence, doctors now call this condition erectile dysfunction.

Estimates of impotence vary so widely that the statistics are nearly meaningless, which says something about truth in reporting when it comes to this delicate subject. By some estimates, only 15 percent of men over the age of 70 are impotent. Other polls put the number nearer 67 percent, which would mean that two out of every three men over the age of 70 are impotent.

Statistics aside, older men do seem to be more prone to erectile problems than younger men. In all likelihood, that's because older men are more apt to have diabetes, atherosclerosis (hardening of the arteries), and other physical ailments that reduce blood flow to the penis. In fact, in men over 50, up to 80 percent of erectile dysfunction is caused by physical problems. But anxiety, depression, and other psychological woes also can contribute to the problem, Dr. Montague says.

Fluff up the pillows. Impotence can be triggered by boredom in the bedroom, says Roger Crenshaw, M.D., psychiatrist and sex therapist in private practice in La Jolla, California. Take a few moments to think about your sex life. Are your nightly patterns with your spouse so predictable that it's difficult to get excited about them? Have you used the same position for years? How do you feel about kissing and foreplay? Where do you have sex? In the bedroom? In the shower?

Often, just changing when, where, and how you

For decades, older men whose sex lives were limp faced some pretty grim choices: go without, use cumbersome vacuum pumps, or inject erection-inducing drugs directly into their penises. Then along came sildenafil citrate (Viagra). It quickly became known for its ability to restore a man's erections even after decades of impotence.

The drugs work wonders for about 80 percent of men, stimulating blood flow to the penis and jump-starting long-lost erections. But for nearly one in three men, particularly those with diabetes and other health conditions that damage nerves in the penis, these medications may not help as much.

Viagra has other downsides as well. Doctors say that you should never use Viagra if you are taking nitroglycerin or related nitrate-containing drugs. When combined, Viagra and nitrates can cause a dangerous drop in blood pressure, and some men have died from this side effect, says Roger Crenshaw, M.D., psychiatrist and sex therapist in private practice in La Jolla, California. Be sure to let your doctor know about any drugs you are taking, including over-the-counter products, prior to taking Viagra.

have sex can be erotic enough to revive your potency, Dr. Crenshaw says. So experiment. Try new positions. Touch your spouse in ways you never have before or try some role-playing games if your spouse is game.

Ask for a healing touch. As men age, they need more physical stimulation to get and maintain erections, explains Dr. Crenshaw. So ask your spouse to

Other drugs are notorious for causing impotence as a side effect. In fact, medications account for about one in every four cases of impotence and may be the single most common cause of sexual dysfunction after age 60, says W. Steven Pray, Ph.D., R.Ph., professor of nonprescription drug products at Southwestern Oklahoma State University in Weatherford. Among the common culprits are:

✦ High blood pressure medications including beta blockers such as propranolol (Inderal), pindolol (Visken), and metoprolol (Lopressor)

✦ Digitalis preparations such as digoxin (Lanoxin), used to strengthen weak heart muscles and correct irregular heartbeats

✦ Antidepressants like clomipramine (Anafranil)

If your erectile dysfunction begins shortly after you begin taking a medication, consult with your physician. You may be able to alleviate the problem by cutting back certain medications or finding substitutes for them. But never reduce or stop your dosage of any drug without your doctor's permission, Dr. Crenshaw warns.

take some time to touch and play with your genitals and other erotic areas of your body.

Turn off the pressure. If you do have difficulty getting an erection, don't dwell on it, Dr. Crenshaw advises. Obsessing about impotence could make you worry so much that you'll have performance anxiety, which leads to impotence, which makes you worry more, which leads to more anxiety. So break the vicious cycle and treat it casually. Shrug it off.

To relieve the tension, avoid having intercourse the next few times you and your partner are intimate, even if you get an erection, Dr. Crenshaw suggests. Instead, hug, kiss, caress, and do other things you enjoy. Satisfy your spouse but avoid touching each other's genitals.

"If intercourse becomes an overarching goal, sex ceases to be fun. And when sex ceases to be fun, that's when you get into trouble," Dr. Crenshaw says.

Clear the smoke. Smoking kills erections, Dr. Montague warns. Each time you light up, you risk damage to arteries; you also restrict blood flow to the penis. And without enough blood, you're not going to be a rocket man. Even if you've been smoking for years, quitting now can help restore your potency.

Stop wining. Alcohol is a depressant that slows down reflexes, including sexual ones. Drink no more than one drink, which is a 12-ounce beer, 5-ounce glass of wine, or 1½-ounce shot of liquor, a day if you want to keep your erections as you get older, Dr. Crenshaw says.

Play hard. The fitter you are, the less likely impotence will be a problem, Dr. Montague says. Regular aerobic exercise such as walking and swimming helps keep arteries healthy and that includes the arteries that supply the penis, says Dr. Montague. Better yet, try to fit some running into your schedule, ideally, 15 to 20 minutes three times a week. Remember to check with your doctor before beginning a new exercise program, he adds.

Slice the fat. Dietary fat contributes to clogged arteries all over the body. So what's good for your heart is also good for your penis, Dr. Montague says. To stay potent, trim the fat in your diet down to about 20

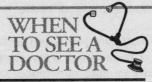

WHEN TO SEE A DOCTOR

If impotence lasts more than two months or is a recurring problem, consult your doctor. Your doctor might also refer you to a sex therapist or physician who specializes in erectile problems, says Roger Crenshaw, M.D., psychiatrist and sex therapist in private practice in La Jolla, California.

More than likely, your doctor will suggest a complete examination and give you a blood test that could rule out physical problems like diabetes and neurological disorders. Blood screenings can also identify low levels of testosterone, the male hormone responsible for sexual response.

Your doctor also may be able to help you cope with stress, anxiety, and other psychological factors that can wilt erections, or refer you to a specialist who can help with these issues.

percent of total calories. If you eat 2,000 calories a day, that means you can eat up to 44 grams of fat, he explains. To get started in the right direction, read food labels, avoid fried foods, look for low-fat and nonfat products, and switch to fat-free milk.

Snooze. Chronic tiredness is anathema to sex, especially for many older men who have difficulty going to sleep and staying asleep through the night, Dr. Crenshaw notes. Try to get at least six to eight hours of sleep a night. If you're tired, even a 30-

minute nap before sex can improve your chances of getting an erection.

Read all about it. There are plenty of tasteful books that can help you learn about sexual techniques, eroticism, and overcoming impotence, Dr. Crenshaw says. For starters, Dr. Crenshaw recommends the timeless classic *The Joy of Sex* by Alex Comfort, M.D. You also may want to check out *A Lifetime of Sex: The Ultimate Manual on Sex, Women, and Relationships for Every Stage of a Man's Life* by Stephen C. George and K. Winston Caine. These and other books can be purchased by mail order or found in a bookstore or library.

Incontinence

If you have a problem with incontinence, it might be a little reassuring to hear that it's a common concern among older people. But is that the kind of reassurance you really want to hear? More likely, you'd like to know that there are things you can do about it.

Well, there are.

"Incontinence is never normal at any age," says Neil Resnick, M.D., chief of gerontology at Brigham and Women's Hospital in Boston and associate professor of medicine at Harvard Medical School. "It's not a function of age nor of gender. Incontinence is almost always treatable and very often curable," he says.

At least 13 million Americans experience urinary incontinence, the involuntary release of urine. And it's not at all fair to both sexes. About 11 million of those 13 million are women. In fact, one out of every three women experiences some degree of urinary incontinence during her lifetime.

In most cases, there are not only solutions your doctor can suggest, there are some methods you can try yourself.

Learn Kegels. Pelvic muscle exercises, also known as Kegel exercises, help many women with the most common kinds of incontinence, says Dr. Resnick.

Kegels strengthen the pelvic floor muscle that supports the bladder. When those muscles are stronger, you can tighten up in the area that controls the release of urine.

To do Kegels, you quickly contract your pelvic floor muscles as if you are stopping a stream of urine. Hold the contraction for about three seconds, then relax the muscles for an equal length of time. This pair of movements should be counted as one exercise. Doing these exercises 45 times each day, divided into three sessions of 15 exercises each for at least six weeks, can help control incontinence, says Dr. Resnick. Just like strengthening biceps or any other muscle-building exercise, it takes time.

The great thing about Kegels is that you can do them anywhere—in the car as you're driving, at a bridge game, while you're washing the dishes—and no one has to know. And they really do work if they're done right, notes Dr. Resnick.

Remember, as with any exercise program, the beneficial effects last only as long as the exercise continues, says Dr. Resnick. One study found that women who practiced Kegels three times a week had the most success, even after five years.

Keep a diary. Before you see your physician, it's a good idea to keep a diary of your urinary habits for two days, advises Dr. Resnick. Write down when you urinate, when you experience leaking, and note activities that may have triggered leaks, such as sneezing, coughing, or exercising. It may also be helpful if you estimate the amount of leakage you experience. Note whether you leaked a few drops of urine, a few teaspoons or tablespoons, or enough to soak a pad or your clothes. Your notes may be able to help your doctor determine what type of incontinence you have and the proper course of treatment.

Time your trips. For people with urge incontinence, bladder drills can help them reassert control, says Phillip Barksdale, M.D., urogynecologist with Woman's Hospital in Baton Rouge, Louisiana.

To do the drills, urinate at set intervals, every hour or two, to keep the bladder from getting too full. After you achieve dryness for a few days, increase the intervals, says Dr. Barksdale. If you pace yourself, you should be able to control urination so you can wait several hours.

Watch what you drink and when. Alcohol and caffeinated beverages like coffee and tea stimulate urine production. Limit your consumption to no more than one or two servings a day or, better yet, eliminate these drinks, suggests Dr. Barksdale. These measures will help you with your bladder drills, reducing the urge to go more often, says Dr. Barksdale. Also, reduce the fluids you have in the evening. Less stress on your bladder will help you remain more comfortable between nighttime bladder drills.

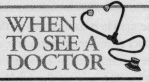

WHEN TO SEE A DOCTOR

Occasionally, incontinence is a symptom of a serious underlying problem, like a brain tumor, urethral blockage, ruptured disc, or multiple sclerosis, according to Neil Resnick, M.D., chief of gerontology at Brigham and Women's Hospital in Boston and associate professor of medicine at Harvard Medical School. In most cases, these conditions are treatable if found early, so you don't want to delay diagnosis.

If your health care provider says nothing can be done about incontinence, don't necessarily accept that as the final word, says Dr. Resnick. Since research into new solutions is being made all the time, you may want to find a doctor who's up-to-date on the subject.

Don't dry yourself out. You may be tempted to drink less throughout the day so you won't have to go as often. But it's important to continue drinking normal amounts of fluids for health reasons, suggests Dr. Barksdale. If you consciously resist drinking when you're thirsty, the deprivation can quickly lead to dehydration, especially when you're a senior.

Timing is everything. Many people with incontinence can be taught by a therapist to contract their pelvic muscles at the moment of physical strain, says Dr. Resnick.

"Usually, you have advance warning that a cough

223

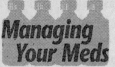

Managing Your Meds

Some muscle relaxants such as the product dantrolene (Dantrium) can cause incontinence by relaxing the muscles that support the bladder, says W. Steven Pray, Ph.D., R.Ph., a professor of nonprescription drug products at Southwestern Oklahoma State University in Weatherford. Caffeine can be a culprit as well, says Dr. Pray. This includes caffeine in aspirin-based analgesics such as Excedrin.

or a sneeze is coming," he says. If you practice doing a Kegel exercise at that exact moment, you can prevent incontinence.

Treat the triggers. Sometimes, treatment of an allergy or cough can "cure" incontinence, says Dr. Barksdale. Once the physical trigger is removed, incontinence often goes away.

Use absorbents wisely. Traditionally, people with incontinence have turned to various absorbent products, like maxipads or disposable adult undergarments.

While absorbent products are still the most widely used means of dealing with incontinence, don't rely on them exclusively. Drs. Resnick and Barksdale stress that they should be used only in addition to a doctor's treatments and your own restraining measures.

Ingrown Toenails

It takes six to nine months for a toenail to grow out. But when that growing toenail takes a wrong turn, you can't wait a minute for relief. That's because ingrown nails, which usually occur in the big toe, cause big-time pain. The nail actually cuts into soft tissue around the top of the toe, and that cutting action produces swelling and redness. Infection sometimes follows.

People with curved toenails are particularly prone to the problem. But whatever the shape of your toenail, you can aggravate the problem by wearing shoes that are too tight around the toe. Even stockings can sock it to you by pressing the nail until it cuts into the tissue around it (called the nail fold). But here's how to nail those nasty ingrown nails and prevent a recurrence.

Cut the nail straight across. Leave the half-moons for cloudy nights. "The best way to cure an ingrown nail and prevent new ones from forming is to always cut your nail straight across, not slightly curved or in a half-moon shape," says William Van Pelt, D.P.M., a Houston podiatrist who is former president of the American Academy of Podiatric Sports Medicine. "You should cut the nail so that it's just higher than the crease of the nail fold."

Give it a soak before a trim. Before cutting—and you should use good-quality, long-handled scissors or nail clippers—soak your foot in warm water to soften the nail and lessen your pain, says Frederick Hass, M.D., a general practitioner in San Rafael, California, and author of *The Foot Book*.

Cut a V and Harm You'll See

It's time to divorce yourself from that old wives' tale that you can treat an ingrown nail by cutting a V-shaped wedge out of its center. (The theory behind this fallacy is the misconception that ingrown toenails are the result of a nail being too big.)

This practice won't prevent an ingrown nail, as some believe. "Chances are the only thing you'll do is hurt yourself," says Houston podiatrist William Van Pelt, D.P.M., former president of the American Academy of Podiatric Sports Medicine.

There are products available over the counter that are made to soften ingrown nails, but read the label before using them. Some cannot be used by those with conditions such as diabetes or impaired circulation.

File the corners. While the nail should be cut straight across, nail corners should be filed and buffed. This eliminates sharp edges. It reduces the pain you get from an ingrown nail cutting into your toe, and it prevents new ingrown nails from forming, says Dr. Van Pelt.

Protect your nail with cotton. An alternative to filing corners is to take a very thin strip, not a wad, of cotton and place it beneath the burrowing edge of your nail, advises Dr. Hass. The cotton helps lift the nail slightly, so it can grow past the tissue it's digging into.

Shun bad shoes. Tight shoes and pointy-toed styles can cause an ingrown toenail and make existing ones worse—especially if your nails tend to curve, says Suzanne M. Levine, D.P.M., clinical assistant podiatrist at Wycoff Heights Medical Center and adjunct clinical instructor at New York College of Podiatric Medicine, both in New York City. You're better off wearing open-toed shoes or sandals—*especially* when you have an ingrown nail.

Use common sense. When working around the house, wear substantial but comfortable shoes, since accidents can also cause ingrown nails, says Dr. Hass. Steel-toed boots should be worn by those doing lots of lifting. And avoid tight panty hose or socks, which can also cause ingrown nails.

Insomnia

Older people need just as much sleep as other adults, about eight hours a night on average. However, their ability to sleep can be compromised for a variety of reasons.

As a natural part of aging, you tend to be more easily roused from slumber. Over time, your sleep cycles can change, too, so suddenly you're feeling more tired earlier in the evening. Insomnia enters the picture when you fight the urge to sleep and stay up later in the evening but then cannot remain asleep in the earlier hours of the morning.

Then there are the times when you will experience an occasional bout of sleeplessness because of stressful and worrisome events in your waking life.

The changing nature of life, adjusting to retirement, or bereavement may cause situational or transient insomnia. The important thing is to keep these periods in perspective, says Michael Vitiello, Ph.D., professor of psychiatry and behavioral sciences at the University of Washington in Seattle.

Insomnia is wearisome, but it's usually not considered a serious hazard to your health. If insomnia lasts for more than two weeks, see your doctor. In the meantime, try practicing these tips to improve your ability to sleep and the quality of the sleep you get.

Reset your clock. The circadian rhythm, the body's internal clock that tells it when to sleep and when to be awake, can be influenced by the body's exposure to the sun. This knowledge can be very useful if you start wanting to sleep at 7:00 P.M. and start waking up at 3:00 A.M. That's a sign that your internal clock may be out of whack and needs some resetting.

To get your body clock adjusted, get as much light exposure as you can toward the end of the day, recommends Sonia Ancoli-Israel, Ph.D., director of the sleep disorders clinic at the Veteran's Affairs Health Care System in San Diego, professor of psychiatry at the University of California, San Diego, and author of *All I Want Is a Good Night's Sleep*. This has the effect of moving your body clock ahead a few hours so you feel like going to bed at your more usual hour. Eat lunch outside, go for a walk in the afternoon, and when you have to spend time outside in the morning, wear sunglasses so your eyes are exposed to a little less light. All of these strategies will move your daylight exposure to later in the day, rather than earlier. You should see results in about two weeks, says Dr. Ancoli-Israel.

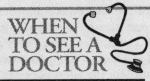
Don't let your clock get cuckoo. Go to bed and get up at the same time of day seven days a week and your body will thank you by becoming accustomed to that rhythm and sleeping during those hours, Dr. Ancoli-Israel explains.

Have a real rest room. Keep your room at a comfortable temperature, advises Dr. Ancoli-Israel. And you'll find it easier to sleep as long as you should if you draw the drapes to block out early-morning light.

Leave your worries at the bedroom doorstep. The bedroom is for sleep and sex, period. Leave eating, working, watching TV, even reading for another room in the house, says Patricia Prinz, Ph.D., professor of behavioral nursing and adjunct professor of psychiatry and behavior sciences at the University of Washington in Seattle.

Tune out that TV thriller. Watching scary, violent, or otherwise disturbing movies or TV programs before you go to bed is not a good idea, says Margaret

Moline, Ph.D., director of the sleep-wake disorders center at the New York Presbyterian Hospital–Cornell Medical Center in White Plains, New York. They're often too stimulating and will keep you up. And don't trade in your remote control for the latest paperback suspense novel. A good page turner can be just as disruptive to your sleep schedule.

Think routine. Any parent will tell you that setting up a bedtime routine for children is important. Guess what? It's important for adults, too. "Grown-ups forget to do that," Dr. Moline says. "But we need routines just like the little kids do, so that we can relax and get ready for sleep." So take a bath, get in your jammies, and spend some time reading (but not in the bedroom) before you climb into bed.

Dim the lights. Exposure to bright light before you sleep may have a stimulating effect and may keep you up, Dr. Moline warns. Keep the lights in the house low as you get nearer to your bedtime.

Get up and bore yourself to sleep. If you do have trouble sleeping, doctors say, you don't want to wallow all night in bed trying to drop off again. Try for 10 minutes and then get up, leave the bedroom, and go do something quiet and dull until you feel sleepy again.

Turn the clock to the wall. If you do wake up in the night, don't focus on your alarm clock. "It doesn't matter if it's 2:30 or 3:30 A.M.," Dr. Moline says. "The more you pay attention to external stimuli when you're awakened in the middle of the night, the more likely it is that you'll have trouble falling back asleep."

Find some ease with the herb valerian. Have some valerian root to help you sleep, suggests Varro E. Tyler, Ph.D., distinguished professor emeritus at

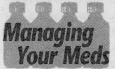

Managing Your Meds

Certain medications that older people may be taking can interfere with their ability to fall asleep, explains Phyllis Zee, M.D., Ph.D., director of the sleep disorders center and associate professor of neurology at Northwestern University Medical School in Chicago. Check with your doctor if you think your medications may be causing insomnia, but never stop taking them without his consent. These can cause problems.

✦ Antidepressants such as fluoxetine (Prozac)

✦ Medications for chronic pulmonary disease and emphysema, such as prednisone (Deltasone), theophylline (Respbid), and beta-blockers like propranolol (Inderal), which can aid breathing but be so stimulating that they interfere with sleep

✦ Diuretics for high blood pressure, which can interfere with sleep indirectly because you'll have to get up in the night to go to the bathroom

Purdue University in West Lafayette, Indiana, and author of *The Honest Herbal*. Valerian is an ancient herb that is helpful in adjusting sleep over a period of time, but you don't need to grow it fresh or grind up the root.

Dr. Tyler recommends buying concentrated valerian and using an amount equivalent to two to three grams of root a day. Valerian is also available in capsule form. Look for a standardized extract (0.8 percent valeric acid) and follow the directions on the label. Do not use valerian with sleep-enhancing or mood-regulating medications such as diazepam (Valium) or amitriptyline (Elavil). If stimulant action occurs, discontinue use. In infrequent cases, it may cause heart palpitations and nervousness in sensitive individuals.

Catch some kava. For acute insomnia such as that brought on by jet lag, you may want to try the herbal remedy kava, says Dr. Tyler. This herb is also prepackaged, but you want to check the label to make sure it has the active constituents kavapyrones or kavalactones.

Take between 60 and 120 milligrams before bedtime to help induce sleep. But because kava has a sedating effect, you shouldn't have it if you're already taking a sedative before bedtime, Dr. Tyler warns. Do not take kava with alcohol or barbiturates. Do not take more than the recommended dose. Use caution when driving or operating equipment, as this herb is a muscle relaxant.

Say no to nicotine. Even though some people feel the need for cigarettes to relax them, the nicotine in cigarettes is a stimulant, says Naomi R. Kramer, M.D., associate director of the sleep disorders center at Rhode Island Hospital in Providence. So it's a bad idea to fight insomnia by lighting up. If you smoke, try to avoid doing it at night. "And if you wake up at night and want to go back to sleep, don't have a cigarette," Dr. Kramer advises.

Watch what you drink. Caffeinated beverages interrupt sleep, so don't drink them after noon. And you'll want to avoid alcoholic drinks before bedtime, too. Alcohol initially has a sedating effect, but as your body turns it into energy, it becomes stimulating, causing wakefulness in the night, Dr. Moline states.

Eat lightly. A big meal late at night might make you sleepy, but then again, it might not. If you are prone to heartburn or gastroesophageal reflux, problems which tend to increase with age, having a huge dinner late will keep you up, says Phyllis Zee, M.D., Ph.D., director of the sleep disorders center and associate professor of neurology at Northwestern University Medical School in Chicago. Try to eat dinner earlier in the evening.

Have some warm tryptophan and cookies. Of course, if you eat an early dinner, it may not be enough to tide you over until you go to sleep. And hunger pangs can certainly keep you awake. Have a light snack to alleviate hunger before bedtime, suggests Dr. Vitiello. He recommends that you include some warm milk in that snack because milk contains tryptophan (a food substance that helps people feel sleepy). Other foods such as turkey, fish, and bananas are also rich in tryptophan.

Plug in a night-light. It's almost inevitable. At some point, you can be pretty sure, you'll have to get up to go to the bathroom. But if you have to turn on a lot of lights, you may overstimulate yourself and find it more difficult to fall back asleep, says Dr. Kramer. If you regularly find yourself in this situation and your eyesight and balance don't cause you any problems, plug in a night-light or even two if it's a long way to the bathroom. Let the small glow light your way.

Limit your sleep. If you are having a difficult time sleeping, you may think that trying to sleep more will help. But this can backfire, making insomnia worse, says Lauren Broch, Ph.D., director of education and training at the sleep-wake disorders center at the New York Presbyterian Hospital–Cornell Medical

Center in White Plains, New York. "You spend a lot more time in bed where you're not sleeping, and you start learning that bed is not a place to sleep—it's a place to ruminate and a place to be frustrated. You start associating your bed with things other than sleep," Dr. Broch explains. As you age, the amount of sleep you need can become very individualized, so in order to fall asleep efficiently, it's important to limit yourself to only an extra half-hour in bed awake. After that, get up.

Confine your sleep to the night. You might think a nap would be good to help combat the effects of insomnia. But any time spent napping actually takes away from the time you'll spend sleeping at night. That only makes insomnia worse. If you feel tired during the day, try to stay awake until bedtime, suggests Dr. Broch. By then, you may find yourself so tired you'll fall right to sleep.

Work it out. Exercise has been shown to help sleep, says Dr. Zee. And it doesn't have to be strenuous aerobic exercise either. In fact, the timing of your exercise is more important than how strenuous it is. Exercise will initially make you more alert. But four to six hours after you exercise, your body temperature and metabolism drop, priming you for sleep, explains Peter Hauri, M.D., co-director of the Mayo Clinic Sleep Disorders Center in Rochester, Minnesota, and author of *No More Sleepless Nights*.

Schedule your workouts for four to six hours before bed, so your body temperature and energy will be declining just about the time you need to get to sleep. Any closer to bedtime and you may be too stimulated to sleep.

Intermittent Claudication

Even in bygone days when doctors were scarce and do-it-yourself medicine was all the rage, some ideas were frankly lame. Take, for instance, this oddball cure for leg pain: "Rub leg with turpentine and sit before the fire until leg begins to tingle." Fortunately, this dubious remedy was just a flash in the pan that never really caught fire—so to speak.

Now there are vastly safer natural remedies for intermittent claudication, a type of persistent leg pain that affects 1 in 10 Americans over age 70. The condition is named for Roman emperor Claudius, who, like many people who have this condition, had a noticeable limp. It is caused by hardening of the arteries supplying blood and oxygen to the lower limbs. High blood pressure, diabetes, smoking, high cholesterol—the very same lifestyle factors that promote heart disease—all contribute to this condition, which can cause a burning, cramped pain in the legs, feet, hips, thighs, or even the buttocks.

The pain typically strikes after a person has walked a short distance, often as little as a block. After you've stopped and rested a few minutes, the pain usually disappears. When you have intermittent claudication, the pain recurs once you begin exerting yourself again. As the arteries become more clogged, the distance you can walk before experiencing pain gradually decreases.

"Intermittent claudication definitely interferes with living well. But up to 90 percent of people who have it never report it to their doctors. Most people consider it just a part of getting old. They think, 'Oh well, I just can't do what I used to do,'" says Steven Santilli, M.D., vascular surgeon at the Veterans Administration Medical Center and assistant professor of surgery at the University of Minnesota, both in Minneapolis.

That fatalistic attitude is unjustified, Dr. Santilli says. "Lifestyle changes like quitting smoking and getting regular exercise can have a huge impact on this condition. There is really no reason you should have to live with intermittent claudication," he says. Here are a few effective ways to put the zing back into your step.

Walk away from it. Walking—the very activity that usually induces the pain associated with claudication—also is one of the surest ways to stop it, doctors say.

"Some people look at me like I'm crazy when I tell them they need to get out there and walk more, not less. They want pills. But the truth is, we really don't have a drug that will treat claudication as effectively as walking," says Jay D. Coffman, M.D., chief of peripheral vascular medicine at Boston University Medical Center.

Walking enhances the ability of your leg muscles to extract oxygen from blood, Dr. Santilli says. So if you walk more, not less, your leg muscles will learn to use oxygen more efficiently, and you'll be less apt to develop cramps and leg pain.

Set aside about an hour a day five days a week for walking, he suggests. As you walk, avoid stopping when you feel the first twinges of pain. Instead, let the pain intensify a bit, then pick out a nearby goal, like

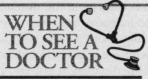

WHEN TO SEE A DOCTOR

Ignoring persistent leg pain can be dangerous, says Jay D. Coffman, M.D., chief of peripheral vascular medicine at Boston University Medical Center. "Many people who have intermittent claudication also have hardening of their coronary arteries and are more susceptible to heart attacks and strokes."

Let your doctor know about any leg pain that happens even when you're not exercising, says Steven Santilli, M.D., vascular surgeon at the Veterans Administration Medical Center and assistant professor of surgery at the University of Minnesota, both in Minneapolis. Also inform your physician if you're suddenly unable to walk as far as you once could or if your legs start to hurt consistently after walking a short distance, he adds.

the next telephone pole, and vow to reach it before you rest. Once the pain subsides, get moving again. When you feel the next surge of pain, set your sights on another goal—say, the length between two telephone poles—that's just a bit more ambitious than the first goal. Keep going on like this for the full hour.

Don't worry about how many times you have to stop or how fast or far you walk, Dr. Santilli says. In the beginning, some people who try this approach have to stop and rest every two to three minutes. That's okay. If you sustain this effort for several weeks, your pain should subside, and the distance between rest stops should increase, he says. In fact, researchers have found that many people with intermittent claudication who use this technique are able to double their walking distance in just two to three months.

Snag a walking buddy. Ask your spouse, a friend, or a co-worker to join you on your strolls, Dr. Coffman suggests. A companion can encourage you to keep moving and reinforce your determination to beat intermittent claudication.

Walk for cover. Rather than ditching your walk on unseasonably hot or cold days, go to an indoor shopping mall where you can do your routine in temperature-controlled comfort, recommends Dr. Coffman.

Corral the Marlboro man. People who smoke are twice as likely to develop intermittent claudication as nonsmokers, Dr. Santilli says. Smoking constricts blood vessels and makes it harder for your leg muscles to work properly. But even if you've lit up for years, quitting now will improve circulation in your legs and help relieve the pain, he says.

Be firm about fat. Eating too much artery-clogging fat will only worsen intermittent claudication, Dr. Santilli explains. That's because a fatty diet can cause hardening of the arteries, which in turn causes intermittent claudication. For every bite of meat, take four bites of fruits, vegetables, beans, and grains. It will help keep you on track for a low-fat lifestyle. If you must, Dr. Santilli says, you can make fatty foods like gravy, bacon, or fried chicken a once-a-month treat.

Kidney Stones

Anyone who has passed a kidney stone can verify that this is an experience he never wants to repeat. The stone has to travel down a passage—the ureter—that easily carries liquid but has a terrible time with a small, grainy, calcified object like a kidney stone.

When it's all over, the stone passer (who is most often male) will breathe a huge, well-deserved sigh of relief. The trouble is, relief may last only for a while.

Usually, once you've had one stone, you're at a higher risk of getting another, says Leroy Nyberg, M.D., director of the urology program at the National Institute of Diabetes and Digestive and Kidney Diseases at the National Institutes of Health in Bethesda, Maryland. And then the risk can *double* after a second stone.

What causes these pebbles of pain? When the concentration of stone-forming minerals such as calcium or oxalate in your urine is too high, you begin to get a buildup of crystals of calcium salts and other minerals that are normally flushed away during urination. The buildup of these crystals in the kidneys eventually begins to form into a hard deposit, similar to a rough pebble. Besides the pain stones cause, you may detect blood in the urine. Only time—and a heck of a lot of water—will help flush a kidney stone. Sometimes a stone must be surgically removed.

Your doctor will need to determine by chemical analysis what kind of kidney stones you have and

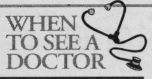

WHEN TO SEE A DOCTOR

Once you pass a stone (thank goodness!), your doctor needs to evaluate it, so you can take measures to reduce your risk of developing another. You should also see your doctor if you're experiencing pain in the groin, lower back, or testicles, or if you see blood in the urine. Any of these signs may indicate that you're getting another stone.

which treatments are appropriate. But here are some ways you can reduce your chances of forming another pain-producing stone.

Drink a lot of water. By increasing fluid intake, you raise urine volume and decrease the concentration of stone-forming elements in the urine. But how much is enough? "I tell my patients to drink enough fluid that they have a urine volume at least equivalent to a two-liter soft-drink bottle every day," says Brad Rovin, M.D., a kidney specialist and assistant professor of medicine and nephrology at Ohio State University College of Medicine in Columbus. To do that, you may have to drink almost a gallon of water a day—especially if you spend a lot of time exercising outdoors.

"It's even more important for people with stones, or who are prone to them, to keep properly hydrated," says Dr. Rovin. And it *is* important to gauge your urine output. Dr. Rovin suggests using an empty milk carton for measuring until you find out how much you have to drink to get at least two liters' worth of urine.

Get plenty of exercise. Regular exercise helps put calcium back into your bones, where it's most needed. "People who are inactive tend to accumulate calcium in the bloodstream," says Dr. Nyberg. A daily workout for at least 30 continuous minutes is advised.

Watch your calcium. Most stones are calcium-based, so it's essential that you avoid excessive intake of milk, butter, cheese, and other calcium-rich dairy foods. "If you've had a kidney stone, you shouldn't have more than one gram of calcium a day—the equivalent of about three glasses of skim milk," says Dr. Rovin.

Monitor protein. But calcium isn't the only no-no. Protein can also raise calcium levels, and it may increase the presence of uric acid and phosphorus in the urine—which may lead to stone formation. So if you've had uric acid or cystine stones, don't exceed six ounces of meat, fish, or other protein-rich foods daily.

Bypass oxalates. If you've had a calcium oxalate stone (your doctor can tell you), then oxalate-rich foods can cause you trouble. So limit your intake of beans, beets, blueberries, celery, chocolate, grapes, nuts, rhubarb, and spinach.

Contain condiment consumption. Table salt and condiments high in sodium should also be avoided. Salt restriction will help decrease the concentration of calcium in the urine. You should reduce your sodium intake to two to three grams per day, according to the National Kidney Foundation. Besides limiting high-salt seasonings such as ketchup and mustard, reduce consumption of processed and pickled foods, luncheon meats, and snack foods such as chips and pretzels.

Beware of stomach antacids. Some antacids are enormously high in calcium, warns Peter D.

Fugelso, M.D., medical director of the kidney stone department at the Hospital of the Good Samaritan and clinical professor of urology at the University of Southern California, both in Los Angeles. If you've had a calcium stone and if you are taking an antacid, check the ingredients listed on the side of the box and make sure the antacid is not calcium-based. If it is, choose another brand.

Be a careful vitamin shopper. Ask your doctor about using certain vitamins to prevent future stones. A daily supplement of magnesium helped stop stone recurrence in nearly all those included in one Swedish study—so it's a good bet that magnesium supplements are beneficial. Also, vitamin B_6 is believed to lower the amount of oxalate in the urine. (But your doctor will probably tell you to avoid supplements that also contain vitamins C and D, since these nutrients increase the risk of calcium-based stones.)

Leg Cramps

Leg cramps are an equal opportunity annoyer—they can strike when you're running, walking, riding a bike, standing up, even sleeping. But what could prompt such intense pain at such diverse times?

If you're a runner, muscle fatigue can be a factor. If you catch a cramp when you're resting, however, poor circulation could be the culprit.

But you don't have to let leg cramps hamper your style. Consider these home remedies.

Pinch away pain. Ready for instant relief? Try this acupressure technique. Grab your upper lip between your thumb and index finger and squeeze for about 30 seconds.

"It's hard to believe, but it works great," says Patrice Morency, a sports injury management specialist in Portland, Oregon, who works with Olympic hopefuls. Although there's no definite explanation for *why* acupressure works, it's a pain relief technique many athletes have found to be effective.

Let your fingers do the massaging. You can use the direct approach, too: Grab the cramping muscle tightly, pushing your fingertips deep into the cramp for about 10 to 15 seconds, then release. You can repeat as often as necessary to relieve the cramp, says Morency.

Contract and relax. Contracting any muscle that opposes a cramping muscle forces the cramped one to relax, says Morency. When you suffer a severe leg cramp in the calf muscle, for example, flex your shin muscle (which opposes your calf muscle) by pulling your toes toward your knee.

Better yet, while you're pulling your toes up, have a friend gently press the top of your foot the other way to provide resistance, says Morency. That maxes out the tension on your shin muscle, which should cause the cramped calf to release.

Stretch toward comfort. After the cramp is gone, stretch out the muscle—but begin slowly and without bouncing on it, says Andy Clary, head trainer for the University of Miami football team in Coral Gables, Florida. Here's a stretch that will ease the hamstring, which lies under the thigh, almost behind the knee: To begin, sit down on the floor and extend the leg. Then reach out and gently pull your toes toward your knee. That applies pressure over the belly of the hamstring muscle, stretching it comfortably. "You simply want to elongate the muscle," says sports injuries specialist Craig Hersh, M.D., of the Sports Medicine Center in Fort Lee, New Jersey.

Water your pain. Drinking a cup of water (about eight ounces) every 20 minutes before, during, and after exercise will help keep your system from dehydrating. And when you prevent dehydration, you prevent cramping, says Dr. Hersh.

Give your electrolyte balance a boost. "People who are maintaining their weight and seem to be well-hydrated but are getting recurrent cramping may have an electrolyte imbalance—too little sodium or potassium in the blood," says Dr. Hersh. He recommends any sports drink that replenishes sodium or potassium. "But you should probably have a blood test to make certain that's the problem," Dr. Hersh adds.

Train harder. Longer runs and walks will teach your muscles to better tolerate fatigue, says Morency.

Loss of Smell and Taste

What do these things have in common?

♦ A crusty loaf of homemade bread just out of the oven

♦ A red Mister Lincoln rose, petals unfurling

♦ A walk in the woods after a spring rain shower

♦ Your grandchild's freshly bathed and powdered little body in your arms

If your answer is that they all still look and feel great but you can no longer smell them, then welcome to one of the most insidious parts of aging: a decline in the ability to smell and taste.

This change profoundly affects your relationship with food as well as many other sensory delights. When the senses of taste and smell are poor, food becomes less interesting. This often causes you to undereat, setting you up for energy and nutrition deficits. Or you might swing too far the other way, overeating in a misguided effort to find something—anything— that tastes good.

The sense of taste is limited to the perception of four basic taste qualities: sweet, sour, salty, and bitter. Smell is what we perceive with our noses. As you chew food, the vapors of the food reach the olfactory

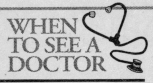

WHEN TO SEE A DOCTOR

If your sense of smell or taste declines so rapidly that you notice it, you may have a problem with some sort of infection or drug interaction. Chronic sinus inflammations or infections have been known to knock your senses for a loop. Because these infections won't go away on their own, you should see a doctor.

Nasal polyps can also form in response to constant irritation of the nasal passages and can interfere with your taste and smell. Difficulty breathing through your nose is an indication of these polyps, which your doctor can treat with steroids or remove surgically.

If your poor sense of taste and smell is accompanied by headache or visual problems, you should see your doctor immediately because there may be a chance that a tumor is causing these symptoms.

(smell) receptors through the nasal cavity. The combined experience of taste, smell, texture, and temperature is called flavor.

When you lose the ability to taste food, it's really because your sense of smell is diminished. This is most often caused by a gradual increase in the obstruction of the nasal passages, as with sinus disease or by sudden viral infections such as a common cold or flu, says Miriam Linschoten, Ph.D., research associate at the University of Colorado's Rocky Mountain Taste and Smell Center in Denver.

Loss of taste and smell is more than just an impediment to gastronomic pleasure. A loss of smell can mean that you don't know when something is burning on the stove.

Fortunately, there are some strategies that you can practice to help make eating a pleasurable, sensory experience again. Likewise, there are precautions you can take to ensure that you are safe in your own home.

Trigger the trigeminal. The trigeminal nerve does not carry taste or smell information. Through its many branches throughout the nose, mouth, and face, it senses touch, warmth, cold, pain, tickle, and itch.

Take advantage of the trigeminal nerve to give you gustatory sensation by adding a little pepper, horseradish, mustard, or hot sauce to your foods.

"It means you take a mouthful of food and get some sensation from it—as opposed to nothing—and that's a positive thing," says Claire Murphy, Ph.D., professor of psychology at the Smell and Taste Clinic at the University of California, San Diego. "If you add hot peppers, then the food becomes appealing in its own right."

Menthol and mint flavors are also felt by the trigeminal nerve, so adding peppermint to cookies and ice cream and using mint in cooking are also good ideas.

Add a little crunch. How your food feels in your mouth becomes more important when taste and smell diminish. Try to vary the textures of foods at meals. "You want one a little spongy, one a little crispy, one a little crunchy, and one a little chewy so that you can get more variety," says Susan Schiffman, Ph.D., professor of medical psychology at Duke University Medical School in Durham, North Carolina. Add croutons or crispy noodles to salads and soups. Sprinkle some chopped nuts over a main course. Toast bread even if you are eating it with dinner.

Give yourself an eyeful. "If you go into a French restaurant and things are served beautifully, that's so appealing," Dr. Murphy says. Contrast that dining experience with the sight of potatoes next to pork or some other light-colored meat with a white vegetable like turnips.

Adding diversity to the color of the foods on your plate goes a long way toward making a meal look good. Chef Janos Wilder, who own Janos Restaurant in Tucson, Arizona, says reds, greens, and yellows actually make food more appealing. So instead of having a pale pork chop with mashed potatoes and turnips, try having it with bright red beets, dark green spinach, and multihued rice pilaf. And then sprinkle on some fresh green herbs such as rosemary and thyme. This not only adds color but also packs an aromatic punch.

Work in contrasts. "The easiest contrast in taste is sweet and sour," says Wilder. But don't limit yourself to contrasts in taste. Serving hot and cold items together, like a dollop of cold salsa on hot soup, Wilder suggests, is a contrast that adds some interest.

Cook in flavorful ways. When certified master chef Ronald De Santis, senior professor at the Culinary Institute of America in Hyde Park, New York, wants to add a flavor punch to food, he thinks about cooking methods. If you're cooking a food by poaching, boiling, or steaming, add herbs, spice seeds, and lemon zest to the water to infuse the food with additional flavor.

Roast and grill foods. These methods of preparation leave a nice browned, caramelized crust on foods that is appealing to the eye. That caramelization and some of the charred flavor found in grilled foods add a further flavor dimension.

Make food the focus. When you sit down to a meal, you want distractions kept to a minimum, says Richard Doty, Ph.D., director of the University of Pennsylvania Smell and Taste Center and professor at the University of Pennsylvania School of Medicine, both in Philadelphia. This means turning off the television and turning on the answering machine. Putting on a little music and lighting a candle makes a meal more of a sensory, leisurely event.

Take a while to thoroughly chew each bite. In addition to making your digestion easier, this little trick helps break down the cells of food and releases more flavor compounds, Dr. Schiffman says.

When serving older people in her own home, Dr. Schiffman likes to keep food covered as she serves it. She puts the plate of food right under the person's nose, then takes the cover off so the first smell is sudden and strong.

Switch-hit around your plate. Imagine walking into a kitchen where bread is being baked. The smell hits you at first, but after a few minutes, you won't notice it any longer. It's called adapting out. "That same thing happens when you eat three bites of food in a row," Dr. Schiffman notes. "The first bite is strong. The next bite is a little weaker. The third is weaker yet." To lessen this phenomenon, change from food to food around your plate as you eat.

Pucker up. The sense of smell is usually more compromised than the sense of taste, which detects sweet, sour, salty, and bitter. So eating foods that appeal to these taste groups can ensure that you have a

Managing Your Meds

Many medicines can affect either the sense of smell or the sense of taste, causing what are called reversible taste perversions that can change the taste of your own saliva as well as the taste of the foods you eat.

Often, drugs affect certain parts of your tastebud palette. "You taste grapefruit and all of a sudden it tastes sweet," says Charles Lacy, Pharm.D., drug information specialist at Cedars-Sinai Medical Center in Los Angeles. This change in the way your tastebuds function leads to a perversion of what food used to taste like.

Some of the drugs commonly used by people older than 60 that can warp the senses of taste and smell are:

✦ Calcium channel blockers (Procardia, Vascor)

✦ Drugs used for Parkinson's disease (Levodopa, Dopar)

---

sensory sensation. Because of the high-fat content in sweets and the risks of too much salt in the diet, it's better to stick with appealing sour and bitter tastes. Doesn't sound appetizing? Beer, seltzer water, coffee, and brussels sprouts are examples of bitter foods that most people have learned to like. Lemons and lemon flavoring, pickles, pickled beets, and pickled eggs are sour foods that you might enjoy. Just know that sour, acidic foods like citrus fruits can eat away at tooth enamel, so it would be a good idea to brush your teeth after consuming them, says Daniel Kurtz, Ph.D., director of the smell and taste disorders clinic at the State University of New York in Syracuse.

✦ Psychiatric drugs such as lithium (Lithane) and fluoxetine (Prozac)

✦ Adrenocorticoids used for nasal allergies and chronic bronchial asthma (Doxycycline)

Over-the-counter drugs such as pseudoephedrine (Sudafed) and aspirin also can affect your senses of taste and smell.

Anything with a high mineral content, including some vitamins, iron tablets, and zinc lozenges for the flu, can alter taste, leading to a metallic flavor in the mouth, Dr. Lacy says.

If your doctor changes your medication to one that has less of an impact on your senses of taste and smell, it may be a while before you experience improvement because the effects of your previous medicine may linger.

Beware of leftovers. "I get quite a few people who lose their senses of smell for one reason or another and then get food poisoning," Dr. Linschoten warns. She suggests that people take freshness dates on foods seriously. Label and date your leftovers. If food has been around for a week or more, just throw it out rather than relying on your sense of smell to tell you if it's still good or not.

Think zinc. A zinc deficiency can affect taste and smell, so taking a zinc supplement may be a good idea, says Laurent Chaix, doctor of naturopathy and supervisor of the teaching clinic at the National College of Naturopathic Medicine in Portland, Oregon.

Also, people who are on dialysis tend to lose zinc, Dr. Kurtz says. Look for a zinc supplement or a multivitamin that provides the Daily Value of 15 milligrams, he suggests. You may also want to talk to your doctor about being tested for a zinc deficiency.

Make sure your dentures fit. Dentures can interfere with eating sensations by covering part of your soft palate and some of the tastebuds there. If your dentures don't fit well, they also could put pressure on and damage the nerves that convey taste information, Dr. Linschoten says. And if dentures aren't kept clean, they are a cause of bacterial growth that could coat your tongue and make the taste receptors harder to reach.

Be honest with yourself and your family. If you think you may be having a sensory loss in the taste and smell department, let your family know, says Dr. Doty. You may be able to call on them to sniff out things in your home that you might be unaware of.

Not surprisingly, people who lose their senses of smell fear that others will detect their body odor. "People become insecure because they don't know whether they need a bath or whether they've put on too much perfume," Dr. Linschoten says.

Honesty is also important when you are cooking for others, because you won't be able to tell if a food is seasoned properly, according to Dr. Kurtz. Ask a friend or family member who will be dining with you to be a taste tester.

Invest in detectors. Smelling gas leaks and smoke from a fire becomes more difficult as the sense of smell declines. Buy smoke alarms and change their batteries twice every year. If you have gas appliances, you can use soapy water to check the gas pipes for leaks, says Dr. Linschoten. Every two months, put the soapy water on the gas pipes in your house. If there's a leak, the water mixture will bubble. But, of course, even that's not foolproof. If you can afford it, replace your gas appliances with electric, Dr. Doty advises.

In addition, it would pay to have a carbon monoxide detector ($30 to $50), Dr. Kurtz says. Carbon monoxide is a colorless, odorless gas that can't be detected even when you have a good sense of smell. But it's usually the by-product of a combustion process, and people take action such as identifying the cause or calling the fire department when they smell something burning. If you are unable to smell those combustion fumes, you are at a greater risk of suffering from carbon monoxide poisoning.

If you have a natural gas source in your home or office, it also makes sense to purchase a natural gas detector ($30 to $50) if your sense of smell is impaired.

Low Blood Pressure

If you've ever experienced low blood pressure after standing up, you probably know the symptoms: You climb out of bed feeling perfectly fine—and then, an instant later, you feel as though you might pass out. This is because when you stand up suddenly, there's a brief period (about a minute or so) when your circulatory system has to adapt to a new body position and may not be sending enough blood to your brain. That's what accounts for the momentary light-headedness, which usually corrects itself after you've been on your feet and moving around a bit.

Low blood pressure symptoms sometimes can also occur after eating a meal or after standing for a long period of time. If you get light-headed under any of these circumstances, you are at risk for falls or fainting, according to Scott L. Mader, M.D., assistant professor of medicine at Case Western Reserve University in Cleveland. If this occurs frequently, you should definitely get a doctor's advice.

Another reason to see the doctor: If you're taking medications for other conditions, these drugs may be *causing* low blood pressure. "Tell your doctor about your symptoms," suggests Mark J. Rosenthal, M.D., associate professor of medicine and geriatrics at the University of California, Los Angeles, School of Medicine and a staff physician at the Geriatric Research, Education, and Clinical Center at the Veterans Administration Medical Center in Sepulveda. It may be possible to reduce your dosage or to switch to a drug with fewer side effects.

In the meantime, here are some other ways to get the pressure up.

Fill 'er up with water. Dehydration reduces blood volume, which can lead to a drop in blood pressure. "I tell my patients to drink liberally," Dr. Rosenthal says. He recommends drinking about one glass (eight ounces) per hour; other doctors suggest eight glasses a day.

Pump your calves. When your blood pressure is low, gravity gets the upper hand. There's too much blood pooling in the lower part of your body. How can you keep it moving?

"If you're standing or sitting for long periods of time, keep blood from pooling in your legs by flexing and pointing your toes, stepping in place, and rhythmically contracting and relaxing your calf muscles," Dr. Rosenthal suggests.

Adopt a flex stance. Standing at attention for a long time seems like an invitation to lower blood pressure. So why don't the guards at Buckingham Palace keel over?

Maybe it's because they don't lock their knees. Dr. Mader suggests keeping your knees slightly flexed rather than locked. "If you flex your knees slightly, you maintain muscle tension in your leg muscles to help pump blood back up to your heart."

Take time to cool down. When you've been exercising vigorously and you suddenly stop, there may be a dizzying drop in blood pressure. "For the next 10 minutes or so following exercising, continue your activity at a slowed down pace," suggests John Duncan, Ph.D., associate director of the exercise physiology department at the Cooper Institute for Aerobics Research in Dallas. That gives your breathing a chance to return to normal and your heart a chance to resume its regular pace.

Stick with nonalcoholic drinks. Alcohol temporarily dilates blood vessels, causing a pleasantly warm flush. But those dilated vessels don't sustain their shape as well as normal, undilated vessels. So when your blood vessels dilate, your blood pressure can hit some dizzying new lows.

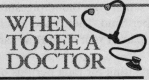

WHEN TO SEE A DOCTOR

Since low blood pressure can contribute to falls, you should see the doctor if you have any blackouts or if you repeatedly feel faint and light-headed during the day. You should also see the doctor if you are taking any medication, since many drugs—especially those for *high* blood pressure—can affect the contraction and dilation of blood vessels. Usually, you can be switched to a different medication that can still treat your condition without causing problems.

In some cases, low blood pressure may be one symptom of diabetes or nervous system diseases, according to Scott L. Mader, M.D., assistant professor of medicine at Case Western Reserve University in Cleveland.

Low blood pressure after standing can be treated. Often a change in diet or activity level will be enough. However, there are more potent therapies available if needed.

Don't restrict salt unless you need to. "I tell a lot of my patients with low blood pressure after standing up to lightly salt their food at each meal," says Dr. Mader. This is only for some people, however. If you've been put on a low-salt diet by your doctor, you shouldn't go off it without his permission.

Lie head-high. Sleeping with your head slightly

elevated may help your body better adjust to an upright position, Dr. Rosenthal says. Try four-inch blocks under the legs at the head of the bed.

Rise and shine . . . slowly. Take lessons from a cat. Stretch before getting up, contracting and relaxing the muscles in your legs, abdomen, and arms. When you sit up, dangle your feet over the side of the bed and flex your calves and arms. "Squeeze your fists and pump your stomach in and out a few times," suggests Dr. Mader. "Arm exercises are particularly effective at raising blood pressure."

Of course, if dizziness is a problem, it's a good idea to keep a chair or handrail by the bed to grasp as you stand.

Eat like a bird, not a boa constrictor. If you feel woozy after a big meal, try eating smaller, more frequent meals, experts recommend. After a big meal, blood rushes to your digestive area, and as a result, there's less blood getting to your brain. By eating smaller, more frequent meals, you're more likely to maintain more constant blood flow.

Walk it off. In one study of older people with low blood pressure after meals, walking afterward restored their blood pressure to normal. "These findings support an old German proverb—'After meals, you should rest or walk a thousand steps,'" says researcher Lewis A. Lipsitz, M.D., director of medical research at the Hebrew Rehabilitation Center for the Aged and assistant professor of medicine at Harvard Medical School, both in Boston.

Lowered Sexual Desire

When she was 30, Eleanor Hamilton, Ph.D., asked a woman in her seventies, "At what age does sexual desire stop?" The woman's eyes twinkled with amusement as she replied, "I'll let you know."

Of course, the woman never did. And Dr. Hamilton, a retired sex therapist now in her late eighties, thinks she knows why.

"Her answer surprised me at the time. But now it doesn't at all. I know full well now that sex can go on until you die," says Dr. Hamilton of West Linn, Oregon.

In fact, studies suggest that up to 74 percent of married men and 56 percent of married women over age 60 are still sexually active. And even after age 80, 63 percent of men and 30 percent of women report having intercourse regularly, researchers say.

"One of the unfortunate myths of our society is that older people aren't sexual and shouldn't want sex anyway. Well, obviously we are sexual, and we do want sex," Dr. Hamilton says.

But sexual desire is also fragile. "It's a real blow to your sex drive when you have problems in the bedroom. Failure doesn't exactly make people want to come back for more," says Fran Kaiser, M.D., adjunct professor of geriatric medicine at St. Louis University

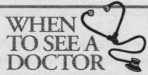

WHEN TO SEE A DOCTOR

If you think that lowered sexual desire is a problem, you may want to seek counseling from a sex therapist, says Eleanor Hamilton, Ph.D., retired sex therapist in West Linn, Oregon. In particular, you should seek help if:

■ You feel angry about or disappointed with your sex life.

■ You and your partner disagree about how often you ought to have sex, to the point that it is eroding mutual respect or hindering communication.

■ You have physical problems that make sex difficult or undesirable, but you don't know how to overcome these barriers.

and senior regional medical director for Merck pharmaceuticals, based in Irving, Texas.

Drops in testosterone production and other hormonal changes, for instance, do decrease sex drive and make it more difficult for older men to get and maintain erections. And without the certainty of success, many older men become skittish about sex, Dr. Kaiser says. As for women, menopause triggers a decline in estrogen production. Without estrogen, vaginal lubrication needs some help because the vagina doesn't get quickly and naturally moistened when foreplay begins. Unless you and your spouse are aware of this, you might attempt intercourse despite vaginal dryness, and that can make the experience painful and, ultimately, less desirable.

Sexual desire also can be derailed by arthritis, heart disease, stroke, osteoporosis, and other ailments associated with aging. "Any chronic disease that causes pain, discomfort, anxiety, or shortness of breath is going to sap your libido. If your body hurts, why would you want to have sex?" Dr. Kaiser asks.

In addition, unreasonable expectations can transform sex into an avoided chore rather than an anticipated pleasure, points out James Semmens, M.D., sex therapist and professor emeritus at the Medical University of South Carolina College of Medicine in Charleston, South Carolina.

"Some older people still think that sex has to be an explosive achievement. If they don't have orgasms, they feel as if they've failed their partners somehow. So they back away from sex altogether. That can place a heavy burden on their relationships," Dr. Semmens says. "It's important to keep sex in proper perspective as you age. Your sexual performance may not be the same as it was in your thirties or forties, but it still can be fun, rewarding, and novel as you get older."

Here are a few ways to keep your sexual flames burning.

Broaden your horizons. Sex is about much more than intercourse. Explore new ways to express your sexuality, Dr. Semmens says. Be sure to give each other lots of hugs, kisses, gentle caresses, and other displays of tenderness. Just the physical act of holding hands can be as fulfilling as traditional sexual activity.

"Learning new ways to play in the sexual sandbox is important in later life," Dr. Semmens says. "Remember, the goal of sex is not always a physical one, it's emotional, too."

Let the hands roam within limits. For a few minutes or longer each day, lend your body to your partner, suggests Karen Martin, program coordinator for the sexuality center at Hillside Hospital of Northshore–Long Island Jewish Health System in New Hyde Park, New York. Your partner can touch you in any way that provides pleasure to either of you, but during this time, the breasts and genitals are off-limits. That will free your spouse to explore different parts of your body without feeling obligated to arouse you. It can also help you feel good about yourself. If a particular touch, such as running a finger down your back, hurts or bothers you in any way, ask your partner not to do it. Allow enough time for each partner to take turns.

This exercise can be emotionally gratifying and can redefine your sexual feelings for each other, Martin says.

Make it a priority. Upgrade the importance of intimacy, Dr. Semmens suggests. Instead of suppressing your desires until all your daily chores are completed, allow lovemaking to be more spontaneous. If you let the moment pass, fatigue, stress, and other pressures of life will extinguish your passion.

Let life imitate art. Provocative television shows, movies, magazine articles, and novels are wonderful icebreakers for older couples, especially for those who are reluctant to discuss their lack of sexual intimacy, Martin says.

"If you're watching television together and a sex scene occurs, you might say to your spouse, 'Gee, that looks like fun. Would you like to try that?' or 'You know, if you touched me like that, I would love it.' You might be surprised by how a simple suggestion like

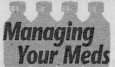

Managing Your Meds

Medications used to treat high blood pressure, including diuretics such as hydrochlorothiazide (HydroDIURIL) and beta blockers like timolol (Timoptic), commonly decrease sex drive, says W. Steven Pray, Ph.D., R.Ph., professor of nonprescription drug products at Southwestern Oklahoma State University in Weatherford. In some cases, estrogens such as estradiol (Estraderm) used in hormone replacement therapy also can lower libido. And there are dozens of other medications that can crimp your sexual desire, including:

✦ Antidepressants such as imipramine (Tofranil)

✦ Haloperidol (Haldol) and other drugs that relieve anxiety and agitation

✦ Allopurinol (Zyloprim) and similar drugs used to treat gout

If your sex drive plunges shortly after you begin taking a medication, consult with your physician. Cutting back on or substituting certain medications often can alleviate the problem. But never stop or reduce your dosage of any drug without your doctor's permission, Dr. Pray warns.

---

this can spark communication and re-ignite your passion for each other," Martin says.

Rediscover romance. Remind your spouse of your love, Dr. Hamilton says. Read a poem, write a love letter, take a moonlit walk, scatter rose petals on the bed. Little romantic gestures can have a big impact on sexual desire.

"My husband always brought me my breakfast in bed and, very often, on the tray there was a love letter, a flower, a pretty seashell, or something else that he thought was delightful,"Dr. Hamilton says. "It was those kinds of things that made me desire him all the more."

Give birth. Plant a garden, build a piece of furniture, make a loaf of bread, paint a landscape, write a novel, or get involved in some other creative activity. It may help rev up your love life, Dr. Hamilton says.

"There is no doubt that creativity and sex are teammates on the vital side of living," Dr. Hamilton says. "Having someone admire something you've done really warms your heart and soul."

Help Mother Nature with some lubrication. Since vaginal dryness is predictable among older women, you probably need some help with lubrication during sex, Dr. Semmens explains. Use a water-soluble lubricant such as Astroglide, K-Y Jelly, or Lubrin to relieve vaginal dryness and pain.

If there's pain, explain. Your spouse can't intuitively know what's painful for you, so you need to tell each other if something makes you uncomfortable. Be sensitive to your partner's physical limitations, Dr. Semmens says. Maybe a sexual position that you used to enjoy is now painful for one of you. If so, experiment and find new sexual positions, Dr. Semmens urges.

If necessary, use pillows to support and protect joints while making love. If the man has arthritis, for instance, the woman should sit astride him or lie beside him, supported by pillows. If the man is on top and the woman has arthritis, he should support his weight with his hands and knees, Dr. Semmens suggests. These simple changes can bring pleasure back into your sex life.

Clean up your act. Poor personal hygiene can make sex less appealing, Dr. Semmens says. Bathe, wash your hair, and brush your teeth or clean your dentures, and your spouse will likely be more receptive to your advances.

Macular Degeneration

About one in four Americans over age 65 and one in three over age 75 will get macular degeneration, the most common cause of vision loss in people over the age of 65, according to the Association for Macular Disease in New York City.

The disease is caused by a breakdown of the macula, a dot-sized part of the retina that allows a person to read, thread a needle, and see other fine details clearly, says Anne Sumers, M.D., ophthalmologist in Ridgewood, New Jersey, and a spokesperson for the American Academy of Ophthalmology. When the macula doesn't work properly, it causes blurriness or darkness in the center of vision.

Macular degeneration may be linked to aging, since it most often strikes in later life. But what really triggers this malfunction is still a mystery, Dr. Sumers says. Some of the suspects include diabetes, family history, atherosclerosis (hardening of the arteries), and ultraviolet light.

There is no cure for macular degeneration. In a few instances, laser surgery can prevent progression of the disease, but it can't restore vision that has already been lost, Dr. Sumers says. Because side vision is usually not affected, people often can continue many of their favorite activities by using low-vision aids such as magnifying glasses.

"Many people with macular degeneration have functional vision for many years, which enables them to see well enough to complete household tasks such as cooking and laundry but may not allow them to read regular print in a newspaper. They might even continue to drive with their doctor's approval," Dr. Sumers says. "It is not necessarily a sentence of blindness. People should not get depressed when they get the diagnosis. There are lots of things you can do to continue living a full and active life despite this disease."

Gaze in the shade. Avoid direct sunlight exposure, which places an additional strain on the retina and damages the light receptors in the eye, says James G. Ravin, M.D., author of *The Eye of the Artist* and a clinical associate professor of ophthalmology at the Medical College of Ohio in Toledo. When you're outside, wear a pair of sunglasses that filters out ultraviolet (UV) rays. "Try to avoid exposure between 10:00 A.M. and 2:00 P.M., when the UV rays are most intense. The closer you live to the equator, the more you need to protect your eyes."

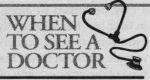

WHEN TO SEE A DOCTOR

There are some signs to be on the lookout for. See your doctor immediately if:

■ You notice irregular patches of dimness in your vision.

■ You have a sudden loss of vision, even if fleeting.

■ You have trouble reading, or words appear blurred on a page.

■ You notice a dark or empty area in the center of your vision.

All these possible symptoms of macular degeneration need to be checked out right away.

Reach for Popeye's favorite dish. Eat five to nine servings of fruits and vegetables daily, including at least one serving of dark green leafy vegetables, says Dr. Sumers. Dark green vegetables, particularly spinach, are the ideal food for the eyes, she says, because they contain an array of nutrients, including zinc, beta-carotene, and magnesium, that may improve blood flow to the eye and protect the retina from the worst effects of macular degeneration.

Normal chemical reactions caused by the effect of light on the macula may activate oxygen and cause macular damage over time. Some vitamins and minerals like beta-carotene function as antioxidants, chemicals that work against this activated oxygen, and perhaps protect the macula from damage. In addition, zinc, one of the most common trace minerals in your body, is highly concentrated in the eye, particularly in the retina and tissues surrounding the macula.

"There's a reason why Popeye always says, 'I'm strong to the finich 'cause I eats me spinach,'" says Stuart P. Richer, O.D., Ph.D., chief optometrist at the Department of Veteran Affairs Medical Center in North Chicago. "Dark green leafy vegetables are very important to the overall health of your eyes. I tell my patients to eat the equivalent of ½ to one cup of frozen spinach a day." That's the same as one-quarter to one-half of a 10-ounce box. For variety, he suggests trying collard greens, kale, and romaine lettuce.

Bigger is better. Large-print books and playing cards, television remote controls with large readable buttons, and other oversized products can help you continue doing activities you enjoy, Dr. Sumers says. Some companies even sell telephones with large numbers and extra-large wall clocks and calculators. Ask your ophthalmologist if these products are available in your area. For a catalog of items designed to make life a little easier for people of low vision, write to Lighthouse International, a nonprofit agency for people who have partial sight or are blind, at 111 East 59th Street, New York, NY 10022. The catalog is available in large-print, braille, and audiotape versions.

Zoom in. A high-quality magnifying glass is a must if you want to read, says Charles R. Fox, O.D., director of vision rehabilitation at the University of Maryland School of Medicine in Baltimore. You don't have to purchase it from a vision rehabilitation center or mail-order service; buy it at Brookstone, the Nature Store, or other gizmo and gadget stores. It can be just as good as one you would get from a low-vision center

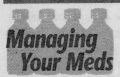

Managing Your Meds

Antimalarial drugs such as chloroquine (Plaquenil), which are also used to treat lupus and rheumatoid arthritis, can spark chloroquine retinopathy, a condition that has many of the same symptoms as macular degeneration, says Samuel L. Pallin, M.D., ophthalmologist and medical director of the Lear Eye Clinic in Sun City, Arizona. The difference is that chloroquine retinopathy is reversible, while macular degeneration is not. If you are on one of these drugs and develop signs of macular degeneration, consult your doctor. In most cases, once you stop taking the offending medication, the symptoms will disappear, and your vision will return to normal.

and often will be cheaper, he notes. To make sure that you get a high-quality magnifier, put the magnifier flat on a piece of lined paper and raise it up until the lines look bigger. It helps to use just one eye for this. The lines should look bigger, but just as sharp. Make sure that there are no distortions, no waves, and no breaks.

Cozy up to your TV. If you have trouble watching television because of macular degeneration, try sitting as close as you can to the set, Dr. Fox suggests. "If the television is far away from you, the black hole in the center of your vision may cover the whole screen. Bring the television closer and closer, and the black hole covers less and less of the screen. So if it helps to sit three feet away from the television, do it."

Light up your life. Switch to 100-watt soft lightbulbs. They will brighten your living space and cut down on glare, Dr. Fox says. Make sure that your lamps or light fixtures can handle the additional wattage. Many have a maximum safe rating of 60 watts, which is usually labeled on the lamp, near the socket that holds the bulb. Get a goosenecked or swing-arm adjustable lamp from a home center or office supply store so you can shine the light directly onto the material you are reading.

Listen to passenger protests. You may feel offended if friends and relatives are reluctant to ride along when you drive. But don't ignore their protests, particularly if their warnings are repeated on a regular basis. Macular degeneration erodes sight slowly, so you may not be aware that your driving skills are impaired because your vision betrays you at times. Consider their concerns about your safety to be a warning sign that it may be time to relinquish the car keys and let someone else slip behind the wheel, Dr. Ravin says.

Weed out cigs before they blindside you. Snuff the smokes, urges Dr. Sumers. People with macular degeneration who continue to smoke are three times more likely to go blind than those who quit, she says. Over-the-counter nicotine patches and gums can help you kick the habit and retain your usable sight.

Menopause

For most women, menopause is a landmark of aging, says Ellen Klutznick, Psy.D., a psychologist in San Francisco who specializes in women's issues. And how women respond to it varies widely. Technically, a woman is considered to be menopausal when she has not menstruated for a year. The average age for menopause in the United States is 51, although women can go through it earlier. For several years prior to actual menopause—a stage called perimenopause—women can experience a whole range of physical changes, including hot flashes, night sweats, sleep difficulties, vaginal dryness, skin changes, hair loss, mood swings, depression, and weight gain.

All of these symptoms as well as the actual cessation of periods are caused by a decrease in levels of the female hormone estrogen. The level of estrogen dips even further after menopause, and that decline can increase the risk of osteoporosis (brittle-bone disease) as well as heart disease.

Unfortunately, you can't avoid menopause. But if you haven't arrived there yet, there are some things that you can do to make the whole experience a little easier. Menopause doesn't have to be a trying time, and it doesn't have to make you look and feel older. Here's what experts recommend.

Get a move on it. Exercise is one of the best things women can do ahead of time in order to fare better during their menopausal years, says Brian

Walsh, M.D., director of the Menopause Clinic at Brigham and Women's Hospital in Boston. Exercise places stress on bone, increasing its density and strength. Since women's bones lose density after menopause—at the rate of 4 to 6 percent in the first four to five years—the stronger they are to start off with, the better. Weight-bearing activities such as walking and running are best, experts say. Exercise also helps keep cholesterol levels down, thus offering protection against heart disease.

Eat right. Eat a nutritious diet low in saturated fat, says Dr. Walsh. This will help reduce cholesterol and the risk of heart disease, he says, both of which go up after menopause. Experts recommend that you keep your fat intake at 25 percent or less of the total calories you consume.

Quit smoking. If you stop smoking, it can help you experience a gentler menopause, says Dr. Walsh. Smokers are more likely than nonsmokers to have menopausal symptoms, he says. Smoking can also cause you to experience menopause earlier, experts say. They think it's because nicotine may somehow contribute to the drop in estrogen. Smokers also have a tendency toward lower bone mass, putting them at greater risk for osteoporosis.

Get your calcium. After age 35, women lose 1 percent of their bone mass per year, so be sure to consume enough calcium. The Daily Value for calcium is 1,000 milligrams, but some experts suggest 1,500 milligrams for postmenopausal women who are not taking hormone replacement therapy and for all women over 65.

Unfortunately, most women consume only about 500 milligrams a day through diet. You can come closer to the protective amounts by adding low-fat dairy products, canned fish such as salmon (with the bones), and soy foods such as tofu to your daily diet.

Get support. "The most valuable thing is gathering together with other women," says Joan Borton, a licensed mental health counselor in private practice in Rockport, Massachusetts, and author of *Drawing from the Women's Well: Reflections on the Life Passage of Menopause*. By talking with other women, either one-on-one or in support groups, you can learn about various symptoms and gather information about doctors and health-care professionals to whom other women go and whom they like and recommend, she says.

"Talking with other women and sharing experiences helps women feel supported and not so isolated," agrees Dr. Klutznick. One option is to join a support group. To find out about groups in your area, call a local hospital or talk to other women.

Find the right doctor. Menopause will bring lots of physical changes and lots of questions, particularly about hormone-replacement therapy (HRT). HRT is recommended to help replace missing estrogen and keep bones strong, but it is also controversial, mainly because it may increase your risk of certain cancers. "The key is to get a doctor who will work with you—one who will honor your decision," says Borton. Ask your friends about their doctors. And don't be afraid to shop around until you find a doctor you like.

Look for a mentor. Find a woman 10 to 15 years older than you who has been through menopause and whom you admire and respect, says Borton. "Spend time with older women, exploring with them what it is that holds meaning in their lives," she says. "Numbers of us feel that doing this has helped us cross the threshold into seeing ourselves as older women and embracing it in a way that feels really wonderful." In addition, look for older women in the public eye whom you can follow and learn from, she says.

Stay lubricated. The decrease in estrogen at menopause can cause vaginal dryness. The elasticity and size of the vagina change, and the walls become thinner and lose their ability to become moist. This can make sex painful or even undesirable, says Dr. Klutznick. Surveys indicate that this happens in 8 to 25 percent of postmenopausal women. While premenopausal women can generally lubricate in 6 to 20 seconds when aroused, it can take one to three minutes for a postmenopausal woman.

Water-based vaginal lubricants such as K-Y Jelly, Replens, and Astroglide, which are available over the counter, are helpful in replacing natural lubrication, says Dr. Klutznick. Steer clear of oil-based lubricants such as petroleum jelly, though, as studies indicate that they don't dissolve as easily in the vagina and can therefore trigger vaginal infections. HRT can also help alleviate dryness, she says.

Stay sexually active. Studies indicate that women who stay sexually active experience fewer vaginal changes than those who don't. Sexual activity promotes circulation in the vaginal area, which helps it stay moist. For women without partners, masturbation helps to promote circulation and moistness in the vagina, Dr. Klutznick says.

Keep it cool. The hot flashes that many women experience during menopause can range from warmth to burning heat that causes flushing and sweating. Experts don't completely understand what causes hot flashes, but they think that the decline in estrogen somehow upsets the body's internal thermometer. It can help to dress in layers and to keep the environment cool, experts say. Some women suck on ice cubes and drink cold liquids or visualize themselves walking in the snow or swimming in a clear lake. Hot liquids and spicy foods can trigger hot flashes, so keep those to a minimum.

Mobility Problems

Mobility is freedom. Each step is a declaration of independence. Each time you stand, you become a statue of liberty.

"Without mobility, your quality of life is greatly diminished," says Sandy O'Brien-Cousins, Ed.D., professor of exercise gerontology at the University of Alberta in Edmonton. Stiffness in your joints doesn't necessarily stop you in your tracks. But it definitely takes more energy to do things; eventually, you will have trouble getting around and may lose your independence.

"We're taught that it is okay to take it easy when you get older," says Wayne Phillips, Ph.D., professor of exercise science at Arizona State University in Tempe. "It's considered the reward for working hard throughout your life. But taking it easy after age 60 isn't a reward. It turns out to be a penalty. It causes much of the loss of mobility that we attribute to aging. You can reduce your risk of these problems if you just stay active. It truly is a matter of move-it-or-lose-it."

Staying active helps you maintain all of the components—your muscles, bones, flexibility, and balance—that you need to remain mobile, Dr. Phillips says.

"Studies have shown that people well into their nineties can improve their mobility. Some of these people were using walkers, canes, and wheelchairs. But when they added strength training and other activities to their daily lives, they were able to rehabilitate themselves and set these assistive devices aside," says Bryant Stamford, Ph.D., director of the health-promotion and wellness center at the University of Louisville in Kentucky.

Be active. Look for ways that you can use more energy and become more active in your life, either by

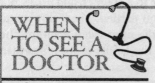

WHEN TO SEE A DOCTOR

Any mobility problem, including walking difficulties, should be evaluated by your physician because it could be a sign of a more serious, underlying condition, says Helen Schilling, M.D., medical director of HealthSouth-Houston Rehabilitation Institute in Texas. It is particularly important to see your doctor as soon as possible if:

■ You have fallen.

■ You have difficulty getting into and out of chairs.

■ You balance yourself on furniture and chairs in order to avoid falling.

■ You are reluctant to go outside without someone to hold on to for balance.

doing things a little faster or a little longer than normal, Dr. Phillips says. "You'll be doing your body a world of good."

For example, if you want to do things faster than normal and it usually takes you 20 minutes to vacuum your house or rake up leaves in your yard, try doing it in 15 minutes, he says.

If you want to use more energy by taking longer than normal to do things, look for ways in which you can break a single task into many. Instead of piling folded clothing on the stairs and letting it sit there until you can carry it up in one trip, take each piece up the stairs as you finish folding it. When you're putting away groceries after shopping, put each item on the table, then move each one to a counter, and finally put it where it belongs. If you garden, kneel down and stand up each time you dig up a weed. Painting the house? Go up and down the ladder more times than necessary.

Be self-reliant. If you have difficulty doing a task, you should be doing it more, not less. So if a friend or relative offers to assist you in getting around, politely refuse, Dr. Stamford suggests.

"Too many people want to rescue older people from difficult situations. If a grandchild sees you struggling with something, she might say, 'Don't worry about carrying those groceries from the car, Grandma. I'll do it for you.' Don't let her do that to you. The only way you're going to get better at lifting and carrying things is to do it," Dr. Stamford says. "If you let others do too many things for you, you'll get weaker. As you get weaker, more things will be a challenge for you."

Take a hike. Walking is moving at its finest, according to Dr. Stamford. It works out all of your mus-

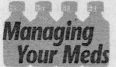

Managing Your Meds

A cornucopia of over-the-counter and prescription drugs can make it harder for you to move about safely, says Helen Schilling, M.D., medical director of HealthSouth-Houston Rehabilitation Institute in Texas. So check with your doctor or pharmacist before taking any drug or drug combinations, she suggests. Be particularly cautious when you are using propoxyphene, acetaminophen, and other prescription pain relievers. These drugs can cause drowsiness and make you less sure-footed. In addition, be wary of:

✦ Alcohol

✦ Prescription antianxiety medications known as benzodiazepines (Valium, Xanax)

✦ Phenothiazines (Thorazine), which are used to treat nervous, mental, and emotional disorders

✦ Antihistamines, including diphenhydramine (Benadryl)

cles and strengthens bones. The more you can do it, the better, he says. Even if you can walk only two to three minutes a day, you'll be moving in the right direction.

Try the bookworm workout. Get in the habit of carrying a box of books from room to room. It will help build the muscle strength you need to stay mobile, Dr. Stamford recommends. Put enough books in the box so that it weighs about as much as a sack of groceries. Every time you leave a room, lift the box from the bottom with two hands, making sure to keep your back straight. Hold the box close at chest level, with your elbows at a 90° angle.

Get out of that chair. Here's a mobility exercise that requires a firm chair with sturdy armrests. Have a seat. Grasp the armrests and push off with your arms and legs, rising to a standing position. Then slowly lower yourself to a sitting position. Do this exercise at least twice each time you sit down, Dr. Stamford suggests.

Hit the floor. Lie with your back flat on the floor and try to get up any way you can. You'll work out virtually every muscle in your body, Dr. Stamford says. Do that three or four times a day. "Most people turn over on their stomachs and do a pushup. It's a great exercise. You're using your hands and knees. You have to balance yourself," he says. "It's really one of my favorites."

Pump some creamed corn. Lift everyday household objects. You'll strengthen your upper body and promote mobility, Dr. Stamford says. Start with an object that you can comfortably lift 10 times, like an 18-ounce jar of peanut butter. Add one lift each day until you reach 25. Then try a slightly higher weight at 10 repetitions and repeat the cycle.

Morning Aches and Pains

Jack LaLanne doesn't feel your pain. "You gotta get up in the morning, count your blessings, and get moving. That's the key to living pain-free," he says.

"I don't even think about morning pain. I just get up and begin living. I kick my butt out of bed every morning, go work out for a couple of hours, and then just do what I have to do," says the octogenarian fitness guru. "Too many people dwell on their aches and pains. Well, don't dwell on them. Get up and do something about it. If you give in to your aches and pains, pretty soon you'll be a goner. Anything in life is possible if you make it happen. God helps those who help themselves. Help the most important person in this world—you!"

Okay, so it may be a lot easier for a real-life man of steel like Jack LaLanne to get going in the morning. And certainly Jack, who once swam 1½ miles while handcuffed, shackled, and towing 70 boats, is more gung ho than most people his age. But his message about being active every day, experts say, is right on target.

"An older person doesn't necessarily have to jump out of bed, dash to the gym, and do a workout every morning. But certainly, if you become more active in your daily life and have a positive attitude about what you are doing, you'll be less prone to joint pain and

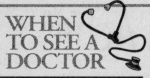

WHEN TO SEE A DOCTOR

Morning pain and stiffness that persist more than an hour after you awaken or that aren't relieved by over-the-counter pain medications like acetaminophen (Tylenol) should be brought to your doctor's attention, says Daniel Fechtner, M.D., assistant professor of rehabilitation medicine at Albert Einstein College of Medicine of Yeshiva University in New York City. In addition, seek medical care if:

■ You have symmetrical pain in both hands or both feet.

■ You have morning pain accompanied by feelings of fatigue or tiredness.

■ You awaken with numbness or tingling that travels down your arms or legs.

■ You have loss of appetite or unexplained weight loss.

muscle stiffness," says Wayne Phillips, Ph.D., professor of exercise science at Arizona State University in Tempe.

Researchers aren't certain how prevalent morning stiffness is among older Americans. If you have it, it could be a sign of overactivity and injury or an underlying illness such as rheumatoid arthritis or other inflammatory conditions of muscles or joints. But in many cases, morning stiffness is merely a stern warning from your body that you may be, in fact, underusing your body in daily activities, says Maria A. Fiatarone Singh, M.D., associate professor of nutrition at Tufts

University and a scientist at the Jean Mayer USDA Human Nutrition Research Center on Aging, also at Tufts in Boston.

In fact, the sedentary lifestyles that many seniors lead can provide an open invitation to morning aches and stiffness. As we age, many of us become less active. As a result, bones become more brittle, tendons lose flexibility, range of motion decreases, and muscles shrink and become weaker. These changes in the musculoskeletal system can make it difficult to do simple daily activities that require stretching, bending, or turning, making you feel like you are stiff all over at times. If your neighbor spends her days lounging by the pool instead of swimming in it, then sleeps on a worn-out mattress all night, you shouldn't be too surprised when she complains about aches and pains in the morning, says Dr. Singh.

Sometimes, simply taking a warm shower or having a massage can ease an occasional morning ache, she says. But if dawn's early light heralds the onset of persistent pains, you'll want to advise your doctor of this symptom. If nothing serious can be found after a medical examination, check out these remedies.

Uncoil tight muscles. Stretching or flexibility exercises can reduce body pain and increase muscular relaxation, which can improve blood circulation, Dr. Phillips says.

Start your day with a gentle stretch in bed. Raise your arms over your head as you curl your toes toward the footboard, Dr. Phillips suggests. Then roll up on your side and sit on the edge of the bed, take a couple of deep breaths, and stretch your hands over your head again.

Get a bungee cord. Some seniors have difficulty doing stretches properly because it is hard for them to bend their arms or legs into certain positions. If you have this problem, try using a bungee cord, suggests Louis Sportelli, D.C., chiropractor in Palmerton, Pennsylvania, and former public affairs spokesperson for the American Chiropractic Association. These cheap elastic cords, available at most hardware stores, can make it easier for you to stretch without overtaxing your muscles and joints. You can also buy specially designed stretch cords for exercising, available at sporting goods stores, he says.

To stretch your hip muscles, for instance, sit in a sturdy chair and make a loop with a bungee cord, interlocking the J-shaped metal loops around a chair leg. Slip your right foot into the circle formed by the bungee. Keeping your thigh flat on the chair seat, press your right foot against this restraint, moving your

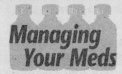

Managing Your Meds

If you consistently wake up feeling as if you've just fallen off an eight-story building, chances are the pain medication you took at bedtime wore off long before dawn's early light, says W. Steven Pray, Ph.D., R.Ph., professor of nonprescription drug products at Southwestern Oklahoma State University in Weatherford.

"If someone, for instance, takes regular-strength ibuprofen (Advil) or acetaminophen (Tylenol) for arthritis pain, it's probably not going to last through the night," Dr. Pray says. "But a longer-acting anti-inflammatory drug like naproxen (Aleve), which you need to take only every eight to 12 hours, should do the trick."

You also might ask your doctor if long-acting prescription pain relievers such as piroxicam (Feldene) or sulindac (Clinoril) might help, Dr. Pray says.

lower leg outward and away from your body until your leg is straight out and parallel with the ground. Hold for a count of 10, then return to the starting position.

Repeat this stretch five times, then switch to your left foot, Dr. Sportelli suggests. Try to do this exercise three times with each leg several times daily. People with arthritis of the knee or ankle, or with hip, knee, or ankle replacements, need to consult their doctors before beginning any exercise program.

To stretch your shoulders, attach the bungee cord to a doorknob and stand with your body perpendicular to and 16 to 18 inches from the door. Pull the cord across your body with your right hand. Hold the cord taut for a count of 10, then return to your starting position. Repeat this stretch five times, then switch to your left hand, Dr. Sportelli says. This exercise also should be done three times with each arm. People with arthritis of the shoulder or with shoulder replacements should check with their doctors before trying to do this exercise.

Rock on. Get a rocker, Dr. Sportelli says. Rocking in a chair helps increase circulation to your legs and may prevent muscle cramps in the morning. The rocking motion from the toe to the heel helps create a milking action that helps return blood to the heart. People who have blood clots should first check with their doctors.

Toss your pillow. If you consistently wake up with neck aches or headaches, your pillow may be the culprit, suggests Dr. Sportelli. If your pillow is too thick, your head and neck might be slightly flexed while you're sleeping. This position straightens your neck and pulls on the muscles and ligaments that support it, causing pain and often morning stiffness and headache. A thin pillow that you can curl under your neck so it supports both your head and neck is a better choice, according to Dr. Sportelli.

Bounce the bed. If your mattress is more than seven years old, consider getting a new one, advises Dr. Sportelli. Even if the covering still looks okay, the springs are probably worn out and not supporting your body as well as they should. So you're more susceptible to morning pain.

When you shop for a new mattress, look for one that has individually wrapped coil springs. It will provide better support than other mattresses, Dr. Sportelli says. It is important to also change your box spring when you change your mattress.

Stretch your imagination, too. Visualizations and imagery are alternative approaches that may help your mind and body work together to conquer morning pain, says Dennis Gersten, M.D., who practices psychiatry and metabolic medicine in the San Diego area and is the author of *Are You Getting Enlightened or Losing Your Mind?* and publisher of *Atlantis: The Online Imagery Newsletter*.

When you awaken, picture your morning pain as a ball that has a particular size, shape, color, and texture, Dr. Gersten says. It may be as small as a marble or as large as a basketball. Allow the ball to grow larger and larger. As it does, your morning pain may momentarily increase. Now let the ball shrink smaller than its original size, but don't let it disappear. As the intensity of the pain changes, allow the ball to change color, too.

Now imagine that the ball turns into a liquid that flows down your arm, drips on the floor, and reforms as a ball. Kick or throw the ball out into space. Watch it disappear. Most of your pain should dissipate as the ball soars off into infinity. Dr. Gersten suggests doing this imagery for 10 minutes twice a day—when you wake up and just before bed.

Muscle Pain

You used to be able to run around all day and wake up the next morning without the faintest trace of muscle soreness. These days, however, overdoing it on the tennis court or even in the garden can cause some unpleasant consequences like sore muscles, a restricted range of motion, or general all-over achiness. These symptoms can make the exercise motto "No pain, no gain" seem like something best left for the grandkids.

But sore muscles actually have a bright side. If you weren't active, you wouldn't get them. It's perfectly normal, says William J. Evans, Ph.D., director of the nutrition, metabolism, and exercise laboratory at the University of Arkansas for Medical Sciences in Little Rock. But, he adds, your symptoms will be much worse if you've exercised too much too quickly.

Since there are so many health benefits to exercise, such as lowering cholesterol and helping to prevent bone and muscle loss, you don't want aches and pains to prevent you from keeping active. The trick is to make sure that exercise doesn't leave you groaning every time you move the day after. And for that, there are plenty of things you can do before, during, and after your workout.

Most of these suggestions apply to dull aches and pains experienced during or after a workout. If you're experiencing acute pain, that's a signal from your body that something is not right. See your doctor if you have sharp pains, says Dr. Evans. Don't try to exercise right through it.

Have an ice day. You may be able to recover from muscle pain more quickly by icing the muscles that are complaining, says Dr. Evans. "Your muscles swell somewhat when you damage them from overuse. Ice can help to reduce the inflammation." Wrap a frozen ice pack in a thin towel and place it on the affected area for no more than 20 minutes each hour. You can repeat as often as necessary until the area is no longer sore. If an ice pack isn't handy, you can use a bag of frozen peas wrapped in a towel instead.

Ask for acetaminophen. Other over-the-counter medications will probably reduce pain, but acetaminophen (Tylenol) is the best choice for muscle pain, says Dr. Evans. Why? Other possible painkillers on the pharmacy shelf—aspirin, ibuprofen (Advil), ketoprofen (Orudis KT), and naproxen (Aleve)—all share a single drawback. These anti-inflammatory drugs block your body's production of chemicals that cause swelling and pain, but in so doing, they interfere with your body's muscle-repair process.

Acetaminophen, on the other hand, blocks pain impulses within the brain itself, allowing the muscle-

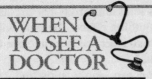

WHEN TO SEE A DOCTOR

Some muscle soreness is routine after a vigorous workout or overdoing it with a new activity, says William J. Evans, Ph.D., director of the nutrition, metabolism, and exercise laboratory at the University of Arkansas for Medical Sciences in Little Rock, but you should be concerned if the pain doesn't go away relatively quickly. "You should report any pain that persists for more than a week to your doctor."

You should also be concerned if the pain is acute, he says. If the pain is sharp or stabbing, you might have a muscle tear or joint injury. This is the sort of thing that can be quite painful and lead to further injury, says Dr. Evans, so you'll want to get checked out right away.

repair process to proceed normally, says Dr. Evans. It's also the pain reliever that causes the least number of side effects when taken in normal amounts. Just make sure to follow the directions on the label and never take more than 12 of the 325-milligram pills in a single day.

Turn up the heat. When the aches and pains are particularly bad the day after you've exercised hard, take a warm bath, says Priscilla Clarkson, Ph.D., professor and associate dean in the department of exercise science at the University of Massachusetts School of Public Health and Health Sciences in Amherst. You can soak for as long as you like, she says. "The warm water helps your muscles relax and promotes circulation, which will have a soothing effect. The pain will come back 15 minutes or so after you get out, but it still makes for a nice break."

Rub it out. Massage can significantly reduce muscle soreness, and it's a safe alternative if you don't want to take over-the-counter medication. In addition, it may decrease levels of cortisol (the stress hormone) and increase production of serotonin, a compound produced in the brain that has a calming, pain-killing effect, says Maria Hernandez-Reif, Ph.D., director of the massage therapy research program and senior research associate at the University of Miami School of Medicine's Touch Research Institute. Here are some self-massage tips from Dr. Hernandez-Reif.

♦ Use a massage oil or lotion to make the experience a lot more pleasant. Put a little oil or lotion on the palm of your hand, then rub your hands together to warm it before beginning the massage. The heat helps loosen muscles more quickly.

♦ Don't skimp on the pressure. You'll know that you're not applying enough pressure if the rubdown feels like light tickling. Ideally, you should cause some muscle stimulation but not so much that you feel pain.

♦ Rub the right way. Cup your hand and glide it along the skin's surface. This is most effective when you can massage a large surface all at once, like the side of your leg from the ankle to the knee. "It's taught in massage therapy classes to rub in one direction toward the heart," says Dr. Hernandez-Reif.

Note: Never apply pressure to any joint area, says Dr. Hernandez-Reif. You might injure that joint.

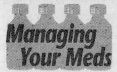

Managing Your Meds

Over-the-counter painkillers can have harmful interactions with some other medications, and they're not good for people with certain health conditions, says William J. Evans, Ph.D., director of the nutrition, metabolism, and exercise laboratory at the University of Arkansas for Medical Sciences in Little Rock. "Acetaminophen (Tylenol) has fewer side effects than any other analgesic," he says, "but taken with alcohol, it can have a toxic effect on the liver." Other than that, acetaminophen has been shown to be remarkably safe. It shouldn't be taken in doses higher than what is recommended on the label, however.

Dr. Evans emphasizes that anti-inflammatory drugs such as aspirin, ibuprofen (Advil), ketoprofen (Orudis KT), and naproxen (Aleve) should be avoided since they interfere with muscle healing. But there are other reasons to avoid them as well. They can occasionally lead to stomach problems, says Dr. Evans, as well as complications with a bleeding condition, kidney disease, or liver disease.

Eat an orange after exercise. Vitamin C after heavy exercise may reduce day-after swelling and pain, reports Dr. Clarkson. When your muscles are damaged by overuse, she says, they produce free radicals, the wide-ranging, highly charged atoms that can damage tissue and age your cells. Antioxidants such as vitamin C may absorb the free radicals before they can cause too many problems, according to Dr. Clarkson. So make sure you're getting the Daily Value

(60 milligrams a day) of vitamin C, she says. You'll find more than that amount in the average orange.

Distract yourself. Another simple way to handle muscle soreness is to just do your best to ignore it until it goes away, says Dr. Clarkson. "Unless you seriously overdid it, the pain will go away within three days." This means that every time you distract yourself with a favorite book or CD or by taking the dog for a walk, you may return from that activity to find that the pain has diminished just a little bit more. (See a doctor if your pain lasts for more than a week.)

Start up slowly. The easiest way to avoid severe muscle pain after exercise is to start slowly any time you try a new activity, says Dr. Evans. Even if it's an activity you're used to, start slowly if you haven't done it in a while, he adds. "Muscle soreness occurs primarily when you force your body to do something it's not accustomed to doing," he says. "If you know you're going to be playing tennis a week from now, do some jogging and light exercises a few days beforehand."

Keep your exercise on an even keel. The key is to keep yourself at a baseline level of fitness where an occasional game or weight-lifting session is no huge shock to your system. If you sit around all winter long and then throw yourself into a day's worth of heavy-duty gardening, you're just asking for trouble, notes Dr. Clarkson. Try to get 30 minutes of aerobic activity such as walking, jogging, or swimming at least three times a week.

Conditioning your body in this way should significantly reduce postexercise muscle pain, says Dr. Evans.

Follow the 10-percent rule. One of the best ways to not overexert yourself is to obey what's called the 10-percent rule, says Dr. Clarkson. Quite simply, it means that you never increase the difficulty of your workout more than 10 percent from week to week. "Because muscle pain usually hits 24 hours after exercising, it's easy to do a lot of damage to your muscles without realizing it at the time," she says. "This rule prevents you from doing that."

How does this translate into your regular exercise routine? Easily. For example, if you take 30-minute power walks three times a week, try to add three extra minutes, but go no further until you're used to the new time frame.

Get ready with a home stretch. When you stretch before exercising, you warm up your muscles, which may help prevent the tiny muscle tears that lead to morning-after pain, says Dr. Clarkson.

Before your next round of vigorous activity, perform this all-around stretching routine, suggests Barbara Sanders, Ph.D., chairperson of the physical therapy department at Southwest Texas State University in San Marcos. Keep in mind that these stretches should be slow and gradual, not bouncy. Don't try to complete any stretch that causes pain.

♦ Shoulder rolls. Stand straight with your head high, your chin in, and your arms at your sides. Rotate your shoulders up, back, down, then forward. Repeat five times.

♦ Side bends. Stand with your right arm above your head, your left arm across in front of your stomach, your knees bent slightly, and your feet about shoulder-width apart. Lean to the left as far as you comfortably can. Hold for five seconds, stand up straight again, then repeat. Now reverse the arm positions and follow the same process, leaning to the right.

♦ **Hip stretch.** Lie on your back with your lower back snugly resting against the floor. Keeping your left leg extended, clasp your right leg with your right hand under the knee and bring it to your chest, letting your knee bend double. Hold for five seconds, release your leg, straighten it, and lower it to the floor. Repeat once, then do the same stretch with your left leg and left hand.

♦ **Hamstring stretch.** Sit on the floor with your right leg relaxed and your right knee bent so that your foot is flat on the floor. Extend your left leg straight in front of you. Now reach for the toes of your left leg with the fingertips of both your hands, feeling the stretch in that hamstring (the long muscle on the back of your thigh). If you can't reach your toes, grab on to your ankles. Stretch for 20 seconds, relax, and then do it again. Now change the position to extend your right leg and repeat the stretch.

♦ **Calf and Achilles tendon stretch.** Stand three to four feet from a wall and lean toward it, supporting yourself with your hands at roughly shoulder level on the wall. Bring your right leg forward, bending at the knee. As you lean forward, keep your left leg straight with your left foot flat on the floor, while pressing your right knee toward the wall until you feel a comfortable stretch in the straight left leg. (Don't arch your back.) Hold for 20 seconds, then repeat with your left leg forward with your knee bent, and your right leg extended behind.

♦ **Shoulder stretch.** Stand straight with your arms extending straight behind your lower back. Grab your left wrist with your right hand and slowly pull both arms back from your spine as far as possible without causing pain, all the time staying as upright as possible.

Keep your neck straight, not arched. Maintain the stretch for a few seconds, relax, then repeat with your left hand grabbing your right wrist.

Muscle Spasms

A human muscle can knot up quicker than an overzealous Boy Scout can tie a figure eight.

Knots occur when your muscle suddenly contracts, or "shortens"—producing immediate and intense pain. Often muscle spasms result when you have overused the muscle while exercising or have injured it in some way.

But muscle spasms are sometimes caused by inactivity, such as sitting in the same position for too long. And you can also get spasms from a pinched nerve. They may even signal a mineral deficiency.

"Most people call these muscle *cramps*, but technically, it's a muscle spasm if the pain is sustained and you can actually feel a lump of muscle tissue under your skin," says sports medicine specialist Charles Norelli, M.D., staff physiatrist at Good Shepherd Rehabilitation Hospital in Allentown, Pennsylvania. But no matter what you call it, here's how to ease a muscle that goes into spasms and prevent the same painful thing from happening again.

S-t-r-e-t-c-h. Logic tells you that pulling on that shortened muscle is the simplest way to get relief.

When you get a muscle spasm, treat it with "gentle, gradual stretching of the affected area," suggests Robert Stephens, Ph.D., chairman of the department of anatomy and director of sports medicine at the University of Health Sciences College of Osteopathic Medicine in Kansas City, Missouri. "Besides pulling on the muscles, stretching helps improve blood flow to the area, which may reduce spasm pain."

If you're in one position too long, muscles tend to shorten. The movement of stretching can prevent this type of spasm.

"A woman who wears high heels all day might get muscle spasms in her feet after she takes off her shoes,"

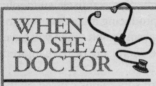

WHEN TO SEE A DOCTOR

Muscle spasms are usually not serious, and the occasional occurrences shouldn't cause you concern. But if you *frequently* get intense leg cramping, it could be a sign that you have restricted blood flow or blood clotting in your legs—both of which can be extremely serious.

Cramping may also signal a nerve injury, says Allan Levy, M.D., director of the department of sports medicine at Pascack Valley Hospital in Westwood, New Jersey, and team physician for the New York Giants professional football team and the New Jersey Nets professional basketball team. The bottom line: If your pain is very severe or if it occurs several times in one week, consult your doctor.

says Dr. Norelli. That's because her feet have been "locked" in the same uncomfortable position all day. "One way to prevent muscle spasms is to stretch your legs and feet after you take off your shoes. Walking around barefoot for a while is usually the best remedy."

Apply moist heat. A hot bath or shower is another way to end muscle spasms. "Like stretching, heat improves blood circulation," says Dr. Stephens. "Heat also helps the connective tissue around the muscles: The warmer that tissue is, the more liquid it is. The colder, the stiffer." In fact, he recommends that you hit the showers *before* your workout to prevent muscle spasms. "I think you'll get your muscles ready for exercise better if you take a hot bath *before* exercise," he says.

Consume more calcium. "Sometimes muscle spasms are the result of a calcium deficiency," says A. J. Hahn, D.C., a chiropractor in Napoleon, Ohio, who specializes in natural remedies. He recommends getting calcium in your diet "if you suffer recurrent muscle spasms that don't result from overactivity." Good sources of calcium include low-fat dairy products such as yogurt, skim milk, and ricotta cheese. Always check with your doctor before adding a calcium supplement.

Say no to acidic foods. Try to limit your intake of acidic foods such as tomatoes and vinegar if you suffer from recurrent muscle spasms, according to Dr. Hahn. That's because these acids can interfere with the body's ability to absorb calcium.

Pump up your potassium. Another nutritional deficiency that's been linked to muscle spasms is inadequate potassium. "Particularly if you're very active—like a long-distance runner or a soccer player—it's very important to make sure you eat plenty of potatoes, bananas, and other foods high in potassium," says Dr. Stephens. Other good sources of potassium include dried peaches, prune juice, and beet greens.

Take it easy. Since most muscle spasms are caused by overusing your muscles, try to give yourself a break every now and then when doing anything physical. "Most people try to work through the pain— and the next morning, they'll pay for it with stiff muscles and intense soreness," says Dr. Hahn. "If you're spading your garden or painting your house when you get a muscle spasm, take a break at the first sign of pain. Rest for 15 minutes or so and *then* resume your work. I think that giving your body a break when it needs it goes a long way toward preventing muscle spasms."

Nausea

Nausea is a universal malady—everyone gets it at one time or another. And depending on the sensitivity of your stomach, it can be caused by just about anything—from the smell of a skunk to (very rarely) appendicitis.

The usual way to end nausea, of course, is to vomit. Fortunately, there are other remedies that aren't so drastic.

Drink a Maalox cocktail. "Put a few drops of

spirits of peppermint into Maalox and mix it with one quart of distilled water," says Christa Farnon, M.D., associate director of Occupational Medical Services for SmithKline Beecham, a pharmaceuticals company in King of Prussia, Pennsylvania. Take a few sips of this to soothe your upset stomach and use the rest later, as needed.

Eat crackers. "In general, when people are slightly nauseated, they will feel better if they can make themselves eat some very plain food," says Robert M. Stern, Ph.D., professor of psychology at Pennsylvania State University in University Park and a researcher on motion sickness and nausea for NASA. "I recommend low-fat foods such as crackers." Don't overdo it, though. A few crackers will ease your nausea, but too much of any food may make you feel even worse.

Exercise your mind. "Sometimes keeping busy can help people," suggests Dr. Stern. "Before they know it, the nausea passes." Play a mental game, read a book, or strike up a conversation with someone to keep the nausea out of your mind.

Rest your body. Astronauts on the first space flights had few complaints about motion-induced nausea. The reason may have been that they were forced to remain still, because the area inside the capsule was so confined. Try not to move around too much, even when your stomach is doing somersaults, recommends Dr. Stern. Most important of all: Try to keep your head still.

Say "I'll pass" on the milk. "Milk and milk products are much more difficult to digest than other foods," says Dr. Farnon. "They contain proteins and fats and create mucus. This means that they are harsher on the stomach." She advises clear liquids such as tea or

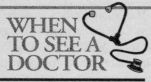

WHEN TO SEE A DOCTOR

Repeated or prolonged nausea can be a symptom of a wide range of conditions, from stomach viruses and food poisoning to intestinal disorders and even tumors.

"If you're nauseated and there's not an obvious reason, you should see a doctor," says Robert M. Stern, Ph.D., professor of psychology at Pennsylvania State University in University Park and a researcher on motion sickness and nausea for NASA. And even if you do know the reason for it—such as car sickness or seasickness—you should see a doctor if the nausea doesn't go away after a day or two.

You should also see a doctor if your nausea is accompanied by fever, especially if you are elderly, according to Dr. Stern.

juices served at room temperature, never cold, when you are trying to recover from nausea.

Try acupressure. Some people find relief from nausea—especially the kind that comes from motion sickness—by applying pressure to the inside of the wrist near the center. Those who practice acupressure believe this is the point that controls things such as nausea and vomiting, says William Grant, Ed.D., vice chairman of the department of family medicine and research associate professor at the State University of New York Health Science Center at Syracuse.

Wrist-wrap with a Sea Band. Sea Bands, special wristbands that put pressure on the inside wrist area, were created for seasickness but are now used for other types of nausea. They can be found at boat dealers, in some sporting goods stores and in most local American Automobile Association offices.

Seek relief in nonprescription drugs. Some over-the-counter medications such as Pepto-Bismol, Maalox, and Mylanta are known to help calm nauseated stomachs. It depends on the cause of nausea, doctors agree, but an irritated stomach may feel better after a couple of spoonfuls.

Don't forget Dramamine. "Some nauseated people might be helped by the anti-motion sickness drugs such as Dramamine," says Dr. Stern. Although he acknowledges that little is known about how Dramamine works to ease nausea, he suggests that you give it a try and keep this over-the-counter medication on hand if it works.

Drink flat soda. "Just open up a carbonated soft drink and let it go flat," says Dr. Grant. He recommends ginger ale, but other soft drinks work just as well. Dr. Farnon suggests the flat syrup of Coca-Cola, available in most drugstores, sipped over cracked ice when your tummy becomes queasy.

Neck Pain

Imagine a jelly doughnut that's been in the microwave too long. While still warm and gooey on the inside, it's lost some of its springy resilience. Now imagine a stack of these doughnuts supporting a 14-pound bowling ball. Doesn't sound like too promising a situation for the doughnuts or the bowling ball.

Your neck and head have been in that situation since adolescence. The human head weighs about the same as the bowling ball and—as we get up there in years—the row of supporting disks are much too much like jelly doughnuts. As people age, disks lose a lot of the fluid that gives them their strength and shock-absorbing ability, says Karen Rucker, M.D., professor in the department of physical medicine and rehabilitation at Virginia Commonwealth University in Richmond. That alone can make people over 60 more prone to stiff, crampy necks.

Couple this with increases in arthritis, osteoporosis, and poor posture, and it's no wonder that neck pain tends to increase as we get older.

Being gentle to your neck and following the rules of good posture go a long way toward lessening neck cricks, twinges, and stiffness. Try these doctors' recommendations.

Give your neck a break. Whatever you're doing, whether it's sitting at a desk or working on a hobby, if you stay in one position for a long period of time, your neck can get stiff, and pain can creep up on you. To prevent this, get a kitchen timer, says Mary

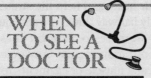

WHEN TO SEE A DOCTOR

If you have neck pain that persists even when you change position and that is also accompanied by any of the following complaints, be sure to call your doctor immediately, says Karen Rucker, M.D., professor in the department of physical medicine and rehabilitation at Virginia Commonwealth University in Richmond.

- Pain shooting down your arms or hands
- Numbness or tingling in your fingers or arms
- Sudden or significant muscle weakness, such as the inability to lift your legs or extend your arms
- Dizziness
- A feeling of pain when you move your jaw, which may be a sign of an abscess or infection
- Onset of fever with a new onset of neck pain and stiffness

Ann Keenan, M.D., director of neuro-orthopedics at Albert Einstein Medical Center in Philadelphia. Set it to go off every half-hour or so to remind you to stand up, do a little stretch, and take a little break.

Get your neck stretched. If tension is causing your pain in the neck, you can relieve it with a little bit of stretching. "Just start by tilting your head from side to side, then rolling it around, first to the right and then to the left," Dr. Keenan says. Next, take your hand, put it on top of your head, and help the stretch by pulling your head gently halfway down toward your shoulder on each side. Be sure to perform these stretches with slow, smooth movements. "Any quick stretch is more likely to tear a muscle or ligament. You need to do it more gradually," Dr. Keenan warns.

Stand and sit up straight. "When you're not using good posture—specifically, you're slumping—all of a sudden your muscles are having to work hard to hold your head up,"Dr. Rucker says. But you can take some of the workload off your neck. Whenever you're sitting or standing, make sure that your shoulders are over your hips and your ears are over your shoulders. Your head should never be tucked under, like a horse in a bridle.

"Think about the top of your head," Dr. Rucker advises. "Try to visualize the top of your head trying to touch the ceiling. You will lengthen, elongate your neck, and get as tall as possible."

Get a chair with a better back. The old clerical chair had nothing more than a seat cushion and an oval pad that you could position somewhere in the middle of your back. If you're still using one of those, retire it in favor of a chair with a back that goes up to shoulder level. With the high-backed chair, your head, neck, and back are kept vertical, and you can lean your head back periodically to give your neck a chance to relax, says Don Chaffin, Ph.D., professor in the center for ergonomics at the University of Michigan in Ann Arbor.

Apply heat or cold. You can apply a hot-water bottle or an ice pack to relieve your neck pain, Dr. Keenan states. It's really your preference. "They both work the same way by increasing the circulation to the area."

Talk on a speakerphone. Wedging a phone in the crook between your tilted head and your

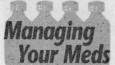

Managing Your Meds

It's not a common reaction, but some blood pressure medications like nifedipine (Procardia) and some anticholesterol medications such as cholestyramine (Questran) can cause muscle aches—including achiness in the neck area. More commonly, if you have stopped taking a sedative drug like diazepam (Valium) or sleep medications such as chlordiazepoxide (Librium) or temazepam (Restoril), you can have an achy neck. "The withdrawal aspect of those medicines will often cause increased pain and muscle tightness all over," says Karen Rucker, M.D., professor in the department of physical medicine and rehabilitation at Virginia Commonwealth University in Richmond. Take these medicines only with close physician supervision, she advises.

---

shoulder can strain your neck. Even phones with headrests can cause pain, Dr. Keenan says. If you have long phone conversations, use a headset or speakerphone. You'll find both at electronics stores or office supply stores.

Buy an athletic bra. If you're a woman with a large bosom, you may not be getting enough support from your bra, and that can surely cause neck, back, and shoulder pain. Try an athletic or jogging bra, Dr. Keenan recommends, because they give more support and have wider straps. Athletic bras are designed to distribute weight more evenly.

Use a fanny pack. Carrying a weighty shoulder-strap purse can put strain on your neck, Dr. Keenan says. A better option would be to switch to a fanny pack, which fits around your waist and doesn't put any strain on your neck at all. You can change to a hand-held purse for more dressy occasions.

Sleep with your neck in line. If you have an old pillow that has become droopy through years of use, throw it out, advises Dr. Keenan. It's time to get a good supportive pillow, she says. You want one that will keep your head in straight alignment with your mid-back (the line from the center of your head down your back to the crease in your buttocks) and your spine when you lie on your back or side. Although pillows have firmness labels that can help, your best bet is to try them out before buying. Throw one on a bed display and lie down on it. Keep testing until you find the right one.

Set up your computer correctly. If you use a computer, make sure it's set up correctly, says Dr. Chaffin. Place the monitor at a distance that is comfortable for reading and at a level where your head is not bent forward or tilted back. Some experts suggest placing the monitor so you are looking at it straight ahead. The keyboard should be positioned so your elbows are at your sides, bent at about a 90° angle, with your wrists straight and level.

Favor the gradual movements. Quick, sharp movements can injure your neck or back. But often, we're reckless about our neck movements until we start to feel pain, notes Dr. Rucker. Treat your neck gingerly, she urges. When you get out of bed in the morning, roll gently onto your side first, rather than sitting bolt upright. And be careful when you're getting in and out of the car. Sit on the car seat first and then rotate your body, bringing your legs around and into the car. Reverse this process when you get out. "We should be using those techniques all the time" to minimize the daily damage that can lead to a big pain in the neck, says Dr. Rucker.

Nicotine Dependency

The good news is that each year a few thousand Americans manage to quit smoking. The bad news is that's a mere fraction of the 50 million Americans who can't. Blame it on nicotine, the active ingredient in cigarette smoke (as well as in snuff and chewing tobacco) that's as addictive as heroin. Seconds after you light up a cigarette, nicotine rushes to the brain, bringing a quiet fix of pleasure and satisfaction—especially to those who have been without a cigarette for an hour or more and may be experiencing withdrawal cravings. But nicotine also quickens the heart rate and constricts blood vessels, impairing normal blood flow, making your heart work harder, and putting you at risk for heart disease.

The pleasure brought on by nicotine quickly convinces the brain to require more, and the smoker soon develops a tolerance for these effects—needing greater "doses" to feel satisfied. Habitual smokers who fail to get a dose of nicotine every 30 minutes or so may show irritability, inability to concentrate, anxiety, confusion, and insomnia.

Quitting is never easy, but the worst part usually comes up front. The physical withdrawal symptoms last a week or two, so getting through that period is usually toughest. Here are some ways to make the rough road a little easier, once you crush out your last butt and retire your habit for good.

Drink orange juice. If you're quitting cold turkey, you'll get over withdrawal symptoms faster if you drink a lot of orange juice. "By making your urine more acidic, you'll clear your body of nicotine faster," says Thomas Cooper, D.D.S., professor of oral health sciences at the University of Kentucky in Lexington and a nicotine-dependency researcher. "However, if you're using the nicotine patch or gum, (which needs a doctor's prescription), then *don't* drink orange juice, because you want to keep nicotine in your body."

Write a letter to a loved one. When the craving to pick up a cigarette hits, pick up a pen instead—and write a letter to loved ones explaining why smoking is more important than they are. "Explain to your grandchildren why cigarettes are so important to you that you would choose to die early rather than live to see them get married and have their own children," according to Robert Van de Castle, Ph.D., professor of behavioral medicine at the University of Virginia Health Sciences Center in Charlottesville.

The letter is realistic, he says, "because that's what is going to happen if you continue to smoke. Certainly heart disease or stroke or lung cancer will get you before you'll be able to share important moments in the lives of your family or loved ones."

When Dr. Van de Castle's patients attempt these

The Only Way to Quit

Many smokers mistakenly think that switching to a low-tar and low-nicotine brand will ease their nicotine addiction, making it easier for them to quit smoking. "Actually, the tobacco is the same in all cigarettes," says Thomas Cooper, D.D.S., professor of oral health sciences at the University of Kentucky in Lexington and a nicotine-dependency researcher. "The only difference is that the 'low' brands have more holes punched into their paper or filters, so you don't get as good a draw when inhaling. But to compensate, people smoking low brands tend to inhale more deeply and take more puffs, so they wind up getting the same amount of nicotine."

Same goes for cutting down the number of cigarettes you smoke. If you smoke fewer every day, "you'll just take longer and more frequent puffs, so you'll still be getting the same amount of nicotine," according to Dr. Cooper. "In studies, I found that the average smoker has 30 cigarettes a day (1½ packs), taking 10 three-second puffs on each butt. When he cuts down to only 10 cigarettes, the number of puffs increases, and each puff becomes longer and more deeply inhaled, up to eight seconds. So cutting down is not an effective way to stop smoking. You have to stop smoking completely."

letters, they usually don't finish writing. "After a while, you begin to feel so foolish, so selfish, and so out of control that you're putting these white sticks ahead of the people who mean most to you that it's often enough to convince you to quit smoking—withdrawal symptoms and all," he explains.

Soak yourself. Another way to distract yourself from the urge to smoke is with a nice hot shower or relaxing bath. And that soothing hot water carries another bonus for the nicotine-dependent: "One of the best ways to deal with pain is to do something relaxing," says Jack E. Henningfield, Ph.D., chief of the clinical pharmacology branch of the Addiction Research Center at the National Institute on Drug Abuse in Baltimore.

Get a lot of exercise. Taking a walk is one of the best ways to walk a mile *away* from a Camel. "Exercise is an excellent method of distraction for people trying to quit," says psychologist Gary DeNelsky, Ph.D., director of the Smoking Cessation Program at the Cleveland Clinic Foundation in Cleveland. "When you exercise, you're not as aware of your internal state. So if you're in the middle of a tennis game, you're not going to think of those cravings; you're focused too much on the game. Besides, the longer you exercise, the more healthy you feel, and many people find that a regular workout psychologically turns them off to smoking."

Most experts, like ex-smoker Dr. DeNelsky, suggest daily exercise when quitting. Some suggest you walk or work out whenever cravings strike.

Drink a baking soda cocktail. If you're not on a low-sodium diet, researchers at the Mayo Clinic in Rochester, Minnesota, say you may get short-term relief from nicotine withdrawal symptoms by dissolving two tablespoons of baking soda—sodium bicarbonate—in a glass of water. Have this drink with every meal. *Note:* This is *not* recommended if you have peptic ulcers.

Pay yourself. A federally funded $1.3 million study on smoking habits found that people who are paid $1 for every day they go without a smoke are more successful at staying off nicotine than other quitters.

"I think the key is to reward yourself quickly," says Doreen Salina, Ph.D., a clinical psychologist and research scientist at DePaul University in Chicago who is the project director of the study. "If you simply put money in a kitty, it won't have the same effect."

Actually, Dr. Salina says *any* reward will do; money is just one option. "Some people allow themselves a nice bath, or they watch a certain TV show they normally wouldn't," says Dr. Salina. Try whatever works, she suggests: "The point is to indulge yourself in some way to compensate for the sacrifice you're making."

Go to the library. "In order to be successful at quitting smoking, you have to prepare to leave situations where smoking is permitted. Modify your activities so that you spend more time in places where smoking is *not* permitted," says Dr. DeNelsky. "Go to the library. Go to church. Visit places where you cannot smoke. It's important to understand that these nicotine cravings will pass, but they will pass more easily if you're someplace where you cannot indulge."

Monitor your vices. "Once you get off cigarettes as a source of nicotine, it's essential that you reduce both your caffeine and alcohol consumption," says Dr. Cooper. "That's because your body loses some of its capacity to process both of these substances as you reduce the amount of nicotine in your body.

"Someone who smokes will process caffeine 2½ times faster than someone who doesn't," Dr. Cooper points out. "That means if you quit smoking, you'll need only about a third as much coffee to get the same 'rush' you got from coffee drinking while still smoking.

And you'll get drunk faster without nicotine in your body, so don't drink as much as before."

Night Vision Problems

Blinded by an explosion, Charles McNider believed that his promising career as a physician and researcher had been hopelessly derailed. Then one evening as he sat alone in his darkened living room, an owl crashed through a window. McNider tore off his bandages and found that he could see in the dark!

Soon he transformed himself into Dr. Mid-nite, a 1940s comic book hero who wore special goggles to see in the light. Armed with blackout bombs that released a pitch-black cloud in which only he could see, Dr. Mid-nite battled evil foes like the Baleful Banshee and the Sky-Raider. "I am blind, yet I can see," Dr. Mid-nite declared. "The city is draped in night, but to me it is always day. There are no dark corners for evil to hide in, no shadows too deep for the ever-vigilant eyes of Dr. Mid-nite to penetrate!"

But in the real world, midnight is hardly prime time for aging eyes. "There are plenty of reasons why virtually every 20-year-old wants to go on a road trip at night and virtually every 60-year-old doesn't," says Anne Sumers, M.D., ophthalmologist in Ridgewood, New Jersey, and a spokesperson for the American Academy of Ophthalmology. "First, as you age, your eyes need more light to work properly. Second, the lenses in your eyes aren't as clear at 60 as they were at 20. Third, as you get older, your pupils don't dilate as well as they used to. And in order to see well at night, your pupils have to get very large. So the overall result is that you have a lot more difficulty focusing on objects and seeing at night as you age."

While none of us will ever match the nocturnal prowess of the fictional Dr. Mid-nite, there are plenty of simple ways to bolster your night vision even at 60, 70, or 80. Here's how.

Lighten up. The average 60-year-old person needs seven times as much light as a 20-year-old to see well in the dark, according to the American Optometric Association. So brighten up the rooms of your home with 60- or 100-watt neodymium lightbulbs, suggests Bruce Rosenthal, O.D., professor and chief of low vision services at the State University of New York College of Optometry in New York City. These bulbs provide higher contrast and produce less glare than regular lightbulbs, so you should be able to see better at night. Neodymium bulbs are available at specialty lighting stores and from some mail-order catalog companies.

For walking in the dark, try using a portable camping lamp to illuminate where you are stepping, says Charles R. Fox, O.D., director of vision rehabilitation at the University of Maryland School of Medicine in Baltimore. Camping lamps, which are available at most sporting goods stores, are better than flashlights because they provide a wider arc of light and make it easier for you to get around, he says.

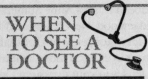

WHEN TO SEE A DOCTOR

Night vision problems could be a symptom of a serious underlying disease such as diabetes, macular degeneration, cataracts, or an inherited disease called retinitis pigmentosa, says Samuel L. Pallin, M.D., ophthalmologist and medical director of the Lear Eye Clinic in Sun City, Arizona. So see your optometrist or ophthalmologist if:

■ You have sudden or increasing difficulty seeing in dim light.

■ You're unable to see stars in the night sky that are visible to others.

■ You are limiting your activities because you're afraid to venture out after dark.

■ You have difficulty driving at night because of glare.

Bend and tilt. Adjustable floor or table lamps that swivel and bend so you can fine-tune the lighting to your needs can help overcome night vision problems, Dr. Rosenthal says.

If you are reading, for instance, adjust the lamp so that it's about 12 inches from the page yet not causing an annoying glare, Dr. Rosenthal suggests. Look for lamps with built-in reflectors that will help increase illumination.

See yourself seeing well. Imagery may help improve your night vision, says Robert-Michael Kaplan, O.D., author of *The Power behind Your Eyes*. Twice a day when natural light is dim—within two hours of sunrise and two hours of sunset—take a moment to close your eyes and move your head slowly to the left and then to the right. As you do this, take five to 10 deep breaths and visualize beams of light streaming into your eyes and activating the portions of your vision that are responsible for seeing well at night. This exercise can be done in less than two minutes a day.

Ease off the gas pedal. Many night vision problems aren't obvious until you get behind the wheel, says Gary Mancil, O.D., adjunct professor at Southern College of Optometry in Memphis.

On low beam, for instance, your headlights illuminate about 100 feet in front of your vehicle, says Steve Creel, California Highway Patrol public affairs officer. And at 65 mph, you're traveling about 100 feet per second. So at that speed, even if you had perfect vision and were driving in perfect conditions, your headlights wouldn't be much help. That's why it's important to slow down at night, particularly in poor weather. As a self-check, pick out an object in the distance and begin counting until you reach the object. A four- to six-second count is an indication that you are driving at a safe speed. If you reach that point in less than two seconds, you would not have been able to stop safely if that sign were in the middle of the road, Creel says. So ease up on the throttle.

"Just because the speed limit is 55 or 65 doesn't mean you have to go that fast. That might not be the safe speed for you, particularly if you have trouble seeing at night," Creel says.

See and be seen. Regularly clean all the lights on your car, especially your headlights, because at night these lights are the only way you can communicate with other drivers, Creel says.

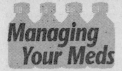

Managing Your Meds

Pilocarpine (Isopto Carpine, Pilocar), beta-adrenergic blocking agents (Betagan), and other medications used to treat glaucoma can cause temporary night vision problems for up to four hours after use, says W. Steven Pray, Ph.D., R.Ph., professor of nonprescription drug products at Southwestern Oklahoma State University in Weatherford. If this dimming of vision is bothersome, ask your doctor if you can switch to another medication that might not cause this side effect. Other drugs that can affect night vision include:

✦ Nasal and eyedrop steroids such as beclomethasone (Vancenase)

✦ Antidepressants containing trazodone (Desyrel), imipramine (Tofranil), or amitriptyline (Elavil)

✦ Antihistamines including over-the-counter products like doxylamine (Nyquil), diphenhydramine (Benadryl), and chlorpheniramine (Chlor-Trimeton)

"If you have night vision problems, you're probably driving slower than some other people on the road. So it's just as important to be seen," Creel says. "One good rule of thumb is if the portions of your windshield that aren't cleaned by your wipers are covered with gunk, it's time to clean all your lights."

Look for landmarks. Street signs are harder to read at night, so when traveling to someplace unfamiliar, get detailed directions that include lots of gas stations, grocery stores, and other landmarks, Dr.

Mancil suggests. Check out a reliable road map before you start out, and take the map with you. If you find yourself on darkened streets, you can always pull over, turn on the overhead light, and check the map.

Don't be a deer in the headlights. When you encounter oncoming traffic, look toward the right and follow the shoulder of the road until the other cars pass, Creel suggests. Diverting your eyes like this will reduce the blinding glare from the approaching headlights.

Break out the shades. Whenever you stop at a gas station, restaurant, or other well-lighted place, put on a pair of sunglasses before getting out of your car, Dr. Fox says. That way you'll have less trouble re-adapting to the darkness once you get back behind the wheel again. Of course, be sure to remove your shades before driving off.

Get a pair of night glasses. Sometimes, poor night vision is merely a sign of increasing nearsightedness, Dr. Sumers says. Ask your optometrist or ophthalmologist if a new pair of glasses that is specifically prescribed for nocturnal activities like driving will help you see better after sundown.

Slash the glare. Ask your vision-care specialist about getting an antireflective coating on your glasses, Dr. Rosenthal suggests. These coatings cut down on glare, increase the amount of available light coming into your eyes, and can improve your night vision.

Nosebleed

Whatever the cause—and there are about a dozen, from allergies to too much nasal spray—a nosebleed can be an alarming experience. In most cases, though, pride is injured more than your nose, since nosebleeds are seldom anything more than a nuisance. In fact, rarely is more than a tablespoon of blood ever shed. But here's how to stop the flow fast.

Gently blow your nose. A gentle honking of your honker can help clear out blood clots that could be preventing a blood vessel from sealing, says Louis D. Lowry, M.D., professor of otolaryngology at Thomas Jefferson University Hospital in Philadelphia.

Pretend you're about to jump into a pool. "Pinch your nostrils the same way you would if you were jumping into the water," recommends Leonard Rappaport, M.D., assistant professor of pediatrics at Harvard Medical School and a senior associate in medicine at Children's Hospital in Boston. "Then hold it that way for five minutes, breathing through your mouth. When you let go and resume nose breathing, *don't* blow your nose."

Stand tall. Sit up straight because lying back or putting your head back causes you to swallow blood, says Alvin Katz, M.D., an otolaryngologist and surgeon director at Manhattan Eye, Ear, Nose, and Throat Hospital in New York City.

Humidify your surroundings. Being in a heated room can dry out mucous membranes, making you more susceptible to nosebleeds. But humidifying your surroundings, especially in winter months, can keep moisture in your home—and your membranes, suggests Paul Edelson, M.D., chief of pediatric infectious diseases at The New York Hospital–Cornell Medical Center in New York City.

Take your vitamins. If you're prone to nosebleeds, consider boosting your iron and vitamin C intake. Iron helps your body rapidly replace the blood supply, says Gilbert Levitt, M.D., an otolaryngologist with the Group Health Cooperative of Puget Sound in Redmond, Washington.

Vitamin C, along with the B-complex vitamins, is necessary for the formation of collagen and free-

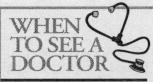

WHEN TO SEE A DOCTOR

If, after blowing out the clots and applying pressure, your nosebleed doesn't stop or slow down after 10 minutes, or if blood flow is severe, you probably need emergency care to help stop the bleeding, says John A. Henderson, M.D., assistant clinical professor of surgery/otolaryngology at the University of California, San Diego, School of Medicine.

If you feel blood running down the back of your throat after you pinch your nostrils, you need medical attention as soon as possible. It means you're losing blood, even if you stop the nosebleed in front, according to Dr. Henderson.

flowing mucus, creating a moist protective lining in your sinuses and nose, adds John A. Henderson, M.D., assistant clinical professor of surgery/otolaryngology at the University of California, San Diego, School of Medicine.

Numbness and Tingling

I magine a four-year-old girl who's sound asleep. Her left arm is contorted behind her neck. Her right hand is twisted into the small of her back. Her head is pinched up against her right shoulder, and her legs are crossed at the ankles.

Yet when she awakens, she won't feel numb. She'll have none of the tingling pins-and-needles sensations that many adults would experience. But give her time—say, 60 years—and her mangled nerves probably won't be so forgiving.

Numbness and tingling become more common as you get older for at least a couple of reasons, says Mark E. Williams, M.D., author of *The American Geriatrics Society's Complete Guide to Aging and Health* and director of the program on aging at the University of North Carolina at Chapel Hill School of Medicine. First,

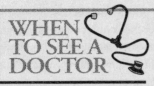

WHEN TO SEE A DOCTOR

Seek emergency treatment if you experience unexplained numbness or tingling or if it's accompanied by any of the following symptoms, which are all warning signs of an impending stroke.

- Blurred vision
- Confusion
- Difficulty speaking
- Loss of movement in your arms or legs
- Dizziness

your body's nerves are an intricate road map comprised of superhighways, side roads, and a maze of intricate paths. These tortured and tangled avenues lead through tiny tunnels between muscles, tendons, and microscopic holes in bone. As you age, many of these spaces shrink, compressing the nerves and making you more susceptible to numbness and tingling. In addition, many seniors tend to develop bone spurs (tiny, hard outgrowths on their bones) that press on nerves and aggravate them, says Dr. Williams.

If a minor problem like pressure on nerves is clearly causing your arm or leg to fall asleep, here's what you can do to wake it up and prevent it from happening again.

Fidget. Okay, so you don't have to be a Rhodes scholar to figure out that if a body part falls asleep, you need to reposition yourself so there is less pressure on

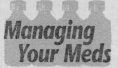

Managing Your Meds

Over-the-counter nasal decongestants such as Sudafed, Dimetapp, Contac, and other products containing phenylpropanolamine can cause tingling, says W. Steven Pray, Ph.D., R.Ph., professor of nonprescription drug products at Southwestern Oklahoma State University in Weatherford. Excessive amounts of vitamin B$_6$ also can cause numbness and tingling in some people. If you take B$_6$ supplements, the National Research Council recommends taking no more than 100 milligrams a day.

In addition, the following prescription medications also can make you feel numb.

✦ Chloroquine (Aralen), used to treat arthritis and lupus

✦ Auranofin (Ridaura), used to treat rheumatoid arthritis

✦ Nitrofurantoin (Macrodantin), used to treat kidney infections

✦ Isoniazid (Rifamate), used to treat tuberculosis

✦ Anticonvulsants such as phenytoin (Dilantin)

the pinched nerve. But what you may not know is how to prevent it from happening in the first place.

The key? Don't allow your arms, legs, and other vulnerable body parts to remain in one position for too long, says Linda Morrow, M.D., medical director of Alexian Brothers Senior Health Center in San Jose, California.

If you're watching television, for instance, take a few moments during each commercial break to uncross your legs, curl your toes, stretch your arms over your head, twirl your wrists, and slowly bend and unbend your fingers into your palms. This routine can prevent compressed nerves and lower your risk of numbness and tingling.

Move the wallet. If you have numbness in a leg, maybe you've been carrying a thick wallet in your back pocket, and its bulk is contributing to the problem, Dr. Williams says. Every time you sit down, that lump in your back pocket puts pressure on the sciatic nerve that runs along your buttocks and continues down the back of your leg. The solution? Find another way to carry your cash and credit cards.

Pop a multivitamin. A variety of vitamin and mineral deficiencies can cause nerve damage in older adults, Dr. Williams says. Take a multivitamin daily that includes zinc, chromium, folic acid, and vitamin B_{12} to help make up for any subtle deficiencies in your diet that may leave you vulnerable to numbness and tingling.

Quit smoking. Smoking reduces blood flow to your extremities and increases the likelihood that you'll feel numbness and tingling in your arms, hands, legs, and feet, Dr. Williams says.

Osteoporosis

As you age, your bones erode a bit. That's normal. But some people lose so much bone that their skeletons become riddled with weak spots. That's osteoporosis, and it causes a lot of hip, spine, and forearm fractures. At its worst, bones become so frail that they crack under the body's own weight!

Anyone can get osteoporosis, but women are more likely to get it than men. They have lighter bones than men, and they lose bone rapidly after menopause, because their bodies are producing less estrogen. But men aren't immune, especially if they drink heavily, smoke, or have taken steroid drugs.

But your bones don't have to crack under the strain of this disease. You can slow, stop, or even reverse bone loss. For women, medical treatment with estrogen-replacement therapy (ERT) is the most effective way to accomplish this. But even if you choose ERT, there are natural methods to help it along. (And not surprisingly, they're the same tips and techniques that can help *prevent* osteoporosis in the first place.)

If you want to step lively and stall bone loss, here are the tactics doctors recommend.

Build those bones. "We suggest, as a minimum, that people follow the American College of Sports Medicine recommendations to exercise aerobically for 20 minutes a day at least three days a week," says Miriam Nelson, Ph.D., an exercise physiologist and research scientist at the U.S. Department of Agriculture

(USDA) Human Nutrition Research Center on Aging at Tufts University in Boston. Exercise actually stimulates bones to lay down new tissue, she explains.

What's the best aerobic exercise for strong bones? "It's one you will continue doing, because if you don't do it *for life*, the bone-building benefits fade," explains Dr. Nelson. In her studies, walking won top ratings—20 minutes a day three or four times a week—but you may prefer running, biking, swimming, or aerobic dance classes.

Walk in water. If you've already had a fracture or two, your best choice of exercise may be walking in chest-deep water, working up to 30 minutes at least three times a week, suggests Sydney Lou Bonnick, M.D., director of Osteoporosis Services at the Cooper Clinic in Dallas. The water will help support your body weight and take stress off bones and joints.

Make your "exercise equipment" a chair and the floor. To complement water walking, do some easy muscle-strengthening exercises in a chair or on the floor, suggests Mehrsheed Sinaki, M.D., a physiatrist in the department of physical medicine and rehabilitation at the Mayo Clinic in Rochester, Minnesota. Such exercises can include abdominal curls, shoulder blade squeezes, and back extensions.

To do back extensions, lie on the floor on your stomach, with a pillow under your hips and your arms at your sides. Using only your back muscles, not your arms, raise your upper body a few inches off the floor. Hold for as long as comfortable, then relax downward. Work up to doing this six to 10 times a day.

Chow down on calcium. Doctors agree that you should try to get 1,000 milligrams a day of calcium, even if you haven't reached menopause. And

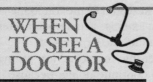

WHEN TO SEE A DOCTOR

To avoid becoming one of the women who first learn that they have osteoporosis while their doctors are setting their broken bones, have a DEXA (dual energy x-ray absorptiometry) scan now. This simple 15-minute test will measure your bone density and tell you whether you're at risk for osteoporosis. In general, you're especially at risk if you:

■ Are thin and small-boned

■ Have a history of eating disorders

■ Have family members with osteoporosis

■ Have generalized bone pain and tenderness

■ Take corticosteroids, anticonvulsants like phenytoin (Dilantin), thyroid medication, or blood thinners

---

they suggest 1,200 to 1,500 milligrams a day for post-menopausal women who are not getting ERT.

Most women consume far less than those amounts. Reaching 1,000 milligrams through diet alone means drinking a quart of skim milk a day or eating two cups of low-fat yogurt or four cups of low-fat cottage cheese.

"Figure out, realistically, how much calcium you can get through your diet, then make up the rest with supplements," says Bess Dawson-Hughes, M.D., chief of the Calcium and Bone Metabolism Laboratory at the USDA Human Nutrition Research Center on Aging at Tufts.

Aim for maximum absorption. Spread your calcium supplements out over the day rather than taking them all at once and take each one with a meal, Dr. Dawson-Hughes suggests. Most doctors recommend calcium carbonate, a relatively inexpensive source of calcium that's fairly well absorbed if taken in divided dosages and with meals.

Get enough vitamin D. For maximum protection, aim for 400 international units (IU) of vitamin D per day (twice the Recommended Dietary Allowance), especially if you don't get much sun, suggests Dr. Dawson-Hughes. "Here in Boston, we tell people they need a more reliable source of vitamin D than the sun, especially during the winter months."

A cup of milk contains about 100 IU of vitamin D, so four cups a day is ideal. But don't count on other dairy products, such as cheese, yogurt, or ice cream, to fulfill your vitamin D needs. Unlike milk, these foods are *not* fortified with vitamin D.

Do not exceed the recommended dosage of 400 IU, however. Vitamin D is toxic in high amounts.

Graze far and wide. Bones are not made from calcium alone. They're an amalgam that includes zinc, boron, and copper, among other minerals. "These trace elements are best gotten through a varied and broad-based diet that includes mostly unprocessed foods, such as whole grains, beans, fresh fruits and vegetables, fish and shellfish, and lean meats," Dr. Dawson-Hughes says.

If you smoke, stop. "Smoking accelerates bone loss," Dr. Dawson-Hughes says. It speeds the rate at which the body metabolizes estrogen, virtually canceling out the bone-beneficial effects of ERT. "And smoking must have other bone-rattling effects, too, because it causes bone loss in men and in post-menopausal women not taking estrogen," she adds.

Monitor your medications. Some drugs can hasten bone loss, says B. Lawrence Riggs, M.D., president of the National Osteoporosis Foundation and professor of medical research at the Mayo Clinic.

Those most likely to cause problems: corticosteroids, which are prescribed for a variety of conditions such as rheumatic disorders, allergic conditions, and respiratory disease; L-thyroxine, a thyroid medication; and furosemide, a diuretic often used against fluid retention associated with high blood pressure and kidney problems.

"Talk with your doctor about this possible side effect," Dr. Riggs suggests. "If you have other risk factors as well, your doctor may want to check your bone density and, if it's low, alter the dosage or stop the drug entirely."

Pass on the pop. Colas and some other carbonated soft drinks get their sharp taste from phosphoric acid, which contains phosphorus, a mineral that in excess amounts causes your body to excrete calcium.

Salt lightly. As with phosphorus, too much salt causes your body to excrete calcium. So go easy on the shaker and check food labels. Avoid products with more than 300 milligrams of salt per serving.

Paroxysmal Atrial Tachycardia

Huh?

That's right, paroxysmal atrial tachycardia. The name may escape you, but it's a condition that's estimated to affect as much as 40 percent of the U.S. population. And if you're among them, it's an experience you'll never forget: Your heart rate suddenly shoots upward to 220 beats a minute, and it feels like it won't slow down. You feel flushed and have body chills. You may also feel nauseated and dizzy and be almost overwhelmed by a sense of panic and doom.

Heart attack? It sure seems like it. But with paroxysmal atrial tachycardia, or PAT, there's no severe, vise-like physical pain in the chest. And another important difference: PAT is *not* fatal.

It's basically a temporary internal "electrical malfunction" that throws the heart's pacemaking system out of sync, causing instantaneous rapid heartbeat and the sudden release of adrenaline. Your heart goes into "high gear" for up to 30 minutes. (If an episode lasts longer, seek *immediate* medical treatment.) "It's the same sort of fight-or-flight reaction you experience if someone sneaks up behind you and yells 'Boo!'" says James Frackelton, M.D., president of the American Institute for Medical Preventics in Cleveland and a PAT researcher.

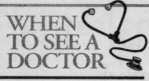

WHEN TO SEE A DOCTOR

Although heart attack and paroxysmal atrial tachycardia (PAT) have similar symptoms, *any time* you feel chest pain you should take it seriously—particularly if you haven't already been told by your doctor that you have PAT. If you have any of these symptoms, seek emergency care.

■ Intense chest pain that lasts 15 minutes or longer (this pain is often described as a feeling of heavy pressure)

■ Pain that could, but doesn't necessarily, extend to the *left* shoulder and arm, back, or jaw

■ Prolonged pain in the upper abdomen

■ Shortness of breath

■ Feeling faint or fainting

■ Nausea, vomiting, and intense sweating along with the pain

And it can be scarier than a Freddy Krueger movie. But this is no nightmare on Elm Street, health-wise. PAT causes no significant tissue damage to the heart—despite a heart rate *three times* that of a normal resting pulse.

Still, the fear of recurrent bouts can be emotionally devastating and may be an early sign that heart-healthy people are stressing their bodies. If you've been diagnosed with PAT, here's what you can do to keep it under control.

Take it easy. "If you can control the stress and anxiety in your life, you're drastically cutting your risk of suffering an attack," according to Michael Crawford, M.D., chief of cardiology at the University of New Mexico School of Medicine in Albuquerque and former chairman of the American Heart Association's council on clinical cardiology. Not surprisingly, PAT often strikes hard-driving, Type A personalities who are easily touched off. So if that's your style, try taking things a bit slower.

Kill that killer instinct. Even during R and R, PAT can strike—especially if you take your playing too seriously and are up against stiff competition. "People notice attacks during competitive exercise, like during a game of tennis, whereas they wouldn't be as likely to get one when running by themselves," says Dr. Crawford. "It's that added factor of psychological stress that makes the difference."

Pass on that second cup of joe. Caffeine can trigger an irregular heartbeat, so some experts suggest that those with PAT limit their daily caffeine intake to about two cups of coffee or tea, says Dr. Frackelton.

Limit the booze, too. "If you drink, even if it's an *occasional* binge, you may experience symptoms," says Dr. Crawford. "I recommend no more than two glasses of beer, wine, or mixed drinks at a time."

Take a cold shower. Cold water helps slow down the heartbeat when you're feeling stressed or having an attack.

Cut down on calcium. PAT, like some other forms of arrhythmia such as irregular heartbeat, is sometimes treated with calcium-blocking drugs. "The theory among preventive medicine specialists is that PAT can be triggered by excess calcium," adds Dr. Frackelton. "Eat less calcium and more magnesium and manganese, found in soy products, leafy vegetables, and nuts. I advise eating more fruits and vegetables, but eat twice as many vegetables as fruits."

Go easy on flour and sugar. "Both can spark the release of adrenaline, triggering an attack," says Dr. Frackelton.

Stock up on potassium. Potassium helps "flush" excess sodium and other harmful substances from the body. It's abundant in fruit juices, raisins, and sardines as well as in bananas and potatoes.

Phlebitis

It's a pain in the leg—or both legs. That's how it begins, anyway. And when the pain doesn't go away, you probably want to pick up the phone and call the doctor.

Well, that's exactly the right thing to do, because anyone with the warning signs of phlebitis needs to find out as soon as possible which *kind* of phlebitis he has. And only a doctor can tell you that.

Phlebitis (the full name is thrombophlebitis) is an inflammation or blood clot in a vein, usually in the leg. There are two kinds. Deep-vein thrombophlebitis is the risky variety. It affects the veins that are deep beneath the skin (that explains the name), and it can be fatal if a blood clot dislodges from the vein and travels to the lungs. So doctors recommend immediate action

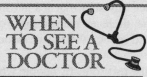

WHEN TO SEE A DOCTOR

If you have been diagnosed with superficial phlebitis, be sure to call your doctor if there's a sudden increase in pain or swelling, if you notice any lumps, or if you develop a fever, suggests Robert Ginsburg, M.D., director of the unit for cardiovascular intervention at the University Hospital in Denver and professor of medicine at the University of Colorado in Boulder.

Increased pain or swelling could be an indication of deep-vein thrombophlebitis, which requires immediate attention. Though it rarely happens, a blood clot could break loose and travel to the lungs. Prompt treatment may include hospitalization and medication with anticoagulants, prescribed drugs that prevent blood clots from forming.

Since fever may be a sign of infection, also see the doctor if you develop a higher-than-normal temperature. Infection can usually be cleared up promptly with antibiotics, but you'll need a physician's diagnosis and prescription.

if an exam turns up any warning signs of deep-vein phlebitis.

More often the problem is superficial thrombophlebitis, which means that you have some blockage in the superficial veins near the surface of the legs. Painful, yes—but not dangerous. Be ready to call the doctor again if you see any sign that it's getting worse. But in the meantime, there are many things you can do to ease the pain and reduce the worry associated with this problem.

The tips here should be used only by people who have been diagnosed with superficial phlebitis and are under a doctor's care. If that means you, here's what you can do to reduce your chances of another bout with pain, redness, tenderness, and itching in your legs.

Take a load off. "Superficial phlebitis can be treated by elevating the leg and applying warm, moist heat," suggests Michael D. Dake, M.D., chief of cardiovascular and interventional radiology at Stanford University Hospital in Stanford, California. Keep legs elevated 6 to 12 inches above the level of the heart and apply a heating pad to the affected area. In fact, it may help to keep your feet up all night long. You can elevate the foot of your bed several inches with wooden blocks.

Put the pressure on. Any kind of exercise, but especially walking, allows you to stay one step ahead of phlebitis. Muscular activity puts pressure on the veins, which helps empty them. Essentially, the walking motion helps prevent pooling of blood in the veins, says Robert Ginsburg, M.D., director of the unit for cardiovascular intervention at the University Hospital in Denver and professor of medicine at the University of Colorado in Boulder.

Pop some aspirin. Besides reducing pain and easing inflammation, aspirin has blood-thinning properties, so it may reduce phlebitis by preventing rapid clot formation. For best results, take aspirin before prolonged periods of bed rest or travel, which are the times when your circulation is most sluggish. And if

Massage Can Be Dangerous

If you have phlebitis, you might be tempted to "massage away" the pain when you have a flare-up. But that's not advisable unless you have explicit permission from your doctor, according to Robert Ginsburg, M.D., director of the unit for cardiovascular intervention at the University Hospital in Denver and professor of medicine at the University of Colorado in Boulder.

Massage can be dangerous for people who have superficial *or* deep-vein phlebitis, because you could dislodge a blood clot and cause a stroke or heart attack. So don't try hands-on healing without your doctor's blessing.

you're phlebitis-prone, your doctor may recommend aspirin before you have any kind of surgery.

But don't down the Pill. "If you've had a history of phlebitis or blood clots, you definitely shouldn't use oral contraceptives," says Jess R. Young, M.D., chairman of the department of vascular medicine at the Cleveland Clinic Foundation in Cleveland. (The incidence of *deep-vein* thrombophlebitis in oral contraceptive users is estimated to be three to four times higher than in nonusers.)

And don't smoke. Another no-no is cigarettes, which can also cause recurring phlebitis in a more complicated circulatory condition called Buerger's disease.

Think of zinc. If itching is a problem, a dab of zinc oxide in the bothersome areas can bring relief, according to Dr. Young. Zinc oxide is sold in most drugstores and doesn't require a prescription.

Sock it to yourself. Many phlebitis sufferers find

that it helps to wear support stockings (the same kind used to beat varicose veins). The rule of thumb: If the stockings ease the discomfort, wear them. However, wearing support hose won't *prevent* a recurrence of phlebitis if you've had it before.

Ease your air travel. "On airplanes, you tend to be confined to your seat a lot more than when traveling by car. So if you've had phlebitis, this is a case where you ought to put on your elastic stockings before boarding, then get out of your seat and walk up and down the aisle every half-hour or so after taking off," advises Dr. Young.

Plantar Warts

They're small, usually less than ¼ inch, but they can be larger. They're slow, often taking months to spread—or even be *noticed*. But plantar warts pack a painful punch.

Plantar warts are caused by a virus that invades the skin through a microscopic cut or abrasion on the sole of the foot. And then they grow inward—under the skin. The pressure of your weight flattens them until they are covered by a callus that sometimes has tiny black dots on the surface. As you walk around, the callus hardens under pressure, and the harder it gets, the worse it feels. When a plantar wart reaches maximum foot-torture stage, it feels as though you're stepping on a tack.

More bad news: Plantar warts are very difficult to

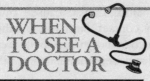

WHEN TO SEE A DOCTOR

Before you treat a wart, make sure that it *is* a wart—not a corn, callus, mole, or cancerous lesion. "Normally you'd think it would be pretty easy to identify a wart, but it's amazing how many people end up treating skin cancers or other growths as warts," observes Alvin Zelickson, M.D., clinical professor of dermatology at the University of Minnesota Medical School in Minneapolis.

So if you have the slightest doubt about what you're dealing with, see a doctor.

treat, because the virus often lies dormant for several months before it reappears. Your podiatrist may wind up having to burn it off with a laser, freeze it off with liquid nitrogen, or cut it off with his trusty scalpel. But first . . . try these do-it-yourself treatments when trouble's afoot.

Give it the corn treatment. "You can use commercial corn remover preparations," says Stephen Weinberg, D.P.M., a podiatrist who specializes in sports medicine at Columbus Hospital in Chicago. The acid in the corn remover irritates the wart and causes it to go into remission. Look for a product, such as Duofilm, that contains salicylic acid.

Avoid them with cleanliness. "Practicing good hygiene is probably the best way to avoid getting plantar warts in the first place," says Robert Diamond, D.P.M., a Pennsylvania podiatrist affiliated with Muhlenberg Hospital Center in Bethlehem and St. Luke's

Hospital of Allentown. "Since they're caused by a virus, they are passed by contact. So if you're using public showers or walking barefoot in any public area, wash your feet afterward and wear thongs."

Poor Concentration

More than 10,000 random thoughts and fleeting images zip through an average person's mind every day. They could include a snippet of a song, a momentary image of an old friend, or a fragment of a joke.

In most cases, these intruders are quickly banished from your mind so you can concentrate on the task at hand. But as you get older, it becomes harder to filter out these distractions and stick to a project, organize your thoughts, or follow the flow of a conversation, says Richard Restak, M.D., clinical professor of neurology at George Washington University School of Medicine and Health Sciences in Washington, D.C., and co-author of *The Longevity Strategy: How to Live to 100 Using the Brain-Body Connection*. Poor concentration also can affect your memory. So if you're doing the laundry, for instance, you may forget all

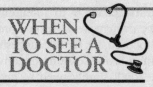

WHEN TO SEE A DOCTOR

Seek medical care if you or others around you notice a significant drop in your attention span or your ability to concentrate, says Richard Restak, M.D., clinical professor of neurology at George Washington University School of Medicine and Health Sciences in Washington, D.C., and co-author of *The Longevity Strategy*. If you find yourself losing track of the subplot in a novel or if you discover that filing your income tax suddenly takes you twice as long, don't simply assume that your mind is failing you. A number of correctable medical problems could be interfering with your ability to concentrate, including:

- Hearing loss
- Vision changes
- Poor blood circulation
- Thyroid diseases
- Severe depression

about a boiling tea kettle in the kitchen until the smoke alarm goes off.

"It's just a natural part of aging," Dr. Restak says. "As you get older, it may take more effort to concentrate on complicated tasks like reading. It doesn't mean you can't do it, you just have to develop some new strategies." Here are a few ideas.

Work in short bursts. Take a 5- to 10-minute rest every 30 minutes when you're working on a project. It will help you stay focused, Dr. Restak suggests. "As we get older, marathon work sessions become more difficult," he says. You'll simply need to take more frequent breaks in order to maintain good concentration.

Do first things first. Do one thing at a time. You're more likely to get distracted if you try to do several things at once, says Michael Chafetz, Ph.D., clinical psychologist in New Orleans and author of *Smart for Life*.

Keep your eye on the prize. Resist the temptation to get distracted. If you're paying bills, for instance, and need to go into another room to get some stamps, do that and immediately go back to your bill paying. If you do find yourself getting distracted while hunting down the stamps, pause, take a deep breath, and ask yourself, "What am I really here for?" Doing that will refocus your attention on what you really need to get done, Dr. Chafetz says. Otherwise, you may still be cleaning out your desk when the post office closes.

Zzzone out. Try to get at least six to eight hours of sleep daily, suggests Laura Slap-Shelton, Ph.D., clinical psychologist with a specialty in neuropsychology at Jeanes Hospital in Philadelphia. When you're tired, you'll have more trouble concentrating. Taking a brief nap in the middle of the day helps some people keep their minds focused on necessary chores and tasks.

Quiet your mind. Meditation is a simple and terrific way to boost your powers of concentration, Dr. Slap-Shelton says. "The mind is a noisy place, talking to itself and responding to all sorts of stimulation in the world around it," she says. "Meditation quiets the

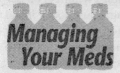
Managing Your Meds

Any medication that causes drowsiness can dampen concentration, says W. Steven Pray, Ph.D., R.Ph., professor of nonprescription drug products at Southwestern Oklahoma State University in Weatherford. In particular, be wary of:

♦ Over-the-counter sleeping tablets that contain diphenhydramine (Nytol, Unisom)

♦ Over-the-counter antihistamines with diphenhydramine (Actifed, Benadryl)

♦ Antipsychotic medications such as risperidone (Risperdal) or haloperidol (Haldol)

♦ Tranquilizers like hydroxyzine (Atarax, Vistaril)

♦ Antidepressants such as imipramine (Tofranil)

♦ Antianxiety medications like diazepam (Valium), chlordiazepoxide (Librium), and other drugs known as benzodiazepines

---

mind and can help filter out all the annoying distractions that make concentration difficult."

To try it, sit in a comfortable chair and begin to slowly breathe in for a count of four to eight seconds, allowing your diaphragm to expand fully, Dr. Slap-Shelton says. Hold your breath for several seconds, and then slowly breathe out as much air as you can. To see if you are breathing from your diaphragm, you can rest your hand on your stomach and feel it expand and contract as you practice your breathing. Whenever a distracting thought pops into your mind, just notice it and let it go, and keep your attention on your breathing. If you do this simple exercise twice a day, your ability to concentrate may improve, Dr. Slap-Shelton says.

Light a candle. Guided imagery can help focus your mind, says Elizabeth Ann Barrett, Ph.D., R.N., professor and coordinator of the Center for Nursing Research at Hunter College of the City College of New York in New York City. To try it, close your eyes and breathe out through your mouth and in through your nose. Breathe out long, slow exhalations and breathe in normally, but with shorter inhalations than exhalations. Notice that you are beginning to relax. Breathe in a feeling of confidence that you can improve your concentration and breathe out the fear that you will be distracted.

Now imagine that you are lighting a candle. Focus on the flame and notice that any distracting thoughts cause the flame to flicker, Dr. Barrett says. Concentrate on seeing the flame burn brightly without flickering. Dismiss all distracting thoughts that create flickering. Each time you see a flicker, return to the steadiness of the flame. Notice how you can keep the flame burning brighter for a longer and longer time with fewer and fewer flickers. Keep watching the flame burning brightly. When you feel ready, open your eyes.

Do this exercise three times a day (morning, noon, and evening) for 21 days, Dr. Barrett suggests. After 21 days, the maximum effectiveness through one episode of repetition is over. Take a break to mark that one cycle is over. After 7 days, begin again. Ideally, this 21-day cycle of guided imagery will become habit-forming.

Clean out the attic. Store just a few bits of information in your head, Dr. Chafetz suggests. The more information you try to keep in your brain, the more distracting thoughts you'll have and the harder it will be to concentrate. So if you haven't done so before, start writing down phone numbers, birthdays, and other facts that you don't need every day.

Play mind games. Give your brain a good workout with chess, checkers, crossword puzzles, or board games like Scrabble at least twice a week, Dr. Chafetz says. These fun, mind-stretching activities can help keep your concentration in tip-top shape.

Prostate Problems

Four of every five men over age 50 develop an enlarged prostate—or, more specifically, a condition called benign prostatic hyperplasia (BPH). One-fourth to one-third of them will experience BPH's uncomfortable and potentially dangerous symptoms.

"BPH causes no pain, but it does make urination more difficult," says Stephen Rous, M.D., professor of surgery at Dartmouth Medical School and a urologist at Dartmouth-Hitchcock Medical Center in Lebanon, New Hampshire. Because the prostate surrounds the urethra, the tube that carries urine from the bladder, it restricts urine flow when it enlarges. This results in a need to urinate more frequently, often with increased difficulty getting started.

With prostate problems, you may also experience

dribbling, because the prostate isn't as strong as it used to be, and you can't urinate with the same force. Some men with this problem are unable to sleep through the night without waking to urinate, while others are completely unable to urinate—an emergency condition.

Surgery to remove the prostate is one alternative, and there are several medications—some of which take months to work—that can reduce an enlarged prostate and improve urination. But for tried-and-true home treatments, here's what the experts recommend.

Cut the caffeine. "Caffeine in any form—coffee, tea, chocolate, or soft drinks—tends to tighten the bladder neck and make it more difficult to pass urine," says urologist Durwood Neal Jr., M.D., associate professor of surgery, urology, microbiology, and internal medicine at the University of Texas Medical Branch at Galveston. "Some of the prostate is made up of smooth muscle, and anything that causes that muscle to constrict will make urination more difficult. Caffeine does this quite a bit."

Don't serve yourself. Alcohol also tightens the bladder neck to hamper urination. And since it's a diuretic, it increases the amount of urine that builds up inside the bladder, adds Dr. Neal. "Drinking alcohol also makes the bladder operate a lot less efficiently. And the more you drink, the more problems you'll likely have."

Give a cold shoulder to cold medicines. Antihistamines and decongestants can cause even more harm to some men. In fact, taking large doses of cold medications occasionally leads to urinary retention—a potentially life-threatening condition in which you completely stop urinating. "Decongestants cause the muscle at the bladder neck to constrict, restricting the

342

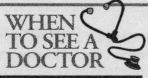

WHEN TO SEE A DOCTOR

An enlarged prostate may cause difficulty urinating, but you shouldn't experience pain. "The only prostate condition that leads to pain or discomfort is prostatitis, a bacterial infection that is treated with antibiotics," says Stephen Rous, M.D., professor of surgery at Dartmouth Medical School and a urologist at Dartmouth-Hitchcock Medical Center in Lebanon, New Hampshire. If you experience painful urination, coupled with lower back pain, fever, and pelvic pain, you may have a prostate or bladder infection. See your doctor.

Of course, it's wise for *all* men over age 50 to see their doctors to be tested for prostate cancer, a leading cancer among middle-aged and older men. And if you can't urinate at all, head straight to the emergency room: Urinary retention is extremely uncomfortable and can be life-threatening if left untreated.

flow of urine," says Peter Nieh, M.D., a urologist at the Lahey Clinic Medical Center in Burlington, Massachusetts. "And antihistamines simply paralyze the bladder."

If you have allergies as well as prostate problems, Dr. Nieh suggests you speak to your doctor about prescribing astemizole (Hismanal) or terfenadine (Seldane), two medications that have no antihistamines. If you must buy over-the-counter medication, take half of the suggested dose. If no problem ensues, move to the full recommended dosage.

Be wary of spicy foods. Spicy and acidic foods bother some men with enlarged prostates, says Dr. Neal. "If you notice more problems after eating salsa, chili, or other spicy or acidic foods, then you're among those men—and you should avoid that cuisine."

Manage your stress. Perhaps the most underrated trigger is unmanaged stress. "Stress plays a major role in prostate-related discomfort, because the bladder neck and prostate are both very rich with nerves that respond to adrenal hormones," says Dr. Neal. "When you're under stress, there are more of those hormones floating around—causing more difficulty in urinating."

Stress also triggers the release of adrenaline in your body, prompting a fight-or-flight response. "Just as it's impossible to get an erection during the fight-or-flight response, it can make urination difficult, too," Dr. Neal adds.

Get more amour. One way urologists help ease urination problems is to massage the prostate. For men with mild to moderate voiding difficulties, an alternative may simply be to have more sex. "Many men notice that the more they ejaculate, the easier it is to urinate," says Dr. Rous. That's because ejaculation helps empty the prostate of secretions that may hamper urination.

Empty your bladder before you go to bed. "Many men get the urge to urinate in the middle of the night, and it can be a real problem," says Dr. Neal. "But if you limit your intake of beverages after 6:00 P.M. and make sure you urinate before going to sleep, you can eliminate much of this problem."

Flee south in the winter. If at all possible, spend winters somewhere in the Sunbelt. "In the urology trade, we usually say that summer is the season to pass kidney stones and winter is the time for urinary problems. I'm not exactly sure why, but people have more trouble urinating and are most likely to go into urinary retention during cold weather. Perhaps this is due to an increase in upper respiratory infections, which many men treat with over-the-counter antihistamines and decongestants. These further aggravate BPH," says Harold Fuselier, M.D., chairman of urology at Ochsner Medical Institutions in New Orleans. "Since an enlarged prostate already makes urinating more difficult, you'll do much better in a warm climate during cold weather."

Psoriasis

If there ever was a medical condition that could convince Sherlock Holmes to get out of the business, it's psoriasis. The clues are obvious—after all, it's hard *not* to notice that maddening itch, the inflammation, and those bothersome silvery scales that usually occur on the elbows, knees, trunk, and scalp. But when it comes to finding its cause or cure, that's even more of a mystery than Watson's first name.

What *is* known about psoriasis is that it causes skin cells to go hyper. A normal skin cell takes about a month to mature, but in those with psoriasis, this process takes only three or four days. These skin cells are poorly developed, and they can't shed fast enough. Instead, they pile up—forming raised, scaly "plaques" that itch and leave skin below red and inflamed.

Psoriasis *isn't* contagious, but beyond that, researchers can't speak about the condition's causes with any degree of certainty. There may be a genetic link, however. In one in three cases, the disorder can be traced through the family, although it sometimes skips a generation. Also, doctors have observed that stress can spark new outbreaks (or make existing cases worse). Other suspected triggers include damage to the skin from injury, dryness or chafing, and reaction to certain drugs and infections (such as strep throat).

But instead of the proverbial heartbreak, there is reason to take heart. While there's no cure as yet, you can control psoriasis and lessen its impact on your life. Your doctor has probably told you about tar shampoos and ultraviolet light treatments, but here are some other ways to keep those plaques from giving you flak.

Look for lactic. All our experts agree that the most important step in controlling psoriasis is to keep skin well-moisturized. "A big problem with psoriasis is scale buildup, and moisturizers are extremely effective at preventing this," says Nicholas J. Lowe, M.D., clinical professor of dermatology at the University of California, Los Angeles, School of Medicine and director of the Skin Research Foundation of California in Santa Monica. "Plain petroleum jelly is a very effective moisturizer. But if you're buying a commercial moisturizer, those that contain lactic acid, such as LactiCare, seem to work better. Also Eucerin cream works well as a moisturizer for those with psoriasis."

Moisturize after bathing. To get the most from your moisturizer, "apply it within three minutes after leaving the shower or bathtub," advises Glennis Mc-Neal, public information director at the National Psoriasis Foundation, headquartered in Portland, Oregon. "We recommend that you pat yourself dry and apply the moisturizer liberally all over your body—*not* just on plaques. That's because even 'clear' skin in people with psoriasis is drier than in people who don't have psoriasis. It's thought that little cracks on dry skin might encourage more psoriasis."

Soak up the sun. Many psoriasis patients are prescribed a specific regimen of ultraviolet light treatments. Getting artificial sunlight from a special lamp or tanning booth can help. An easier and less expensive method is simply to hit the Great Outdoors. "We know that exposure to sunlight is extremely helpful for treating psoriasis," says David Kalin, M.D., a family practitioner in Largo, Florida. A moderate amount of sunlight enhances the production of vitamin D, which may be effective in controlling psoriasis.

But don't soak up the booze. Doctors are still trying to find out for sure why alcohol exacerbates psoriasis. They suspect that alcohol increases activity of a certain kind of white blood cell that's found in psoriasis patients but not in other people. (But it's also possible that drinkers are just more highly stressed—and therefore more prone to psoriasis.)

"Alcohol is a definite problem," according to Stephen M. Purcell, D.O., chairman of the department of dermatology at Philadelphia College of Osteopathic Medicine and assistant clinical professor at Hahnemann University School of Medicine in Philadelphia. "It's best to not drink at all if you have psoriasis."

Spice up your bath. Bathing is often a catch-22 for those with psoriasis. That's because soaking in warm water helps soften psoriasis plaques, but it sometimes dries skin and worsens itching. "One way to get the benefits of a bath without the dryness is to add a couple of capfuls of vegetable oil to your bath," says McNeal. "The best way to do it is to get in the tub first, so your body soaks up the water, and then add the oil." Another alternative suggested by McNeal: Mix two teaspoons of olive oil in a large glass of milk and add that to your bath.

Be extra careful stepping out of the tub, since oils can make surfaces very slippery. (Be sure to scrub the tub afterward.)

Head to the kitchen to soothe that itchin'. To soothe itching caused by dry skin and psoriasis, dissolve ⅓ cup of baking soda in a gallon of water. Soak a washcloth in the solution, wring it out, and then it apply to the itchy area. Or add a cup of apple cider vinegar to the water and apply that to the skin.

Cover the cracks with cow cream. If your skin is cracked because of psoriasis—which can cause itching and more plaques—do what dairymen do. "They found that Bag Balm, a product originally used to relieve cracking in cow udders, worked just as well on their cracked hands," says McNeal. "Then people with psoriasis found it worked *great* on their dry or cracked skin." Bag Balm is available at most feed stores; some drugstores may have it or be able to order it.

Take care of mind and body. Stress is a known trigger of psoriasis, so managing your mental state— through exercise, relaxation techniques, or whatever mellows you out—is one way to keep your condition under control.

Guard against infection and injury. "Infection may lead to an outbreak or worsen your condition, so it's important to try to avoid infectious disease," says Dr. Kalin. New lesions may also appear on injured skin, so try to avoid cuts and scrapes.

Watch what you eat. "Although there are no specific links that have been proven, it appears a diet high in oily fish—such as tuna, mackerel, sardines, and salmon—helps reduce the itching and inflammation of psoriasis," says Dr. Lowe.

Avoid certain foods. "Some anecdotal reports suggest patients do better when they reduce or eliminate tomatoes and tomato-based dishes—possibly because of high acidity levels," says Dr. Kalin. "Also, some of my patients with psoriasis have noticed a decrease in plaques by avoiding or limiting their intake of pork products and other fatty meats as well as caffeine."

Go electric. If you have plaques on your face, neck, legs, or other areas that require shaving, use an electric razor instead of a blade. "An electric razor won't cut skin as easily, and every time you cut yourself, you risk new lesions," says dermatologist John F. Romano, M.D., clinical assistant professor of dermatology at New York Hospital–Cornell Medical Center in New York City.

Reading Problems

S ince you're reading the words on this page, you have the vision power that it takes, and maybe you can zip along just as fast as you did when you were in your twenties or thirties. But many of us have to slow down. And after a while, almost without noticing, reading becomes more of a problem.

It helps to accept the fact that your eyesight is less than it was—and, therefore, reading adjustments have to be made. "Your ability to focus deteriorates in a straight line from birth to death, but most people don't notice until their forties," says Joseph Kubacki, M.D., professor and chairman of the ophthalmology department and assistant dean for medical affairs at Temple University School of Medicine in Philadelphia.

You can do a number of things to make your reading environment as easy on your eyes as possible, whether you're reading for pleasure, using your computer, or searching for signs and labels. Here are some ideas.

Get a bright light. Aging eyes need more light on the page, which means that the light needs to be brighter, says Pamela R. Oliver, O.D., director of the low-vision rehabilitative service at the Eye Institute at Nova Southeastern University and chairwoman of the low-vision subcommittee of the Florida Optometric Association in Fort Lauderdale, Florida.

The amount of light needed depends on the type of lightbulb as well as on the wattage of the bulb. If you've been using 60-watt bulbs, you might want to

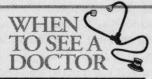

WHEN TO SEE A DOCTOR

Since a whole host of eye diseases could cause reading problems—from cataracts to macular degeneration to glaucoma—you should see an eye doctor any time you notice a change in vision. Also, try to get a checkup eye exam every one to two years.

continue to use the same wattage but select a different kind of bulb, suggests Eleanor E. Faye, M.D., ophthalmologic consultant to Lighthouse International, a vision rehabilitation organization, and ophthalmologist in New York City. Instead of buying "soft white" or similar bulbs that are for general lighting, look for the bulbs that are "indoor floodlights." Such bulbs don't use more electricity, but they provide double the illumination, explains Dr. Faye.

Play with positioning. You'll get the most benefit from a bright light if it's positioned so it shines directly on your page. And the closer the light is to what you're reading, the easier it will be for you to see, says Dr. Oliver. Place your reading light over and behind your shoulder to eliminate shadows, she suggests. Then angle it so it shines directly onto your reading material.

Buy large print. The larger the print, the easier it is to read. You can get large-print versions of many books, ranging from cookbooks, dictionaries, and the Bible to the latest romance novel. For large-print versions, contact the following organizations: American Bible Society, New York City; American Printing House for the Blind, Louisville, Kentucky; Doubleday Large-Print Home Library, Indianapolis; G. K. Hall and Company, Unity, Maine; and the National Association for Visually Handicapped, New York City.

Get help from cutouts. If you need to read line by line to follow the text, you can make a simple focusing device, suggests Dr. Faye. Cut a thin rectangle in a piece of black construction paper or cardboard. The rectangle should be just as wide and tall as a single line of type. As you're reading, place this paper over the page, allowing just one line of text to show, moving it down line by line as you read.

Raise your computer font. Font refers to the type size. Every word processing program has easy ways to make the font larger or smaller on the screen. If you use the computer frequently and would like larger-size type on the screen, check your manual or call the toll-free number listed in your manual to find out how to increase the font size. You'll have an easier time reading electronic mail or using a word processing program if you make the font size at least 13 or 14, says Dr. Faye.

Consider a screen change. See if you can change the colors on the computer screen. For easiest reading, choose a black background with yellow or white letters, advises Dr. Faye.

Wear tinted glasses. When you're trying to read food packages at grocery stores or road signs as you travel, lightly tinted lenses can eliminate some of the irritating glare, suggests Dr. Faye. These glasses are especially helpful if you have cataracts or another eye condition that makes sign-reading difficult. For the grocery store, choose light amber- or yellow-tinted lenses. For the outdoors, you want polarized gray- or amber-tinted lenses, Dr. Faye says.

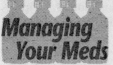

Managing Your Meds

Chances are, your reading problem is not related to any medications you're taking. The following medications, however, may cause blurred vision, which can make reading difficult. It is important to keep in mind that most vision changes are transient, says W. Steven Pray, Ph.D., R.Ph., professor of nonprescription drug products at Southwestern Oklahoma State University in Weatherford.

✦ Antiarthritis medications such as acetaminophen (Tylenol)

✦ Anti-inflammatory medications such as ibuprofen (Advil)

✦ Antidepressants such as amitriptyline (Elavil)

✦ Ophthalmic drugs used to dilate the pupil of the eye, such as pilocarpine (Isopto Carpine)

✦ Antibacterial treatment for the eye, such as ciprofloxacin (Cipro)

✦ Cortisone-like drugs such as prednisone (Deltasone)

✦ Medicines that treat severe psoriasis, such as etretinate (Tegison)

✦ Antibiotics used to treat eye infections, such as norfloxacin (Chibroxin)

✦ Anticonvulsants such as phenytoin (Dilantin)

Use a big black pen. Whenever you write a note to yourself—a phone number, address, recipe—use a black marker that makes a thick line. Dr. Faye recommends Sharpies, which are available at most hardware and art supply stores.

Mark your medications. Do you have trouble reading the labels on medicine bottles? That can be risky because you can easily get your pills mixed up if you can't make out the small print on the labels. To avoid confusion, mark the bottles clearly with a black marker like a Sharpie, suggests Dr. Faye. For instance, put "BP" on blood pressure medication and "HR" on hormone replacement pills.

Rectal Itching

O kay, so it doesn't warrant the same awe-inspiring stories as that knee injury you got when you made the winning touchdown in the Big Game or that shrapnel you took while saving everyone in your platoon during the war. "So, Bob, there I was on this important job interview when, all of a sudden, I got the most uncontrollable, embarrassing itch. . . ."

While rectal itching may be the butt of many locker room jokes, it isn't at all funny. In fact, it takes real endurance to put up with the aggravation. But here's how you can reduce the discomfort—or banish it.

De-yeast it with yogurt. "Many times, rectal itching is caused by a yeast infection, and when that's the case, applying plain, unflavored yogurt will do the trick," says Jerome Z. Litt, M.D., assistant clinical professor of dermatology at Case Western Reserve University School of Medicine in Cleveland. "Yogurt with active cultures has bacteria that compete with the growth of yeast; the bacteria literally kill the yeast. The best way to apply it is to sit in a tray of yogurt for about an hour, but you can also apply it with a handkerchief. It's very soothing."

Sit in sitz. "People with hemorrhoids often have rectal itch because they can't clean the area as effectively, and that soil is what causes the itch," says D'Anne Kleinsmith, M.D., a cosmetic dermatologist at William Beaumont Hospital in Royal Oak, Michigan. "Taking sitz baths, or just taking a lot of baths in general, helps stop the itch."

Cast that witch hazel spell. Witch hazel, applied with a cotton ball or hanky, provides cool relief for some. An application also helps dry out the infected area, adds Dr. Kleinsmith. (Medicated pads such as Tucks are also recommended.)

Use a drugstore-bought cleanser. "A product called Balneol, available at your local drugstore, is very good," says Dr. Kleinsmith. "It's very mild and should be used after you go to the bathroom."

Restless Legs Syndrome

Elizabeth Tunison struggles to sit still as she talks on the telephone in her Whittier, California, home. "I'm massaging my right leg with my right hand right now. It helps relax my leg muscles a bit and keeps me still for a few moments," she says. "But I'm eventually going to have to get up and move. I can't help it. My legs just don't know how to stop."

Tunison, a retired college professor in her seventies, is one of the estimated 3 percent of Americans—many of them over 60—who have restless legs syndrome (RLS), a condition that causes odd sensations of creeping, crawling, or tingling in the legs. For many, walking provides the only relief. They don't have to walk far to rid themselves of the sensation. A stroll down the hallway or around the living room may be enough. But they often must do it over and over again. Because it usually worsens while lying down, people who have this syndrome seldom sleep well.

Restless legs syndrome typically starts at the onset of sleep, says Wayne Hening, M.D., Ph.D., research neurologist at the University of Medicine and Dentistry at Rutgers University in New Brunswick, New Jersey, and member of the Restless Legs Foundation's medical advisory board. In severe cases, it may be impossible to sleep. Even more unusual are in-

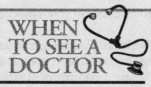

WHEN TO SEE A DOCTOR

See your doctor if:

■ You have frequent "crawling" or other types of discomfort in your legs, occurring typically in the evening.

■ You feel an overwhelming urge to move your legs or body to relieve the sensations.

■ You find that the symptoms get worse in the late afternoon and keep you awake until the wee hours of the morning.

■ You notice that the symptoms worsen when you sit or lie down.

stances where the movements are noticeable enough to wake a person. Typically, the "wiggles" will subside within minutes.

Doctors aren't certain what causes RLS, but it may have a genetic link since the condition tends to run in families, says Ralph Pascualy, M.D., medical director of the Sleep Disorders Center at Providence Medical Center in Seattle. Some researchers also suspect that RLS may be caused by low levels of dopamine, a neurotransmitter in the brain that helps regulate the body's nervous system. In fact, doctors have discovered that drugs like levodopa (Larodopa) and dopamine substitutes like pergolide mesylate (Permax), which are used to treat Parkinson's disease (also linked to low dopamine levels), can relieve RLS. Pain medications, sedatives, and certain drugs for high blood pressure also can dampen the symptoms. In addition, these natural remedies can help you handcuff this sleep thief.

Maintain a regular bedtime. Fatigue aggravates RLS, says Dr. Hening. Getting all of the shut-eye you can is important, particularly if you have a mild case of RLS that only flares up once or twice a month. Hit the sack at the same time each evening, he suggests. Even if you have to get up several times during the night to stretch your legs, a consistent bedtime should help you get an adequate amount of sleep. After all, adds Dr. Hening, a regular bedtime is known to generally promote better sleep, and clinical experience has shown that waiting for fatigue to set in before going to bed may actually worsen the condition.

Splish and splash. Sitting in a warm bath or hot tub for 10 to 15 minutes just before bedtime sometimes helps relieve RLS, Dr. Hening says. If you have difficulty getting into a tub, stand in a shower and let the warm water gently pour over your back and legs.

Sleep in. If necessary, sleep late, suggests Virginia N. Wilson, co-founder of the Restless Legs Syndrome Foundation and author of *Sleep Thief, Restless Legs Syndrome*, a guide to coping with RLS. Because RLS is usually worse at night, many people who have it don't get to sleep until 3:00 or 4:00 A.M. So avoid early-morning appointments because, odds are, you'll be groggy and irritable, she says. Wilson, for instance, usually sleeps until at least 10:00 A.M. and rarely schedules any activities before noon.

Zone out. Some people report that engaging in mentally absorbing games and activities like building jigsaw puzzles or solving logic problems stifles their attacks of RLS, Dr. Hening says. If you find an engaging hobby that requires intense concentration, it may help you control this condition, he says.

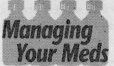
Managing Your Meds

Any drug that reduces or blocks activity of the brain chemical dopamine, responsible for the transmission of nerve impulses, can worsen the symptoms of restless legs syndrome, says Wayne Hening, M.D., Ph.D., research neurologist at the University of Medicine and Dentistry at Rutgers University in New Brunswick, New Jersey, and member of the Restless Legs Foundation's medical advisory board. In particular, be wary of prescription neuroleptic tranquilizers including haloperidol (Haldol) and chlorpromazine (Thorazine). In addition, avoid:

✦ Alcohol

✦ Caffeine

✦ Prescription antinausea drugs containing metoclopramide (Reglan)

✦ Prescription tricyclic antidepressants such as amitriptylene (Elavil)

Find an aisle land. Ask for an aisle seat in the back of the theater when you attend a play or concert, Wilson suggests. If your legs begin to bother you, you will be able to stand up and walk around without blocking the view of other patrons.

Likewise, ask for an aisle seat when making airplane reservations. Try booking a flight that has one or two stops before your destination, so you can get off the plane and stretch your legs for a few minutes during each layover, Wilson says.

Dr. Hening advises scheduling a morning flight, when discomfort is less likely. He also suggests asking your doctor if medication will help.

Sciatica

If you've ever run a vacuum, cared for children, or tossed a few baseballs in the school yard, you've probably experienced a lower-back ache or two. Most people do.

But sometimes, lower-back pain isn't confined to the spine. It radiates, producing shooting pain or numbness into your buttocks and down your leg, below your knee, even into your foot and toes. When it does, you may be experiencing sciatica.

Sciatica is no respecter of circumstances, which is why its onset usually comes as a complete surprise. Maybe you've been weeding in the garden. As you rise to your feet, you suddenly feel as though someone has shot darts at your leg. Or perhaps you've been relaxing for an evening in your favorite reading chair with a cup of tea in one hand and a new novel in the other. But when you get up to refill that teacup, your lower-back pinches and your foot feels tingly. Either scenario portrays the beginnings of sciatica.

If you have sciatica, your symptoms are caused by irritation of the nerve that runs across your buttocks and into your thigh, calf, and foot, says John E.

Thomassy, D.C., chiropractor in private practice in Virginia Beach, Virginia.

Sometimes, the rubbery disks between the back bones, or vertebrae, bulge and then press on a nerve root. This bulge may be referred to as a herniated, or slipped, disk. Poor posture, improper technique when lifting, and injuries may be contributing factors in this condition.

Over time, the disks experience more wear and tear. So by the time you reach retirement age, they're eager for some kid-glove treatment. As wear and tear catches up with you during your senior citizen years, the disks become compressed, vertebrae grow bony

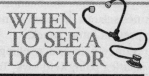

WHEN TO SEE A DOCTOR

If you have shooting pains down your legs, don't just assume that you have sciatica, says Steven Mandel, M.D., clinical professor of neurology at Thomas Jefferson University Hospital in Philadelphia. Any time back pain is accompanied by radiating, burning, or tingling, see your doctor. Several conditions can cause that kind of pain, including stroke, diabetes, and vitamin B_{12} deficiency. It could even be caused by osteoarthritis, which afflicts more of us as we get older. Or you may have a fracture caused by osteoporosis (thinning bones). Since there are so many possible explanations, it's best to let a doctor determine what the problem is, says Dr. Mandel.

spurs, and nerve irritation becomes more likely, explains Dr. Thomassy.

The discomfort may be worse when you sit, and the pain in your leg or knee may be more severe than the one in your back, says Steven Mandel, M.D., clinical professor of neurology at Thomas Jefferson University Hospital in Philadelphia.

Forty percent of people will experience sciatica some time in their lives. For most, the pain will subside on its own, often within one month, says Dr. Mandel.

As a rule, anytime you have back pain for more than two to three days, you should see your doctor to rule out serious illness or injury, suggests Sheila Reid, therapy coordinator at the Spine Institute of New England in Williston, Vermont. But once your doctor rules out other things and positively identifies sciatica, here are some ways to find relief and help prevent future attacks.

Get a chill. To help reduce pain and swelling, apply ice where you feel sciatica pain, Reid says. To protect your skin, place a towel between your back and the ice pack. Ice may be used for 15 to 20 minutes every hour. Or switch to the warmth of a heating pad, shower, or bath, she says. Heat relaxes muscles.

Please sit up. Prolonged sitting may aggravate your discomfort because it reverses the normal curve in your back, Dr. Thomassy says. Sitting may compress disks and weaken lower-back ligaments and muscles. When you sit, maintain good posture. Don't slouch. Keep your knees level with your hips, your feet flat on the floor, and your back straight.

Get the angles right. If you are working at a desk or computer, adjust your chair so your elbows can be positioned at a 90° angle, with your forearms parallel to the floor, advises Dr. Thomassy. Tuck a small

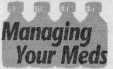

Managing Your Meds

Although it's very rare, one drug may cause sciatica, says W. Steven Pray, Ph.D., R.Ph., professor of nonprescription drug products at Southwestern Oklahoma State University in Weatherford. Talk with your doctor or pharmacist if you experience sciatic pain while taking Zolpidem (Ambien), which is prescribed for insomnia.

To help with your sciatica pain, your doctor may recommend that you take acetaminophen (Tylenol), aspirin, or nonsteroidal anti-inflammatory drugs (NSAIDs) such as ibuprofen (Advil). These types of medicines may interact with other drugs. Make sure to tell your doctor about any drugs that you are taking.

pillow behind your back to help you sit up straight and promote the normal curves in your spine.

Break things up. Take frequent breaks when you're working, Reid says. Get up and walk around every half-hour. If you're traveling in a car, avoid prolonged time behind the wheel or even in the passenger seat. Make frequent rest stops at least every hour or so.

Reach over the counter. Nonprescription pain relievers such as acetaminophen (Tylenol), ibuprofen (Advil), or naproxen (Aleve) may help relieve temporary discomfort, Dr. Mandel says. But be sure to ask your physician first. Even over-the-counter medicines can have side effects.

Step right down. Wear comfortable, low-heeled shoes, Dr. Thomassy urges. Heels that are higher than

1 to 1½ inches push your body weight forward and your spine out of alignment.

Get some Z. Try the Z position, suggests Augustus A. White III, M.D., professor of orthopaedics surgery at Harvard Medical School, in the booklet "Back Care: How to Relieve and Prevent Pain from Low Back Problems."

Lie on your back on a rug or exercise cushion with your knees bent and your feet propped on a low table or chair. Your thighs should be nearly parallel to the floor. To get more comfortable, put a thin cushion under your buttocks and a pillow under your head. Then relax.

This relaxing position often provides quick relief, writes Dr. White.

Stretch it out. For sciatica pain, try this stretch from Dr. White. Stand with your feet apart and your hands on your buttocks. Push your hips forward and gently bend backward while looking up. Keep your knees straight. Hold for several seconds, relax, and repeat. You can do this several times a day, and it's especially helpful after sitting.

Lift safely. Even if your back feels better after an episode of back pain, you'll need to lift correctly to prevent a relapse. "Lifting is when most people are injured," Dr. Thomassy says. Whether you're lifting a laundry basket or toolbox, make sure your feet are square to the object, then crouch with your knees and hips bent and your back straight. Bring the object close to your body and when you rise, continue to keep your back straight. If you have to twist, bend forward, or reach out for an object, take the time to get into the proper position before you try lifting. If that's not possible, get help.

Sleep sideways. If you want to minimize or stave off back pain and sciatica, don't sleep on your stomach, Dr. Thomassy cautions. Instead, lie on your side, curl your legs, and slip a pillow between your knees. Or go belly-up with a pillow or rolled towel under your knees. If you like to sleep with a pillow under your head, don't strain your neck with a big one. Instead, use a smaller one that keeps your head and neck in line with your upper back.

Get around. Stay as active as you can while you're recovering from sciatica, even if you only walk around the house, Reid says.

After pain subsides, try gentle stretches and, later, mild aerobic exercise, Dr. Mandel suggests. Swimming and walking, for example, will help strengthen and condition your back and whole body. They may even make you less vulnerable to injury. "If people stretch and exercise," Dr. Mandel says, "they will reduce their chances of having back problems."

Seasonal Affective Disorder

For most people, the old "winter blues" simply mean that we feel a little run-down and melancholy in the season when we should be jolly. But for those who experience seasonal affective disorder (SAD) at its most extreme, the blues hit harder than a flat ote on a slide trombone. "We're talking about a condition that may compromise your life so seriously that you can't work or cope with your family, something that leaves you so lethargic that you can barely get out of bed," says George Brainard, Ph.D., associate professor of neurology and pharmacology at Jefferson Medical College of Thomas Jefferson University in Philadelphia and a researcher on the benefits of light therapy for SAD.

Research is being done on the causes of SAD, with no definite conclusions as yet, according to Norman E. Rosenthal, M.D., chief of environmental psychiatry at the National Institute of Mental Health in

Lighten Up Your Mood

A surefire way to lighten up winter depression caused by seasonal affective disorder (SAD) is to undergo at-home therapy with a special lighting fixture. The most common type is known as a light box. This is a square fixture, usually a little larger than a briefcase, that stands upright on a desk or table. Other devices for treating SAD are configured as workstations, head-mounted visors, or dawn simulators. Prices range from $200 to $500.

What's so special about a light box? "It's not so much that there's a magic bulb that works," explains SAD light therapy researcher George Brainard, Ph.D., associate professor of neurology and pharmacology at Jefferson Medical College of Thomas Jefferson University in Philadelphia. "What's more important is the *dosage* emitted and the fact that it's emitted at *eye level*." The dosage is about five to 10 times that of

Bethesda, Maryland, and a pioneer in SAD research. Even though the mechanism is not known, however, most doctors are in agreement that light therapy definitely helps those who have SAD.

Symptoms of SAD may include a tendency to overeat, oversleep, and even become disinterested in sex. But it doesn't have to get that far. Here's what to do to beat a major case of the blues.

Go with the glow. Although the *best* treatment for SAD is daily light therapy using a specially designed "light box," exposure to any type of bright light may help some people. "Flooding the room with bright,

---

normal indoor lighting, and according to Dr. Brainard, you have to look repeatedly at the light; just having it fall on your skin isn't enough.

"The general prescription is two hours a day at 2,500 lux—a unit of light intensity," according to Dr. Brainard. He recommends that you set the light box in a position so that you can glance for a few seconds directly into the light. Glance at the light box about once a minute over the two hours. "Alternatively, some people use a 10,000-lux box for 30 minutes a day," says Dr. Brainard.

But before you plunk down your money, one last piece of advice: "First see a qualified physician or therapist and make sure you are diagnosed with SAD," says Dr. Brainard. "These lights won't work if you're just depressed; they'll only work if you have SAD." Your health professional can also advise you about reputable mail-order companies that sell light boxes.

but not harsh, light actually helps some people," says Maria Simonson, Ph.D., Sc.D., professor emeritus and director of the Health, Weight, and Stress Program at Johns Hopkins Medical Institutions in Baltimore. A word of caution: *Staring* into bright light emitted from lamps and overhead fixtures may harm your eyes, so don't stare at a bulb as a substitute for the light box.

Head for the Great Outdoors. The days are shorter in the winter, but you can still take advantage of what little sunlight there is. "*Any* exposure to sunlight will help," says Henry Lahmeyer, M.D., professor of psychiatry and behavioral sciences at Northwestern University Medical School and co-director of the Sleep Program at Northwestern Memorial Hospital, both in Chicago. "You should try to spend about an hour outdoors every day—even on days when it's not particularly bright and sunny."

Stroll in the dawn. "Research in Switzerland found that SAD patients who took an outdoor 30-minute walk at sunrise showed a lot of improvement," says Dr. Brainard. "We're not sure whether it's the exercise, the sunlight, or even the cold that invigorates them, but whatever it is, it seems to help."

Use your yoga. "Our research seems to indicate that some of the specific meditations in yoga may act on the pineal gland (which controls circadian and seasonal rhythms)," says Eric Leskowitz, M.D., a psychiatrist and SAD researcher at Spaulding Rehabilitation Hospital in Boston. "Yoga also provides a general energizing effect and offers great stress release. I think practicing yoga is a great way to start off the day if you have SAD."

Take milk for all its worth. A form of vitamin D called soltriol that's found in milk may help keep us in sync with the sun, according to the theory based on a study by Walter E. Stumpf, M.D., Ph.D., a researcher at the University of North Carolina in Chapel Hill. The theory is that soltriol may trigger the release of "stimulating" hormones that keep our body clocks on track.

Keep consistent sleeping habits. "Having a regular sleep schedule and sticking to it is very helpful to all people, including those with SAD," says Alex Clerk, M.D., director of the Sleep Disorders Clinic at Stanford University in Stanford, California. "The tendency is to sleep more with winter SAD, but your body doesn't need more sleep. You'll be much better off keeping a consistent sleeping schedule."

Shingles

If you had chicken pox as a child, you probably thought the virus that caused that itchy, blistering rash was gone for good. While it's true that you won't get chicken pox again, you may get its relative: herpes zoster, or shingles.

The virus that causes both chicken pox and shingles hides in the nervous system of anyone who's had chicken pox, which is the majority of American adults. About 20 percent of us also will get shingles later in life. When that happens, the virus awakens with a vengeance, producing an oozing, blistering, short-lived rash and pain that can linger for months or years, long after the skin itself heals, says Karl R. Beutner, M.D., Ph.D., associate clinical professor and researcher in the department of dermatology at the University of California, San Francisco.

It is not known what causes the virus to reawaken. Stress, poor nutrition, and another illness may be triggers. "Attacks tend to occur during times of great stress," says Richard P. Huemer, M.D., holistic practitioner in Lancaster, California.

As the years roll by, your chances of shingles roll upward. Shingles is most common in people over 50, and about half of people over 80 will get the illness.

This condition is a trickster. The burning and stabbing pain often precedes the rash by one to three days, so many people don't realize the two are connected, Dr. Beutner says. Other early symptoms may

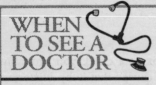

WHEN TO SEE A DOCTOR

If you think you have shingles, you really need to see a doctor, says Karl R. Beutner, M.D., Ph.D., associate clinical professor and researcher in the department of dermatology at the University of California, San Francisco. Your doctor can determine if you have it by assessing the nature of your pain and the appearance of any rash. He can also give you an antiviral medicine that may reduce the length of your outbreak. The medicine is most potent if given early on, often before that telltale rash appears, Dr. Beutner says.

include tingling, extreme sensitivity, or a dull ache on one side of the body, usually the trunk, buttock, or thigh. You may have fever, headache, or other flulike symptoms. If you have these symptoms, see a doctor right away. With a prompt diagnosis, you have the advantage of an opportunity for early treatment.

The rash occurs in the same area as the pain and quickly turns into pus-filled blisters that look much like the chicken pox you tried so hard to forget. The blisters themselves aren't painful, Dr. Beutner says. Although they may occasionally scar the skin, the blisters crust over and fade in about two to three weeks.

The pain, which emanates from nerve bundles, may not fade nearly as fast. In people over 60, symptoms may be more pronounced or prolonged. What's more, the pain can be severe enough to disrupt sleep and daily activities.

If you have symptoms of shingles, you need to see a doctor. But while you're at home, here are some additional ways you can keep discomfort at bay or even prevent shingles from paying you an unwelcome visit.

Stay dry. You can't do a lot to get rid of the shingles rash; it must run its course. But you can help dry the oozing blisters, Dr. Beutner says. Apply calamine lotion or use Burrow's solution made from Domeboro tablets, both available in drugstores. As the wet solutions evaporate from your skin, they also steal moisture from the blisters.

Say "aloe-ahhh." The thin milky liquid inside the leaves of the aloe vera plant may help soothe the blisters, Dr. Huemer says. If you have an aloe houseplant, cut a leaf and smooth the liquid over your skin. Or try an over-the-counter aloe lotion.

Get into a lather. Wash your hands regularly, Dr. Beutner says, especially if you have an oozing rash

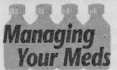

Managing Your Meds

Oral corticosteroids such as prednisone (Deltasone), taken for certain types of arthritis, allergies, and skin conditions, may weaken the immune system, causing shingles to appear, says W. Steven Pray, Ph.D., R.Ph., professor of nonprescription drug products at Southwestern Oklahoma State University in Weatherford. Also, using a nonprescription topical steroid such as hydrocortisone (Cortaid) on an area of skin affected by shingles could cause the lesions to spread further and last longer.

from shingles. The blisters contain varicella virus, so you could unknowingly infect someone with chicken pox. You also can cover the blisters with an antibiotic ointment, such as Polysporin, and wrap the area with gauze.

Pull the reins on pain. With your physician's okay, reach for acetaminophen (Tylenol) or another mild over-the-counter pain reliever such as ibuprofen (Advil), Dr. Beutner says. Your doctor can prescribe stronger medicine for more serious discomfort.

Pack some heat. If your pain remains after the rash, you can smooth a capsaicin cream on the affected area three or four times a day, Dr. Beutner says. But be sure you have no more rash. Capsaicin cream is made from the extract of hot pepper. "On an open rash, it really hurts," he says. Capsaicin cream usually begins to work within two to four weeks, but it must be applied three or four times a day, every day. If the product is not used in this way, pain may recur in a few days or weeks. When you first apply capsaicin cream, you may feel a burning sensation on your skin, which should subside within a few weeks.

Take care of you. Because stress is a factor in developing shingles, relaxation is important. "Pace yourself," Dr. Beutner says. Stop and put your feet up or take an afternoon nap, especially if you don't feel well. "People should listen to their bodies and rest when they feel tired," he says.

Since the pain of shingles can interrupt your normal night's sleep, try to make up for lost rest at other times during the day, Dr. Beutner says. Getting plenty of rest will keep you healthier overall and may help you mend more quickly.

Eat to your health. "Probably the best prevention is a healthy lifestyle and immune system," Dr. Huemer says. Poor nutrition contributes to weakened immunity. The American Dietetic Association recommends eating at least five servings of vegetables and fruits daily, along with an array of whole grains, dairy products, lean meats and fish, and small amounts of fat.

Look to lysine. Your diet also should include an amino acid called lysine, says Dr. Huemer. This amino acid, which prevents viruses from growing and spreading, may bring your bout with shingles to a quicker end. You can boost your lysine intake by drinking milk and eating potatoes and chicken. They are good sources of lysine, Dr. Huemer says.

It's hard to get enough lysine to prevent shingles outbreaks through diet alone. Luckily, lysine also is sold at stores. Take 500 to 1,000 milligrams three times a day during an outbreak, Dr. Huemer says. For prevention, use 1,000 milligrams a day.

Do Bs and more Bs. Vitamin B_{12} can boost your immune system and help you fight a shingles outbreak,

Dr. Huemer says. A daily 500-microgram sublingual lozenge, which melts under your tongue, probably is worth trying, he says.

Bring in some big doses. For super immunity during an outbreak, Dr. Huemer recommends a daily regimen of:

♦ 10,000 international units (IU) vitamin A

♦ 10,000 milligrams vitamin C

♦ 800 IU vitamin E

♦ 50 milligrams B complex

♦ 100 to 200 milligrams pantothenic acid

♦ 25,000 IU beta-carotene

♦ 200 micrograms selenium

♦ 60 milligrams coenzyme Q_{10}

♦ 25 milligrams zinc

Since most of these doses are way over the Daily Values for these nutrients, and supplements may cause problems at these high levels, these supplement levels should be monitored by a doctor. High doses of vitamin C, for example, can cause diarrhea in some people. Also, although vitamin E is generally sold in doses of 400 IU, one small study showed a possible risk of stroke in dosages higher than 200 IU. Consult with your doctor if you are at high risk for stroke.

See something completely different. When you're in pain, it's easy to wonder if it will ever go away, says Emmett Miller, M.D., mind-body specialist and author in Nevada City, California. That can make your perception of the pain worse, he says. Dr. Miller teaches patients to use visualization to see and feel their pain differently.

First, take a deep breath and let yourself relax as you slowly release it. Close your eyes and allow an image that represents your pain to arise in your mind. Is it hot or cold? Is it moving? What color is it? Perhaps you see a twisting red-hot poker, Dr. Miller says.

Now, create a parallel image of something that would remove that object's harmful quality—and put it to use. You might picture a fire hose extinguishing the hot poker or an Eskimo with a bucket of snow, Dr. Miller says. If you can learn to transform your mental image of pain, he says, you may feel less affected by it physically.

Shoulder Pain

Even Atlas got a break every now and then from carrying the weight of the world on his shoulders—and you can bet he didn't use his free time painting the kitchen ceiling or trying to relive his youth on a tennis court.

But you? If you're like the majority of Americans these days, you have so many responsibilities to juggle that it's a wonder Ringling Brothers hasn't offered you a job. But all that stress and strain is no clowning matter: It can give you high-powered shoulder pain as a main-ring event. Along with your knees, your shoulders are the most used joints in your body—and are commonly abused and injured.

Most shoulder pain usually results from one of two causes: Muscles and tendons may be injured from prolonged overuse, as can happen when you paint or garden for too long. Or they can get pinched between bones or ligaments, a process called impingement that frequently results from activities that require power strokes or throwing, such as swimming, tennis, or softball. Whatever the cause, you may get symptoms that involve a steady aching pain, with intermittent bursts of sharper pain when you're in certain positions.

Moderating or stopping the offending activity—at least for a while—is the first step on the road to recovery. But in addition, here are some other ways to ease shoulder pain and help prevent a recurrence.

Exercise after your workout. "Shoulder pain often results from repetitive motion—whether it's caused by your job or by playing a sport such as tennis or softball," says Robert Stephens, Ph.D., chairman of the department of anatomy and director of sports medicine at the University of Health Sciences College of Osteopathic Medicine in Kansas City, Missouri. "One of the best ways to remedy this problem, and help prevent it in the future, is to perform full range-of-motion stretching and strengthening exercises to compensate for these repetitive movements. For instance, if you have shoulder pain after playing tennis, perform some gentle stretching exercises such as rotating your arm inward and outward and doing slow, full arm circles (like the backstroke and crawl stroke) in both directions.

"Stretching the muscles associated with the movement that's causing you the pain may help pre-

Try to Find the Cause

All shoulder pain might hurt like the dickens, but not all the pain comes from the same source. To determine the probable cause of your problem, sports medicine specialist Charles Norelli, M.D., staff physiatrist at Good Shepherd Rehabilitation Hospital in Allentown, Pennsylvania, suggests you try these exercises.

■ Hold your arm out and twist your wrist as though you were emptying a soda can, then raise your arm. If this causes pain, your problem is probably tendinitis.

■ If the pain is in your right shoulder, grab your right elbow with your left hand and pull it across your body. If this causes pain, that might be a signal that something in the bone or muscle is getting in the way. This problem may be remedied with specific range-of-motion exercises and light weight lifting.

Dr. Norelli points out that any severe shoulder pain requires professional medical attention. Heart attack pain, for example, can sometimes be transferred to the shoulder. While these quick "diagnostics" can give you a clue in many cases, if the pain is severe, be sure to see your doctor for a more thorough examination.

vent muscle imbalances and ease the tension on the joints," says Dr. Stephens.

Use heat, but don't rely on it. Applying heat to a sore shoulder will help ease your pain, but it won't cure it.

"A heating pad is to shoulder pain what a microwave oven is to a bad sandwich: The sandwich tastes better warm, but if you let it cool down again, it'll taste just as bad as it did before you warmed it," says sports medicine specialist Charles Norelli, M.D., staff physiatrist at Good Shepherd Rehabilitation Hospital in Allentown, Pennsylvania. "In other words, you'll feel better while you have heat on your shoulder, but unless you fix the problem, you'll feel just as bad once you remove the heat."

Hoist some barbells. How do you "fix" shoulder pain? Besides practicing full range-of-motion exercises, lifting weights often helps, adds Dr. Norelli. "You want to strengthen rotator cuff muscles (behind the shoulder), and lifting weights is the best way to do that," he says. "Take a two- to six-pound barbell and lift it sideways, keeping your arm straight and your thumb pointing up. It's important to keep your thumb pointing up, because if it points down, you could be impinging your tendon."

Wear a muffler. If you notice more shoulder pain in the winter, then Mother Nature might be more to blame than an active lifestyle.

"A lot of times, people get shoulder pain because they're breathing cold air. The pain they feel is really referred pain from the lungs taking in freezing air," says A. J. Hahn, D.C., a chiropractor in Napoleon, Ohio, who specializes in natural remedies. "The answer is to wear a muffler or scarf during the cold months."

Slowed Reaction Time

Her slap shot doesn't zing off the stick anymore. She can't skate as fast as she once did. But Mickey Walker, a woman in her eighties, is still in the game. She believes that age is only a number and that seniors should think young and stay active. "We don't have to get old," she says.

"I've been playing hockey since the 1920s, and I'm still a good enough skater and stick handler to play recreational hockey every Monday night with people half my age and younger," says Walker, the oldest registered female hockey player in Canada. "I just love this game."

In a game that requires quick feet, quick thinking, and quick reactions, she is still swift enough to play—and win. "My reflexes are still real fast, and hockey has helped keep them that way," says Walker, who plays center for Mickey's Mares of Bala, Ontario. "I can take a deck of cards, put the edge of the cards over the edge of a table, tip them up, and catch them in mid-air. That's how fast my reflexes still are."

Okay, Mickey Walker is an extraordinary woman. But her nimbleness is well within the reach of all of us, says Charles Richman, Ph.D., professor of psychology and director of the martial arts program at Wake Forest University in Winston-Salem, North Carolina.

Granted, Mickey has maintained her physical and

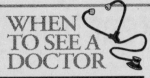

WHEN TO SEE A DOCTOR

Seek immediate medical care if you notice that one side of your body is reacting much more slowly than the other, says Harry Jaffe, M.D., professor of internal medicine at Northwestern University Medical School in Chicago. It may be a warning sign of a stroke.

In addition, consult your doctor if:

■ You are suddenly more clumsy or accident-prone.

■ You have a sudden onset of headaches that are unlike any that you've had in the past.

■ You have sudden hearing loss in one ear, which might indicate wax that has plugged the canal, an infection, or a more serious condition.

---

mental abilities through an inordinate amount of practice and exercise. "But I presume that anyone can do that. We all have the capability to slow down the processes that diminish reaction time as we age," Dr. Richman says.

In a sense, almost everything we do is a reaction. If you feel cold, you grab a blanket. If you see a pot boiling over, you instinctively reach for it. But as you age, your sensory organs—eyes, ears, nose, mouth, and skin—that help your brain stay in touch with the outside world all gradually wear down. Eyesight dims, hearing fades, smells and tastes become less distinct, and your sense of touch becomes less refined.

Meanwhile, the nerves that relay this sensory information to your brain and activate your muscles to get you moving become less efficient. As a result, it takes you longer to gather and process information about the world around you and then react to it, says Augustine DiGiovanna, Ph.D., author of *Human Aging: Biological Perspectives* and professor of biology at Salisbury State University in Maryland.

Even when we're in peak condition, reaction time slows about 6 percent every 10 years, starting at about age 30, Dr. Richman says. So by the time you get to age 80, even if you are in terrific health like Mickey Walker, you've lost about 30 percent of your ability to react quickly.

"As we get older, we become less competitive and stop doing the very things—like exercising and eating well—that would help us maintain good reaction time," Dr. Richman says. "We become grandmothers and grandfathers. The problem is that we assume our time is over. We sit back and allow whatever happens to happen. We shouldn't. We are still able to make things happen."

But even grandparents can have better than average reaction times for their ages, says Harry Jaffe, M.D., professor of internal medicine at Northwestern University Medical School in Chicago. Here are a few ways to keep your reflexes in tip-top condition.

Keep your motor running. Swimming, walking, stretching, and other forms of exercise are probably the best ways to slash your reaction time, Dr. Jaffe says.

"The better conditioned you are, the better your muscles are going to work, and the better your reaction time will be," Dr. Jaffe says. "It's hard to ask a muscle to do something quickly if you've been sitting in a chair for 15 years."

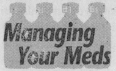

Managing Your Meds

Avoid using sleeping pills, tranquilizers, and excessive amounts of alcohol. They can dangerously slow your reaction time in a crisis, says Gisele Wolf-Klein, M.D., chief of geriatric medicine at Long Island Jewish Medical Center in New Hyde Park, New York.

It's particularly vital for seniors to avoid these numbing influences. When your body is older, you don't metabolize drugs the way you did when you were younger, so they linger longer in your body, slowing down your reflexes. In fact, the effects of a drug like diazepam (Valium) can linger for up to three days after an older person takes it, Dr. Wolf-Klein says.

If you drink, limit yourself to one 12-ounce beer, one 4-ounce glass of wine, or a 1-ounce shot of liquor a day, she advises.

He recommends doing a physical activity you enjoy—like ballroom dancing or gardening—for at least 20 minutes a day, three times a week.

Visit the pyramid. Nerve and muscle cells work better and react faster if you eat a well-balanced diet, Dr. Jaffe says. The U.S. Department of Agriculture's Food Guide Pyramid recommends 6 to 11 servings of grains, rice, and pasta, 3 to 5 servings of vegetables, 2 to 4 servings of fruit, 2 to 3 servings of milk and other dairy products, and 2 to 3 servings of meat or fish daily.

See the sights, hear the crowd. Hearing and vision problems account for up to 80 percent of problems with reaction time, Dr. Jaffe says. So get your eyesight and hearing checked at least once a year after age 60.

Bridge the gap. Chess, jigsaw puzzles, and other

challenging mind games not only keep your brain alert but may shave your reaction time, says Gisele Wolf-Klein, M.D., chief of geriatric medicine at Long Island Jewish Medical Center in New Hyde Park, New York.

"Even card games like bridge can help because you have to think quickly, you have to add quickly, and you have to move quickly to play," Dr. Wolf-Klein says.

Jack be nimble. Playing jacks, Ping-Pong, and other games involving hand-eye coordination can improve your reflexes, too, says Jim Buskirk, licensed physical therapist at Balance Centers of America in Chicago.

Play ball. Just playing paddleball for one to two minutes twice a day can help speed your reaction time, Buskirk says.

You also could cut out a variety of letters, small shapes, and colored pieces of paper and tape them to a wall. Then bounce the ball off the wall. As you do this, spot and call out one or more of the colors, shapes, or letters before you catch it, Buskirk suggests.

Earn a belt. Martial arts are a terrific way for seniors to improve their reflexes, Dr. Richman says. These ancient Eastern techniques build muscle strength, improve flexibility and concentration, and force you to react quickly.

"One of my tae kwon do instructors is 67 years old, and his reaction time is great. It's not as good as some of the young football players in his class, but he certainly has better reflexes than most 40-year-olds," Dr. Richman says.

If you are over age 60, Dr. Richman recommends that you try tai chi, aikido, kung fu, or any other low-impact martial arts that focus on developing fluid, dancelike movements. Check your phone directory to locate a martial arts school near you.

Slow Healing

If it seems as if your latest injury is taking a long time to heal, don't despair. With a few changes in diet and lifestyle, you can strengthen your healing forces and speed your recovery.

It's true, however, that your body's wounds are slower to heal when you're old than they were when you first bled in life's battles. "That's why it's so important for seniors to take good care of themselves, especially with their nutrition and activity levels," says Larry Millikan, M.D., chairman of the department of dermatology at Tulane University School of Medicine in New Orleans.

There are several reasons for this slowdown in healing. In women, hormones are a factor. Research has shown that women do not heal as rapidly after they pass through menopause and stop producing estrogen at their premenopausal levels. When women take estrogen replacement therapy (ERT) after menopause, they tend to heal at a faster rate—and that change can be attributed to the increase in estrogen. For men, the slowdown in healing is more often the result of chronically poor health and diabetes—and these are large factors for some women as well.

Once you have adequately cleaned and cared for your wound or injury, there are several things you can do to speed healing and recovery. If you're looking for a good place to begin boosting your wound-healing power, start with the dining room table.

Heal with your meals. Even though you may not be as active or have as much appetite as you used to, your body still needs a regular supply of nutritious foods if it's going to be able to stay healthy and make speedy repairs. "All too often, seniors eat only one meal a day. Let's say it's dinner, but they've skipped breakfast and had a candy bar for lunch. That's going to weaken their immune systems and slow down their healing," says Dr. Millikan. Try instead to eat three nutritious meals a day.

Put in the protein. Your body requires about 45 grams of protein a day to repair damaged tissues. A three-ounce serving (about the size of a deck of cards) of fish, chicken, or turkey or a serving of cheese will provide about 21 grams of protein. A cup of milk will

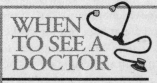

WHEN TO SEE A DOCTOR

Some injuries take longer to mend than others. If a simple cut takes longer than a week to heal or if the cut becomes red and swollen, though, see your doctor, says Larry Millikan, M.D., chairman of the department of dermatology at Tulane University School of Medicine in New Orleans. Slow healing is often the sign of some other problem—a cold, an infection, or some more serious ailment—that is interfering with your body's ability to heal quickly and properly. If your doctor can identify the real problem, there's a good chance he can correct that and speed your healing along.

give you 8 grams of protein, and a half-cup of beans will provide about 7 grams.

Boost immunity with antioxidants. Vitamins C and E as well as beta-carotene (a vitamin A precursor) are all antioxidants, which means they're particularly beneficial in boosting your immune system, helping to fight infection, and promoting more rapid healing, says Frederic Haberman, M.D., assistant clinical professor of medicine (dermatology) at Albert Einstein College of Medicine in New York City and director of the Haberman Dermatology Institute in Ridgewood, New Jersey.

"I tell people to take 500 to 1,000 milligrams of vitamin C, about 400 international units (IU) of E, and up to 2,000 IU of vitamin A after surgery," Dr. Haberman says. "They should also take about 70 micrograms of selenium." Although vitamin E is generally sold in doses of 400 IU, one small study showed a possible risk of stroke in dosages higher than 200 IU. Consult with your doctor if you are at high risk for stroke.

Be zealous about zinc. When it comes to wounds, the mineral zinc has strong healing power, according to Eleanor Young, R.D., Ph.D., a licensed dietitian and professor in the department of medicine at the University of Texas Health Sciences Center in San Antonio.

Dr. Haberman recommends 15 milligrams of zinc per day. You can get it in supplement form, and it's also in foods like steamed oysters and most meat dishes.

Make multis part of a healthy diet. Take a multivitamin and mineral supplement, such as Centrum, says Dr. Millikan.

"The supplement provides the antioxidants and minerals they need to promote a stronger immune response," says Dr. Haberman.

Go for aloe. Buy an aloe plant to keep on the shelf as a houseplant, suggests Dr. Millikan. The next time you cut yourself, break off a leaf, split it lengthwise, and use the juice to speed healing. "Many of my patients firmly believe that this is a great help," he says. Research has shown that aloe can penetrate and numb tissue, prevent the growth of harmful bacteria, fungi, and virus, reduce swelling, and improve blood flow.

Walk your wounds off. People who exercise regularly tend to heal more rapidly and are more likely to have stronger immune systems. "The key is good blood circulation," says Dr. Millikan. As long as your tissues get enough blood, they're also getting adequate oxygen, nutrients, and immune cells—all the ingredients they need in order to heal. "On the other hand, people who have circulatory disorders tend to heal more slowly and can suffer from more infections," Dr. Millikan observes. One circulation problem that can slow healing is atherosclerosis, or hardening of the arteries, a condition that impedes blood flow. Another is diabetes—the inability to incorporate blood sugar, which leaves body cells deprived of nutrition and wounds more susceptible to infection.

For most seniors, the best exercise is walking, says Dr. Millikan. "You shouldn't adopt an exercise program, even walking, without first consulting your doctor to see how much exercise you can do safely. Once your doctor gives you the okay, walking is an ideal way to promote circulation and more rapid healing."

Stiff Neck

Maybe it's just to remind us that our lives are full of stress. Or it could be a punishment for sleeping with the windows open on a cool autumn night. Or because we didn't fix the shocks on the car. Now we have to pay the price in aches and pains.

Sometimes, the proverbial pain in the neck does have a physical basis. Stress—physical or otherwise—tenses the muscles in your neck, and you wake up one morning with a neck that sends complaint messages flashing through your nervous system.

A stiff neck is a common, usually harmless, problem that lasts just a few painful days. Whether you already have a stiff neck or you've had it before and want to avoid an encore, try these helpful hints.

Roll a towel into a collar. "Take a dry towel, roll it up, fasten it with a safety pin in the front or back, and use it as a soft collar to support your head," says Christa Farnon, M.D., associate director of Occupational Medical Services for SmithKline Beecham, a pharmaceuticals company in King of Prussia, Pennsylvania. "This supports your head in place and limits the movements that you make with your neck." If you would prefer a ready-made collar, check with a medical supply store; ask for a soft cervical collar.

Dunk a terry towel. Dr. Farnon recommends a moist, hot compress, using a towel. "Dunk the towel into hot water, wring it out, and apply it to the back of

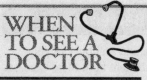

WHEN TO SEE A DOCTOR

"If neck pain gets worse or if it doesn't improve within 24 hours and is associated with headache, drowsiness, confusion, or fever, people really need to be seen by a physician," says Christa Farnon, M.D., associate director of Occupational Medical Services for SmithKline Beecham, a pharmaceuticals company in King of Prussia, Pennsylvania. "Sometimes a stiff neck is a sign of meningitis, a very serious illness that is treated with high dosages of antibiotics.

"Also, if the pain radiates into an arm and the arm becomes numb and increasingly dysfunctional, a stiff neck could be an indication of a slipped disk," Dr. Farnon adds.

your neck," she says. "It's better than dry heat." If a moist compress is impractical, a hot water bottle or heating pad works almost as well. Place the bottle or pad on your neck for 30 minutes three or four times each day.

Shower away pain. "A hot shower will also help relieve the tension in your neck muscles," says Ron Plamondon, D.C., director of member services for the American Chiropractic Association in Arlington, Virginia. The hot shower gently massages your neck muscles while providing deep heat.

Try a pain reliever. Reach for the aspirin: Two pills every four hours will reduce the swelling and pain of a stiff neck. If aspirin doesn't agree with your

Building a Better Neck

Strength and flexibility training isn't only for your arms. Even your neck can benefit from these exercises to prevent and treat neck pain, if you remember two simple rules: Never exercise if the pain is intense and never allow someone else to twist your neck for you.

Go isotonic. Isotonic exercise strengthens your muscles and prevents injury. Take your right hand and hold it against your right temple, then press your head against the palm of your hand, tightening the neck muscle. Hold for five seconds, relax, and repeat. You can move your hand to the left, front, and back of your head, putting pressure on different sides to strengthen the neck muscles all around.

Increase flexibility. Let your head hang forward so that the weight of your head draws your neck into a curve, suggests Bill Connington, board chairman and president of the American Center for the Alexander Technique in New York City. This position will gently stretch the muscles in the back of your neck. When you are finished, imagine that you are building the neck up again, vertebra by vertebra, until

stomach, try another pain reliever recommended by your doctor. Also remember not to give aspirin to children because of the risk of Reye's syndrome.

Sleep on your back. To avoid morning neckaches, try to fall asleep on your back, with a pillow under the curvature of your spine, suggests Joseph J. Biundo Jr., M.D., professor of medicine and chief of physical medicine and rehabilitation at Louisiana State University Medical Center in New Orleans.

your head is balanced on top of your spine. Next, watch yourself in a mirror as you let your head tilt toward one shoulder. Bring your head straight, then let your head tilt toward the other shoulder. Don't force it; allow the weight of your head to do the work.

Try out your range of motion. Allow your neck to relax so that your head is poised on top of your spine. Move your head slowly from side to side as if you're saying no. Keeping your neck relaxed, nod your head up and down as if you're saying yes. If you find that there are places where it is harder to move your head, keep breathing evenly and remind yourself to relax the neck.

Practice releasing and relaxing. Lying on the ground with your knees bent, your feet flat, and a paperback book underneath your head for support, try this relaxation technique: Imagine your muscles releasing and your head unlocking from your spine. Ask the muscles at the base of your skull to soften. Let your back spread out against the floor and feel your breathing deepen. A few minutes each day will ease chronic neck pain.

Avoid the draft. Older people are especially prone to stiff necks caused by open car or bedroom windows, says Dr. Farnon. Do not sleep in a draft, and when driving, keep the window closed on your side.

Fix your car's shocks. The condition of your car may be playing a role in your stiff neck. Good shock absorbers will make both your car and your body run more smoothly, says Susan Zahalsky, M.D., former director of medical services at the Comprehensive Spine Center at Midway Hospital Center in Los Angeles.

Walk around. Is your workplace giving you a pain in the neck? If your muscles are "locked" in the same position, you'll begin to ache. "If you're doing desk work every day, get up every 20 minutes or so and walk around to keep your muscles alive," says Deborah Caplan, a physical therapist and founding member of the American Center for the Alexander Technique in New York City. She suggests stretching exercises: Make large circles with your arms to extend your muscles. And look around the room—up, down, and to the side—to get the kinks out of your neck.

Look forward to your work. Computers and reading materials should be placed directly in front of you, at eye level. For computer users, Dr. Zahalsky suggests purchasing a book stand; check art supply stores. If you are in a jam, a pillow placed under your book may also work.

Keep your phone off your shoulder. The telephone is often the greatest pain in the neck for workers. If you spend time on the phone, Caplan recommends getting a headset that will hold it in place.

Stomachache

You've long since graduated from using stomachache as an excuse to get out of having to go to school. But you're probably still learning a thing or two about how to avoid this brand of midsection misery—such as bypassing the blue plate special during your next visit to the local diner.

Actually, food is only one cause of stomachache. "In fact, you're probably more likely to get a stomachache when your stomach is empty, as the result of stomach acid," says Michael Oppenheim, M.D., a Los Angeles family practitioner and author of *The Complete Book of Better Digestion*. He points to stomach acid as one cause. "Anxiety is also another common cause, especially among children," he adds.

For the stomachache, doctors say it's okay to simply gut it out. But there are some things you can do to stop your bellyaching a bit quicker.

Take an antacid. "If the pain occurs when your stomach is empty, food can't be the cause," says Dr. Oppenheim. "Most likely, it's stomach acid—so taking an antacid is the answer."

Almost any antacid can help neutralize stomach acid, but it can also have other effects on digestion, depending on the kind you choose. "The basic thing to look for in an antacid is the amount of calcium or magnesium it contains," says William B. Ruderman, M.D., chairman of the department of gastroenterology at the Cleveland Clinic-Florida in Fort Lauderdale. "If you tend

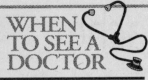

WHEN TO SEE A DOCTOR

"Most stomachaches are minor and don't require a doctor's assistance," says William B. Ruderman, M.D., chairman of the department of gastroenterology at the Cleveland Clinic–Florida in Fort Lauderdale. "But if pain becomes intolerable or if there's vomiting, fever, excessive nausea, or abdominal cramping in an otherwise healthy person, you probably should notify your doctor." This could indicate food poisoning or a more severe abdominal condition such as appendicitis or stomach ulcers.

If your stomachache lasts longer than 24 hours, call your doctor for advice, adds Dr. Ruderman. Prolonged pain could be a sign of something more serious.

to have trouble with constipation, then pick a brand that lists magnesium first on the label. If you're more prone to diarrhea, pick a brand listing calcium first."

Have a snack. A light snack can also absorb stomach acid if your stomachache isn't the result of overeating.

"A bland diet with soft foods is best—things such as bananas or crackers," says Dr. Ruderman. "Apple juice is an excellent choice. But stay away from overly sweet juices such as strawberry or raspberry as well as acidic beverages such as orange juice." He points out that the acidic drinks can actually *aggravate* stomach acid.

Drink to burp. If that stomachache is the result of overeating, then a good burp is usually the quickest way to get relief. Adults may turn toward a product like Alka-Seltzer, but children usually prefer a better-tasting remedy.

"My approach to treating mild stomachache is the same as what my mother did—with flat ginger ale or cola," says Perri Elizabeth Klass, M.D., a pediatrician in Boston and author of *Baby Doctor*. "The carbonation in the soda helps stir things up, so you burp and feel better. And I believe that if soda is a little flat, it has a slightly medicinal taste, which probably helps on a psychological level."

Hey, relax. Mom was only half right when she suggested a nice hot cup of tea. "Tea, particularly peppermint tea, can calm down your stomach, but it should be warm—not hot," says Dr. Ruderman. "You're also better off with lukewarm beverages. Something too hot or too cold can induce a spastic response in your stomach, which increases pressure and pain."

What Causes Stomach Gurgling?

A rumbly stomach may get your attention, but should it demand your concern? "You can't do much about stomach gurgling—and there's no need to," says William B. Ruderman, M.D., chairman of the department of gastroenterology at the Cleveland Clinic–Florida in Fort Lauderdale.

"To understand this condition—called borborygmus—think of your stomach as a giant Mixmaster. When you eat, your stomach grinds up and mixes the food you've eaten to help digestion. The gurgling you hear is the noise created as the intestines squeeze this solution through."

Feast on fiber. Studies show that the incidence of stomachache was halved among a group of children who ate high-fiber cookies at the first sign of stomachache. "Popcorn is also an effective source of fiber," says William Feldman, M.D., head of the division of general pediatrics at the Hospital for Sick Children in Toronto. "Eating prunes, and fruits in general, can help a lot," adds Dr. Klass.

Stomach Cramps

Most of us have had a muscle cramp somewhere in our body at one time or another. A calf muscle may tighten up into a hard knot, a hand may "freeze." Even your little toe can cramp up if you stretch your foot the wrong way.

The point is, muscle cramps can happen anywhere you have muscles, and that includes your stomach, where a cramp may be mistaken for a "generic" bellyache, indigestion, upset stomach, or side stitch.

Muscle cramps can occur when a muscle isn't getting enough oxygen carrying blood to meet its needs. Your stomach can become the fall guy for cramping when stress, overindulgence, or heavy exercise after a big meal sets the stage. Your first line of defense? Stomach-soothing over-the-counter drugs. Your best long-term strategy? Avoid tummy-knotting situations. Here's what you need to know.

Try a smooth coating. Several over-the-counter drugs are designed specifically to relieve the stomach pain that's caused by overindulgence, says Thomas Gossel, Ph.D., R.Ph., professor of pharmacology and toxicology and associate dean at Ohio Northern University College of Pharmacy in Ada.

"For first-line treatment, I'd recommend Pepto-Bismol. It relieves many minor stomach upsets," Dr. Gossel says. Antacids and sodium bicarbonate (Alka-Seltzer) may also help some people, he adds, especially if the cramping is compounded by heartburn.

Forgo feeding frenzies. Eat slowly, chew your food well, and don't guzzle down drinks. Food that's chewed well first and mixed with saliva is easier to digest, according to John C. Johnson, M.D., director of Emergency Medical Services at Porter Memorial Hospital in Valparaiso, Indiana, and a past president of the American College of Emergency Physicians.

Graze, don't gorge. Stomachs are very sensitive to overstuffing. "A distended stomach can cause sharp pain and can be very uncomfortable for some people," says Dr. Johnson. If you're one whose stomach cramps up when you just dig right in, try eating smaller, more frequent meals.

Hold off on eating if you're upset. Anxiety and eating don't mix. "When you're tense, the blood supply to your digestive system is reduced, making it hard to digest food," says Steven Fahrion, Ph.D., a clinical psychologist and director of the Center for Applied Psychophysiology at the Menninger Clinic in Topeka, Kansas. While there are many ways to relax, one of the fastest and easiest is with deep, slow, deliberate breathing, Dr. Fahrion says. As you exhale, imagine tension leaving your body.

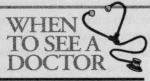

WHEN TO SEE A DOCTOR

Pain that seems to be in your stomach can be caused by countless things, including some that don't have anything to do with your digestive tract, says John C. Johnson, M.D., director of Emergency Medical Services at Porter Memorial Hospital in Valparaiso, Indiana, and past president of the American College of Emergency Physicians.

If your "stomach cramp" persists for more than 30 minutes or if it seems to be increasing in intensity, see a doctor. You may have an obstruction, a twist in your intestines or inflammation.

Heart attacks are often mistaken, early on, for attacks of indigestion. That mistake can be fatal. If your pain includes a feeling of pressure, nausea or vomiting, sweating, chest pain, or trouble breathing, don't wait to see if it goes away. Get to an emergency room fast!

Stick with noncaffeinated drinks. Coffee and colas make a tense stomach worse, Dr. Johnson says. Try water, fruit juices, or a tummy-taming herbal tea.

Go easy on cold fluids. Leave chugalugging for the fraternity boys. Too much of your favorite icy cold beverage, downed too fast, can send your stomach into temporary but painful spasms.

Fill up on fiber. In one study of bellyache-prone kids, two high-fiber cookies a day (providing 10 grams of fiber) cut episodes of stomach pain in half.

"Fiber helps food move through the digestive system more quickly and so may reduce stomach and intestinal cramping," says William Feldman, M.D., head of the division of general pediatrics at the Hospital for Sick Children in Toronto.

Give your guts a time-out. Allow a half-hour or more for big meals to move through your stomach before you engage in heavy-duty activities, recommends Dr. Johnson.

"Exercise diverts blood from your digestive system to your arms and legs, increasing your chances for stomach and intestinal cramps," he explains.

Then speed things up with a little walk. If you're feeling full after a sumptuous repast, try "walking it off" before you resort to antacids. Light exercise, especially walking, helps speed the movement of digested food through your bowels. "This may reduce stomach cramps by allowing the stomach to empty faster," Dr. Johnson says.

Stress

The images in the retirement-community ads certainly are alluring. A man fishing with his grandson. Golf seven days a week. A leisurely afternoon siesta. No worries, no problems, no stresses.

Dream on.

For many people who dream of such a stress-free

nirvana, there may be a surprise waiting by the hammock. Stress doesn't retire. It can follow you like the flu. In fact, the retirement years often are among the most stressful in a person's life, says George T. Grossberg, M.D., director of geriatric psychiatry at St. Louis University School of Medicine. "Late life is a time of tremendous stress. You face numerous strains that you probably have never faced before, like the loss of loved ones, loneliness, disability, and unanticipated financial strain. And when you're 85, you're not going to bounce back from these stresses as quickly as a 25-year-old would," he says. "Consequently, the chances that stress will lead to chronic illness are much greater."

Researchers suspect that stress contributes to a multitude of physical and emotional disorders, including high blood pressure, muscle spasms, chronic fatigue, insomnia, obesity, heart disease, digestive problems, anxiety, phobias, and depression. But it is particularly harmful after age 60, because the body can't physically adapt to the strain as well as it once did, explains Dr. Grossberg.

Under stress, for instance, an older person's blood pressure rises more rapidly and stays higher longer than a younger person's, because the older person's blood vessel walls may have lost some elasticity, increasing the risk of a heart attack or stroke, Dr. Grossberg warns.

Stress may take a greater toll as you get older because of a chemical imbalance—the body continues to crank out stress hormones at a steady pace, while the production of the hormones that counteract it declines dramatically as you age, according to Dr. Grossberg.

The result is like overinflating a balloon. You'll likely feel stretched—nearly to the limit. And that pressure can affect your mind, body, or spirit, says Frieda

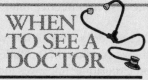

R. Butler, Ph.D., professor of gerontology at George Mason University in Fairfax, Virginia.

But it is never too late to learn how to deflate stress, Dr. Butler says. In fact, even if you've managed to corral stress in the past, you may have to develop new coping skills because the ones you used at 30 may not work as well at 70.

"As you get older, it takes longer to get yourself together after facing a stressful situation. So you'll have to adapt to maintain a healthy balance," she says. "Some of the old strategies may still work, but also you will have to take on new, more effective ones." Try these.

Take it in stride. "Exercise does more to relieve stress than a lot of other things combined," Dr. Butler says. "It helps get the blood circulating, improves mobility and muscle strength, and boosts morale. If you can move without pain, it changes your whole outlook on life. Exercise also has been shown to have a positive effect on mental abilities such as memory and in relieving anxiety."

Exercise also can improve your energy reserves so you'll feel more vigorous, says Robert E. Thayer, Ph.D., author of *The Origin of Everyday Moods* and professor of psychology at California State University, Long Beach. And the more energized you feel, the better you'll be able to cope with stress. If you feel slightly blue or worried, he recommends taking a brisk 10-minute walk at a pace as if you were late for an important appointment, but don't tense up as if you really were late.

Stop peddling the news cycle. Computers, television, radios, and other forms of media offer staggering amounts of information instantaneously. But do you really need to know it all? Of course not, Dr. Butler says. In fact, letting go of news and information you don't need is one of the best stress busters for a person over 60.

"If you feel pressured to keep up with the world, then you may begin to feel stressed out. But who says you have to keep up with the latest music or styles anymore? Who says you have to read the newspaper or watch the evening news every day anymore? You don't. Only hold on to the information that is relevant for your new lifestyle. So if you golf, you may want to know who won the Senior

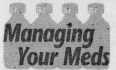

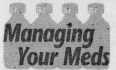
Managing Your Meds

Caffeine, a prime ingredient in coffee, tea, cola drinks, and chocolate, is a stimulant that has a greater effect on the body after age 60, says George T. Grossberg, M.D., director of geriatric psychiatry at St. Louis University School of Medicine. Drink no more than one eight-ounce cup or glass a day to avoid feeling jittery and stressed out, he advises. Five ounces of dark, bittersweet chocolate has almost the same amount of caffeine as an eight-ounce cup of coffee. Milk chocolate has considerably less. Caffeine also is a major component of over-the-counter (OTC) stimulants such as No-Doz. Check with your doctor before using these drugs. Here are a few other common medications that can heighten feelings of stress or irritability.

✦ OTC sleep aids or cold and allergy medications such as diphenhydramine (Tylenol PM, Benadryl) and clemastine (Tavist)

✦ OTC decongestants, antihistamines, or antihistamine/decongestant combinations like pseudoephedrine (Sudafed), triprolidine and pseudoephedrine (Actifed), and clemastine and phenylpropanolamine (Tavist-D)

✦ Antihistamines found in some analgesics such as phenyltoloxamine (Percogesic)

✦ Antidepressants such as fluoxetine (Prozac), paroxetine (Paxil), and Zoloft (sertraline)

✦ Prescription and OTC asthma inhalants containing epinephrine (Primatene)

Open but not give a hoot about movies or politics. That's fine."

Get cozy. As you age, your natural ability to regulate body temperature declines, so you'll be more prone to stress in extreme cold or heat, according to Dr. Butler. Keep the temperatures in your house well within your comfort zone and avoid venturing out on unusually frigid or sultry days, she suggests.

Inhale relief. Deep breathing is one of the simplest ways to keep stress under wraps, says Dr. Butler. Practice it by doing the following:

1. Sit in a comfortable chair with your back straight.

2. Slowly breathe in and feel your lungs filling from the bottom to the top.

3. Focus your attention on your belly; let it expand as you breathe. It should feel as if your diaphragm, a muscular membrane separating your lungs from your abdomen, is being pulled down, as if it were attached to a string in your belly.

4. Slowly exhale, emptying your lungs from top to bottom.

5. Feel your diaphragm relax into its natural position. Then take another deep breath and repeat.

Do this exercise twice a day for five minutes, Dr. Butler suggests.

Anticipate power surges. Energy levels tend to be higher at certain times of the day than at others, Dr. Thayer says. Being aware of this cycle is very important because when you have low energy, you'll be more susceptible to stress. Every two to three hours for three days, jot down on a notepad whether your energy levels feel high, moderately high, moderately low, or low. You should see patterns emerge that will help you make decisions, schedule appointments, and run errands at times when your energy levels are high and you are less apt to feel stressed, he says. So if you find yourself feeling drained around 2:00 P.M. each day, take a nap instead of balancing your checkbook or playing a chess game.

"This technique works particularly well for people over 60, who tend to not have the energy reserves that they once had," according to Dr. Thayer.

Head for the showers. Plunging into a steaming shower, bath, or hot-tub is an excellent way to relieve stress, Dr. Thayer says. But don't stay in too long. Staying in warm hot-tub–like water for more than 10 minutes actually increases tension and can dampen your mood, he says.

Swelling

Eyes, nose, thumbs, toes—just about any body part can swell up. It happens for lots of different reasons, and the sensations that go along with swelling can be painful, itchy, or annoying. And while there are many general remedies for swelling, some body parts require their own special treatments.

Swelling often accompanies injury, for instance, as fluid normally flowing through blood vessels seeps out into the surrounding tissue. That may happen when blood vessels are injured by a bump, by a muscle or ligament tear, or by a fracture.

Swelling can also happen slowly, without an injury, as the result of pooled blood in an arm or leg. Through a process called effusion, fluid seeps from the blood vessels into tissue. It's this kind of swelling that occurs when you notice your hands puffing up while you walk or your feet getting a shoe size bigger when you've been standing around for a long time. (Because varicose veins impede the return of blood to the heart via the veins, they can cause this kind of swelling.)

Hives, welts, and the itchy bumps caused by mosquitoes and other blood-sucking parasites are other examples of swelling. So are the stuffy, runny nose and scratchy, puffy eyes that accompany hay fever.

"The more a body part swells, the more blood circulation is slowed. And poor blood circulation slows healing," says Clayton Holmes, an athletic trainer and assistant professor of physical therapy at the University of Texas Health Science Center at San Antonio. For serious injuries, you'll want to see the doctor and follow his recommendations. But here are some all-purpose ways to keep swelling down.

Try an over-the-counter antihistamine. These drugs help counteract the swelling caused by insect stings and many kinds of allergic reactions, says Thomas Platts-Mills, M.D., Ph.D., head of the division of allergy and clinical immunology at the University of Virginia Health Sciences Center in Charlottesville. Antihistamines are contained in some liquid medications, but Dr. Platts-Mills recommends the faster-acting chew-

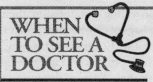

WHEN TO SEE A DOCTOR

Many injuries that cause swelling deserve a doctor's prompt attention. That's because ligament or muscle tears, fractures, or cartilage damage may be hiding under all that puffiness.

If you think you might have an ankle, foot, or leg fracture, don't try to remove your shoe. Let the doctor do that. First-aid treatment is different for each kind of fracture, but generally you want to keep the limb from moving around until the doctor can treat it.

Also, if swelling is the result of an insect bite or sting and is accompanied by severe reactions such as chest tightness, dizziness, or fainting, seek medical help at once. These are signs of potentially deadly anaphylactic shock.

able tablet. "Take the dosage suggested on the box as soon as you are stung," he says. (That way, the drug gets into your system quickly.) Take the antihistamine at recommended intervals as long as the swelling continues. *Note:* Antihistamines are useless for injury-related swelling.

Remember RICE. Not the long-grain variety but a proven first-aid method for injured ankles, knees, and elbows: rest, ice, compression, and elevation. "The sooner you do all four, the better," says Holmes.

If you want to reduce swelling in a leg, for instance, do RICE in this order. Wet a four- to six-inch-wide elastic bandage in ice water. Firmly wrap it a few times around the injured ankle or knee, providing compression, then apply two quart-size plastic bags of crushed ice, so they completely surround the joint. Continue wrapping, using the bandage to hold the ice in place. Leave the ice on for no longer than 20 minutes. Take off the ice and rewrap the injury. Wait an hour before you ice again.

While you're icing, elevate the injured part above the level of your heart.

Rest the injured part by immobilizing it. If it's an ankle or knee that's hurt, don't try to hobble around. Get some assistance when you walk, or use crutches.

Step in place. Standing motionless for long periods of time may cause swelling. That's because up to a quart of blood pools in your legs and feet, and fluid may seep out of blood vessels into tissue. That not only makes your legs feel like lead but also makes your feet a size bigger. So walk in place, lifting your knees and pointing your toes downward. That helps your muscles pump blood upward. If you must stand still, keep your knees slightly flexed. Don't lock them, experts say.

Stay active after exercise. If you stop suddenly after hard exercise, blood can pool in your legs, resulting in swelling and sometimes low blood pressure as well. Instead of stopping abruptly after a run or swim, cool down with lighter activity for 10 minutes or so. That keeps your circulation going but at a less intense pace, suggests John Duncan, Ph.D., associate director of the exercise physiology department at the Cooper Institute for Aerobics Research in Dallas. This gradual slowdown is especially important for people taking heart medications such as beta-blockers.

Bend and pump. Swinging your arms while you walk is a good way to loosen up, but the centrifugal force it creates can make blood pool in your hands,

Stuck Ring?
Dental Floss to the Rescue!

A ring may be a symbol of wedded bliss, but it can pose real danger when it's stuck on a swelling finger. Because it can cut off blood circulation just as surely as a tourniquet, that band of gold has got to come off—the sooner, the better.

If your joint has swollen and is already too big to slip the ring over, try this trick using dental floss. (Better yet, use waxed dental tape.) Used by emergency medical technicians, the technique is recommended by John C. Johnson, M.D., past president of the American College of Emergency Physicians and director of Emergency Medical Services at Porter Memorial Hospital in Valparaiso, Indiana.

Take a long piece of floss (two to three feet is not too long). Starting at the tip of the finger, closely wrap the floss around the finger, spiraling down toward the ring. Keep the encirclements $\frac{1}{8}$ inch apart or less. When you get to the ring, slip the end of the floss under the ring and pull it toward your palm. Lift that end of the floss over the top of the ring and pull up toward the tip of your finger. As the floss unwinds, it will ease the ring up and off the finger.

To make this even easier, grease the floss-wrapped finger with petroleum jelly before you remove the ring.

causing swelling. "Try bending your arms 90 degrees at the elbows and use them as pistons," suggests Dr. Duncan. "Raise them up higher than you normally would and swing with the cadence of your walking gait." While you're doing that, keep your hands loosely open. Although you can occasionally clench your hands to squeeze out fluid, continual clenching interferes with the flow of fluid through the arm and will make your lower arm swell.

Keep a loose grip on your bike. Do your lower arms swell when you're bicycling? Unless you're barreling down some potholed road, you shouldn't have to grip the handlebars of your bike so tightly that you cut off circulation in your arms. But that's exactly what some people do, even while they're riding stationary bicycles indoors, Dr. Duncan says. "A healthy person might not notice it, but someone who already has circulation problems will see his lower arms swelling," he says. So keep a loose grip, he suggests, and shift from the upper to lower bars occasionally. Or simply move your hands. Padded gloves can help, too.

Tinnitus

For most people, the rhythmic sound of ocean waves caressing the shore is as soothing as a mother's lullaby. But if that splish-splash-hiss-crash is *inside* your ears, it's a different story. Tinnitus, or "ringing in the ears," is the name of that lullaby. And it's anything but soothing!

Tinnitus is not a disease, and it doesn't cause hearing disorders. It's any kind of swishing, hissing, whirring, ringing, whistling, buzzing, or chirping that goes on inside your head.

The causes? Tinnitus can be a sign of hearing loss, or it can result from head injuries, ear infections, or diseases that range from the common cold to diabetes. People who work with noisy equipment, such as power tools, can also get it. Or tinnitus may be initiated by a single loud noise, such as a gunshot or an explosion.

Sometimes tinnitus is only temporary. If you have a ringing in your ears for only a few days (perhaps after listening to loud music), take it as a warning sign. Tone down your listening habits, or tinnitus may become permanent.

Even when tinnitus moves in to stay, there are still things you can do about it. The first move is a medical checkup. After that, here are some ways to make it easier to live with.

Tone down sound around you. "Never expose your ears to loud sounds, because they simply make tinnitus worse," says Jack Vernon, Ph.D., professor of otolaryngology at Oregon Health Sciences University and director of the Oregon Hearing Research Center, both in Portland. "If you have to raise your voice to be heard, then the sound around you is too loud. That includes vacuum cleaners, dishwashers, lawn mowers, and so forth."

So wear earplugs whenever noise abounds. Pharmacies carry foam, rubber, and moldable wax plugs as well as headphones you wear like earmuffs.

Try a little night static. Some people don't notice their tinnitus in the daytime, but as soon as the lights go out, they're up to their inner ears in bells and buzzers. "For those folks, I recommend detuning an FM radio to static between stations," says Dr. Vernon. If you keep the radio near the bed, just loud enough to be audible, the static will mask the sounds in your head and let you fall

411

asleep. Other sounds that might be the key to dreamland: a fan running all night or a bit of soft music.

Play that shower! In the "mask that sound" department: "Some people can't hear their tinnitus when they take showers," says Dr. Vernon. Of course, you can't stay in the shower all day, but you *can* carry shower sounds around with you. Dr. Vernon suggests making a long-playing tape of a running shower. When the tinnitus gets bad, listen to the tape through headphones, he recommends. (The idea is to find a band of tones that includes your tinnitus tone but is more acceptable to listen to.)

Breathe deeply to dismiss distress. "Reducing stress often reduces tinnitus," says Robert E. Brummett, Ph.D., a pharmacologist at the Oregon Hearing Research Center. Deep, slow breathing is one safe way to ease tension any time you feel it creeping up on you, according to Dr. Vernon. But he cautions that this may not be enough. See a counselor if you're having difficulty dealing with stress in your life and your tinnitus is becoming worse because of it.

Skip the smokes and drinks. "Restrict the nicotine, alcohol, tonic water, and caffeine you consume," Dr. Brummett suggests. If you find that it helps to cut out one or all of these, consider a permanent vacation from the noise provoker.

Don't take aspirin. People with tinnitus who take aspirin daily (for arthritis, for example) should try a different anti-inflammatory drug if possible, suggests Dr. Brummett. Aspirin can cause or worsen tinnitus. Some of the other anti-inflammatory drugs can also cause or worsen tinnitus, but not in everyone. By working with your doctor, you can try some of the alternative drugs until you find one that you can tolerate.

Give yourself a dose of distraction. "Getting distracted from tinnitus surely will help," says Dr. Vernon. "Focus on some outside things: Help other people. Join some volunteer groups. Don't retire!" he suggests. "People with tinnitus need to enrich rather than restrict their lives."

Toothache

Atoothache is usually an early sign of a cavity. But it also can be caused by inflammation of the gums, an abscess (an infection that develops in the tooth root or between the tooth and gum), a cracked tooth, or a dislodged filling. Each of these problems can cause different types of toothache, says Flora Parsa Stay, D.D.S., dentist in Oxnard, California, and author of *The Complete Book of Dental Remedies*. Your dentist will probably suspect that you have a cracked tooth, for instance, if you have pressure and pain while chewing. Severe pain accompanied by sensitivity to hot and cold could be a sign that a cavity has reached the nerve of the tooth.

The following remedies can help soothe your tooth pain while you're waiting for an appointment with your dentist.

String it up. Sometimes, a toothache is caused by something as simple as trapped food between the teeth. These food particles actually irritate the gums, but the pain can radiate into the surrounding teeth, Dr. Stay says. So try rinsing your mouth with warm water to loosen any food particles. Then floss or use a water-irrigating device to clean between your teeth. But even if this technique relieves your pain, you should still consult a dentist to make sure other more complex dental problems aren't contributing to your toothache, she says.

Gnaw a knot of cloves. Take a couple of cloves from a spice rack and place them between your aching tooth and your cheek—much like you'd use chewing tobacco. They can help soothe the pain, says Richard D. Fischer, D.D.S., dentist in Annandale, Virginia, and past president of the International Academy of Oral Medicine and Toxicology. Let the hard seedlike cloves soak in your mouth's saliva for several minutes to soften them up. Then gently chew on them—like you would on a toothpick—so the soothing oils within the cloves are released into the area surrounding your aching tooth. Leave the cloves in place for about 30 minutes or until the pain subsides. Continue this treatment as needed until you can see a dentist, he suggests.

Lay on the ointment. If gnashing on cloves is unappetizing, then consider using an over-the-counter tooth-pain ointment such as Anbesol or Orajel, Dr. Fischer suggests. Be sure to follow the directions on the label.

Make some waves. Swishing warm saltwater around in your mouth can help reduce gum swelling, disinfect abscesses, and relieve tooth pain. Mix a teaspoon of salt into an eight-ounce glass of warm water and use as needed for discomfort, Dr. Fischer says. Swish each mouthful for 10 to 30 seconds, focusing the saltwater on the painful area as much as possible. Repeat until the glass is empty. Do this as needed throughout the day, he suggests.

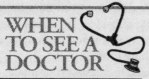

WHEN TO SEE A DOCTOR

Seek dental care for a toothache even if the pain diminishes or disappears completely, advises Richard D. Fischer, D.D.S., dentist in Annandale, Virginia, and past president of the International Academy of Oral Medicine and Toxicology. Although it may not still be provoking pain, an abscess or other underlying cause of your toothache could still be damaging your teeth and gums.

If you have high blood pressure and are on a sodium-restricted diet, use Epsom salt instead of table salt, he says. Epsom salts are made with magnesium and, unlike table salt, shouldn't adversely affect your blood pressure.

Pop a pain reliever. Simply taking a 325-milligram aspirin tablet every four to six hours can dampen a lot of tooth pain and gum inflammation, says Robert Henry, D.M.D., dentist in Lexington, Kentucky, and past president of the American Society for Geriatric Dentistry. If you can't tolerate aspirin, then try taking 200 milligrams of ibuprofen (Advil) every four hours, Dr. Henry suggests. Ibuprofen is a potent anti-inflammatory that is gentler on the stomach than aspirin.

If you do use aspirin, never put it directly on the tooth or gums, Dr. Henry urges. Remember, aspirin is an acid. Keeping it in your mouth for more than a few seconds can cause a painful burn that will only complicate the treatment of your toothache.

Chill out. Wrap an ice pack in a towel and apply

it to the outside of your mouth for 15 to 20 minutes every hour until your pain subsides, Dr. Fischer suggests. The ice will reduce swelling and calm agitated nerve endings in your aching tooth.

Load up on minerals. Increasing your intake of calcium and magnesium can help soothe nerves and temporarily ease tooth pain, Dr. Fischer says. He suggests taking 500 milligrams of calcium and 200 to 300 milligrams of magnesium at the first sign of a toothache.

Note: People with heart or kidney problems should check with their doctor before taking supplemental magnesium.

Invite your teeth to tea. Herbal teas made with chamomile or echinacea often can quell mild toothache pain, Dr. Stay says.

To prepare a chamomile tea, add two tablespoons of dried chamomile flowers to two cups of boiling water and steep for 10 minutes. As for echinacea, add four tablespoons of the dried herb to eight cups of boiling water and steep for 10 minutes. After they have been strained, you can drink either of these teas as needed for pain, Dr. Stay says. You can also buy these teas premade in the tea section at your health food store. They may not be as strong as the do-it-yourself versions, but they're a little more convenient.

Note: Very rarely, chamomile can cause an allergic reaction when ingested. People allergic to closely related plants such as ragweed, asters, and chrysanthemums should drink the tea with caution. Don't use echinacea if you have autoimmune conditions such as lupus, tuberculosis, or multiple sclerosis. Don't use it if you're allergic to plants in the daisy family, such as chamomile and marigold.

Picture yourself pain-free. Your imagination is

a powerful healer that can help you dampen tooth pain, Dr. Fischer says.

To try it, imagine swimming in ice-cold water or playing in the snow. Feel the chill of the water or snow penetrating your hands and feet so that they are almost numb. Now imagine that feeling of numbness enveloping your aching tooth, soothing it as if you were rubbing it with snow until all of the pain is gone, says Deena Margetis, certified clinical hypnotherapist specializing in dental care in Annandale, Virginia. Doing this imagery for one to two minutes as needed may relieve much of your pain, she says.

Ulcers

Ulcers were once seen as the scourge of stressed Type A executives and older people with weak constitutions. Now, revolutionary discoveries are changing the way doctors think about and treat painful ulcers. Unfortunately, the news hasn't made it to everyone who has ulcers.

Despite what many have thought for years, anyone at any age can get ulcers, and roughly 25 million Americans have them. The problem starts when a chronic sore develops either in the protective lining of the stomach or in the part of the intestine just below the stomach, which is called the duodenum. When your stomach's caustic acid seeps over this sore, you will know it by the

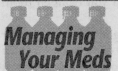

Managing Your Meds

Ironically, agonizing ulcers not caused by *Helicobacter pylori* bacteria often develop from the use of common pain relievers. "The family of drugs known as nonsteroidal anti-inflammatory drugs (NSAIDs) interferes with the body's ability to maintain its protective lining in the stomach and intestine," says W. Steven Pray, Ph.D., R.Ph., professor of nonprescription drug products at Southwestern Oklahoma State University in Weatherford. NSAID-related ulcers occur more frequently among people over the age of 60 because they use these drugs more often than younger people do. If you need a pain reliever and you have an ulcer, are recovering from one, or simply want to avoid problems with ulcers, ask your doctor if acetaminophen (Tylenol) would be suitable, says Dr. Pray. Popularly used over-the-counter and prescription NSAIDs include aspirin, ibuprofen (Advil), naproxen (Aleve), ketoprofen (Orudis KT), diclofenac (Voltaren), etodolac (Lodine), and oxaprozin (Daypro).

burning pain you feel, says Martin Brotman, M.D., gastroenterologist at the California Pacific Medical Center in San Francisco. As you age, you can be at further risk for this problem, too. Taking too many painkillers like aspirin or ibuprofen (Advil) can irritate your stomach lining and put you at greater risk. What's more, aging adults have a higher incidence of infection by a bacteria called *Helicobacter pylori (H. pylori)*, which is associated with virtually all duodenal ulcers. About 60 percent of Americans age 60 and over have *H. pylori*.

If you have burning abdominal pain—especially when your stomach is empty—or if you are awakened at night by this pain, see your doctor. He can determine what the problem is. If it is an ulcer, he will need to figure out where it is and what is causing it in order to treat it properly. He may, for example, order a blood test for the *H. pylori* bacteria. Whatever the cause, ulcers require prompt, supervised medical treatment to be healed properly, says Dr. Brotman. And while your ulcer is mending, use these tips to speed the healing process and to keep from irritating the sore spot in your stomach.

Eat small. Although you might notice acid pain most when you have an empty stomach, the act of eating also signals the stomach to secrete acid to digest food. To keep that acid at manageable levels, try to eat smaller, more frequent meals rather than three big meals, says Roger L. Gebhard, M.D., gastroenterologist at the Veterans Affairs Medical Center and professor of medicine in the division of gastroenterology at the University of Minnesota, both in Minneapolis.

Don't hold the onions. As a precautionary measure, add onions to your sandwiches, salads, and other meals. A study in the Netherlands found that the odorous sulfur compounds found in onions help fight the *H. pylori* bacteria linked with ulcers and stomach cancer.

Perk up with pink. Over-the-counter stomach remedies like Pepto-Bismol can coat your stomach and provide temporary relief from acid, says Dr. Gebhard. Follow the instructions on the bottle when using any bismuth product such as this, as excessive use can be harmful, he says.

Be smoke-free. If you smoke, you have yet another reason to quit. Not only can smoking delay the healing of existing ulcers but also help cause them, says Melissa Palmer, M.D., gastroenterologist and liver specialist in private practice in New York City.

Can the citrus. Avoid high-acid citrus foods and juices; they may aggravate ulcer symptoms, says Marie L. Borum, M.D., assistant professor of medicine in the division of gastroenterology and nutrition at George Washington University Medical Center in Washington, D.C.

Abstain from alcohol. If you like a cocktail or a glass of wine with dinner, scratch it from your diet while your ulcer is mending, says Dr. Brotman. Alcohol stimulates acid production. What's more, alcohol can irritate your stomach lining.

Go easy on the milk. Dairy products, such as milk and yogurt, used to be recommended for those with ulcers. It is now known that they stimulate acid secretion, so it is probably not good to use them to soothe ulcer pain, says Dr. Gebhard.

For pain, take acetaminophen. If you have been taking aspirin or other over-the-counter anti-inflammatory medication for pain, switch to acetaminophen (Tylenol). Aspirin and other anti-inflammatories such as ibuprofen can increase your risk of ulcer and irritate your stomach lining, says Dr. Brotman.

Feel great with ginger. Ginger is considered an herbal remedy to help protect against ulcers. Take it in capsules, in root form, or as tea, says Mindy Green, director of education services at the Herb Research Foundation in Boulder, Colorado. You will find ginger in these forms at many drugstores and natural food stores. Fresh ginger is available in most grocery stores. To make tea from fresh ginger, cut a quarter-inch slice of a one-inch-round chunk of ginger, place it in a pot containing a cup of water, and simmer it for 10 to 15

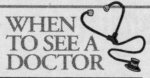

WHEN TO SEE A DOCTOR

Any ulcer should be checked by a doctor. If you have stomach or abdominal pain that is eased by eating or if the pain wakes you up at night, call your doctor.

An untreated ulcer may bleed, leading to vomiting of blood or blood in your stools. If you are vomiting material that looks like coffee grounds or if your stools have turned black, get to a doctor as soon as possible, says Chesley Hines, M.D., a gastroenterologist at the Center for Digestive Diseases in New Orleans.

minutes. While fresh ginger is safe when used as a spice, some forms of ginger aren't recommended for everyone. Ginger may increase bile secretion, so if you have gallstones, do not use therapeutic amounts of dried ginger or ginger powder without guidance from a health-care practitioner.

Choose vegetables for your vittles. Fiber and vitamin A from vegetables and fresh fruits may help protect against ulcers. Researchers at the Harvard School of Public Health studied the relationship of dietary factors and ulcer risk in nearly 50,000 men ages 40 to 75 years. Those with a higher consumption of fruits and vegetables were found to be less likely to develop ulcers than men who didn't add those foods to their fare. How fiber is of benefit in the reduction of ulcer risk is not yet understood, but the researchers believe that vitamin A may help protect the lining of the stomach and duodenum by increasing mucus production there.

Underweight

For many of us, the fun house at a carnival was a real treat. Especially the mirror that made a rather rotund person look tall and skinny. It was an instant, effortless, and ever-so-momentary diet.

Now, decades later, you may have noticed that you *really* are losing weight. If the undistorted image in the mirror tells you that you are beginning to look a bit gaunt—and you are not trying to lose weight—should you be concerned?

Perhaps, says Jan I. Maby, D.O., director of the Geriatric Medical Home Care program at Mount Sinai Medical Center in New York City.

Weight usually peaks in the early forties for men and in the fifties for women, says Dr. Maby. Then as a person creeps toward 60, the amount of muscle in the body naturally drops. By age 70, a typical woman has lost about 11 pounds of muscle, and an average man has lost about 26 pounds of it.

But a weight plunge may not stop there. Add in chewing difficulties, mobility problems, chronic intestinal upset, alcohol abuse, loneliness, and financial woes that hamper your ability to buy food and you could be facing a major health problem, Dr. Maby says. In fact, involuntary weight loss or being severely underweight can touch off a host of related problems. As your body loses weight, your bones are also deprived, so bone loss, or osteoporosis, is accelerated. Other possible complications include liver problems, nutritional deficiencies, heart disease, slow wound healing, and arthritis. If you are severely underweight, the deprivation might impair your ability to think clearly, and it can contribute to dry, flaky skin and skin sores.

If you are 15 percent or more below your ideal weight or if you have lost 5 percent of your body weight in a month without really trying, see your doctor for an evaluation, Dr. Maby says. Once you have done that, here are a few tips that can help you regain your appetite.

Beef up your diet. Although low-calorie, low-fat meals are great for younger people, they may not be all that terrific for seniors who are underweight, says David A. Lipschitz, M.D., Ph.D., chairman and professor of geriatrics at the University of Arkansas for Medical Sciences in Little Rock. In fact, for seniors who are underweight, the health risks of a low-calorie diet may exceed the perils of being a bit more lax in your eating habits, according to Dr. Lipschitz.

"The rules of good nutrition still apply here—you just need to consume more calories," says Marilyn Cerino, R.D., marketing director for Allegheny University Executive Health and Wellness Program in Philadelphia. "Carbohydrates are an excellent source of calories and can be combined with lean protein sources and limited amounts of unsaturated fats to help fill the void. Try mixing fat-free milk, fat-free milk powder, low-fat frozen yogurt, and bananas or strawberries in a blender for a high-protein, high-carbohydrate, low-fat drink. A bowl of cereal with fat-free milk and raisins can be a calorie booster as well," she says.

In conjunction with your doctor or dietitian, choose calorie-rich foods that are also loaded with nutrients, like red meats, pork, milk, and ice cream. Bagels, cornbread, and biscuits also can help you pack on some

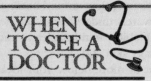

WHEN TO SEE A DOCTOR

See a doctor if you experience any of the following symptoms or life circumstances.

■ You notice that your clothing is becoming loose, and you can't explain why.

■ You have an illness or condition that has changed the kind or amount of food you eat.

■ You eat fewer than two meals a day.

■ You have three or more drinks of beer, liquor, or wine almost daily.

■ You have tooth or mouth problems that make it hard for you to eat.

■ You don't always have enough money to buy the food you need.

■ You aren't always physically able to shop, cook, or feed yourself.

pounds. Also, consider eating regular portions of potatoes, avocados, nuts, eggs, peanut butter, kidney beans, puddings, custards, fruits such as peaches canned in syrup, and other foods high in calories, Cerino says.

"For a senior seeking to recover from a weight loss that is the result of an illness, you may want to relax the rigid rules of good nutrition during the initial recovery period and indulge in some of the foods that you normally limit to an occasional basis. Milk shakes, cheesecake, full-fat cheeses, and whole milk may appeal to a poor appetite. While they are not the recommended foods for everyday use, I would not deny them to someone who is attempting to recover a lost appetite. Oftentimes, you need to eat to get an appetite, and it is most important to at least get started—no matter what you initially choose. Of course, if there are medical conditions that require some dietary constraints, you must take those into consideration," Cerino says.

Shoot for six. Frequent small feedings may help the depressed appetite, Cerino says. So instead of the traditional breakfast, lunch, and dinner, try eating six small meals a day, she says.

For instance, you might start your day with an omelet or poached eggs and a piece of toast, then have a midmorning snack like fruit. For lunch, you might have a bowl of soup with added pieces of chopped chicken or lean beef and rice, and a glass of low-fat or whole milk with some milk powder mixed in. In the afternoon, try having some rice pudding with a glass of juice. A good dinner might comprise a pork chop, a baked potato with butter and sour cream, squash or another vegetable, and milk as a beverage. Then finish off your day with an early evening snack like peanut butter crackers and milk, Cerino advises.

Use a timely reminder. Carry a small pocket alarm clock and set it to go off every three to four hours as a reminder to eat. Even if you have only a piece of bread or fruit, the alarm may help you establish regular eating times and tweak your appetite, Cerino says. If you wait for your brain to tell you to eat, you will lose even more weight, she adds.

Maximize each mouthful. Adding extra calories and nutrients to your favorite meals is actually quite easy, Cerino says. Here are some suggestions.

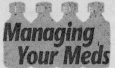

Managing Your Meds

When you see your doctor about your condition, be sure to take with you any medications—including over-the-counter preparations. It may help your physician pinpoint the cause of your weight loss or underweight problems, says Jan I. Maby, D.O., director of the Geriatric Medical Home Care program at Mount Sinai Medical Center in New York City. Possible side effects of many medications include cramping, nausea, diarrhea, malabsorption, and anorexia. A doctor's close examination could help evaluate the cause of your weight loss.

Drugs that can contribute to unintentional weight loss include:

✦ Certain prescription antidepressants such as fluoxetine (Prozac) and other serotonin uptake inhibitors

✦ Over-the-counter decongestants that contain phenylpropanolamine or pseudoephedrine, such as NyQuil, Contac, and Dimetapp

✦ Nonsteroidal anti-inflammatory drugs (NSAIDs) including over-the-counter products like ibuprofen (Advil), naproxen (Aleve), or ketoprofen (Orudis KT), which can cause stomach upset and can indirectly lead to suppressed appetite and significant weight loss

◆ Use milk in place of water in soups and sauces.

◆ Sprinkle milk powder into regular milk, casseroles, and meat loaf.

◆ Use pureed tofu in spaghetti sauce.

♦ Mix nuts, wheat germ, beans, cheeses, or cooked or chopped meat into pastas, casseroles, and side dishes.

♦ Top oatmeal and other hot cereals with melted margarine, pureed fruit, or vanilla ice cream.

Pack in the protein. Your appetite may diminish, as it often does after age 60, even if you are not ill. If that happens, increase the amount of protein in your diet to help your body retain lean muscle and keep your heart and other muscles working efficiently, Dr. Maby says.

She recommends that all adults, unless otherwise directed by their doctors, have at least 1.2 grams of protein for every 2 pounds of body weight. Protein content is listed in grams on all packaged foods. If you weigh 110 pounds, for instance, you need about 66 grams a day of protein from animal products such as milk, cheese, yogurt, and other dairy products; meats like beef and pork tenderloin; and tuna fish. Other protein-rich foods include kidney beans and soy products like tofu and soy milk, Dr. Maby says.

Forget the rules. Who says that you must have bran flakes for breakfast? If you want leftover lasagna for breakfast, have it, Cerino says. Don't lock yourself into eating certain foods at certain times of the day. Let your cravings reign until you regain your appetite.

Tune in. One in every three older people lives alone, and loneliness can shrink your waistline, Cerino says. So try watching television or reading an interesting book or magazine while you are eating if there is no one to share your meal with, she says.

Have a before-dinner nip. In moderation, alcohol stimulates hunger, Cerino says. So if you drink, prime your digestive tract by having no more than two ounces of wine or four ounces of beer about 20 minutes before you are going to eat.

Don't forget the appetizers. Low-fat tortilla chips dipped in low-fat guacamole are a great way to get extra calories into your diet and tweak your appetite for other foods, Cerino says. Plus, low-fat tortilla chips are a good source of fiber.

Eat with your eyes. Pay attention to how a meal looks, because it really matters, especially after age 60 when senses of taste and smell begin to wane a bit, Cerino says. Use colorful plates, place mats, and napkins. "Make an effort to vary the colors and textures of the foods you eat."

Spice up your life. If you have noticed a change in your ability to smell, then spice up your foods. Increase the flavor, says Cerino. "A great deal of the food-flavor connection comes from the ability to smell. Use a heavy hand with the seasonings to compensate." Also, warm foods will taste better than cold foods since the flavors are transmitted better when foods are warm, she says.

Urinary Tract Infections

You have a nearly uncontrollable urge to go. But once in the bathroom, you have very little success, just lots of burning and pain. And almost as soon as you go back to what you were doing before you were so rudely interrupted, that insistent impulse is back again. Sound familiar? It could be a urinary tract infection (UTI).

UTIs are a common malady, especially as you age, accounting for about eight million doctor visits a year. They are caused when bacteria enter the urethra, or urine tube. If the bacterial infection stays in the urethra, it is called urethritis. If the infection travels farther up the urinary tract into the bladder, as it often does, it is called cystitis (or a bladder infection). Unless treated promptly, a bladder infection can move to the kidneys, leading to a serious condition called pyelonephritis.

Women are especially prone to UTIs. In fact, one in every five women experiences a UTI during her life. The reason is partly structural. Since a woman's urethra is shorter than a man's, bacteria can travel up to her bladder quickly.

Even though men are less susceptible in general, their odds of getting UTIs increase as they get older. In men, however, the problems usually stem from some urinary obstruction—such as a kidney stone or an enlarged prostate—or from a medical procedure involving a catheter. In fact, any abnormality of the urinary tract that obstructs the flow of urine sets the stage for an infection.

People with diabetes also have a higher risk of UTIs because of changes in their immune systems. Any disorder that suppresses the immune system raises the risk of a urinary infection.

Not everyone with a UTI has symptoms. But if you do, you may have a frequent urge to urinate. Or you may experience a painful burning feeling in the area of your bladder or urethra during urination. It is

---

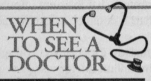

WHEN TO SEE A DOCTOR

Antibiotics can clear up most urinary tract infections, says Dorothy M. Barbo, M.D., professor of obstetrics and gynecology and director of the Center for Women's Health at the University of New Mexico in Albuquerque.

But occasionally, a urinary tract infection can develop into a more serious problem with the kidneys. Call your doctor if antibiotics don't relieve the symptoms within 72 hours, says Dr. Barbo, or if you experience any of the following danger signs.

- Blood in the urine
- Pain in the lower back or flank
- Fever
- Nausea or vomiting

---

not unusual to feel bad all over—tired, shaky, washed out—and to feel pain even when you are not urinating, says Dorothy M. Barbo, M.D., professor of obstetrics and gynecology and director of the Center for Women's Health at the University of New Mexico in Albuquerque.

If you suspect that you have a UTI, you should see a doctor as soon as possible. A prescription of antibiotics will help kill the infection, says Dr. Barbo. But there are also some actions you can take yourself to help ease your discomfort and minimize the problem. The first few tips are for both men and women, but the rest apply to women.

Flush the system. Many doctors suggest that you drink plenty of water when you are in the throes of a UTI.

Eight to 10 glasses a day of any caffeine- or alcohol-free fluid will cleanse the bladder and wash bacteria out of the urinary tract, says Phillip Barksdale, M.D., urogynecologist at Woman's Hospital in Baton Rouge, Louisiana. "Drinking plenty of water flushes out the system, reducing the amount of irritating bacteria." To pace yourself, have an eight-ounce glass of water every hour throughout the day, he advises. Drink enough water so that your urine is light yellow. Yellow- or amber-colored urine is a sign that you aren't consuming enough fluid, he says.

Even more fluid is needed if you are in a hot environment or exercise strenuously, says Dr. Barbo.

Ward it off with cranberries. Cranberry juice—a popular home remedy for UTIs—actually can prevent bacteria from sticking to cells that line the urinary tract. A study by Mark Monane, M.D., gerontologist and director of Merck-Medco Managed Care in Boston, found that women who downed a 10-ounce glass of cranberry juice every day for six months had fewer UTIs than those who drank other fluids.

Apart from clinical research, plenty of anecdotal evidence shows that cranberry juice helps, says Dr. Barbo. "I know it works for my patients," she says. The juice increases the acidic quality of urine, which, in turn, reduces bacteria levels.

Dr. Barbo recommends drinking four ounces of diluted cranberry juice two or three times a day. If you have diabetes, be sure to select low-calorie cranberry juice, which Dr. Barbo says is safer for diabetics.

Avoid irritants. Certain foods and beverages can magnify UTI discomfort. The worst of the offenders are coffee, alcohol, spicy foods, citrus, and chocolate. Avoid them until the infection clears up, says Dr. Barksdale.

Don't hold it. Even though it might be painful to urinate when you have a UTI, don't resist the urge, says Dr. Barbo. In general, you should try to empty your bladder completely every three to four hours. "It's a wise way to prevent bacterial infection and to hasten recovery if you already have one," she says. Urinating frequently helps to eliminate bacteria before they have a chance to multiply.

Have a seat after sex. Women should urinate after they have sexual intercourse, says Dr. Barbo. During sexual intercourse, bacteria may enter the urethra. By urinating, you help wash out the invaders right away.

Soothe with heat. To relieve the pain and cramping that are sometimes associated with a UTI, try a warm sitz bath, says Dr. Barksdale. Fill your bathtub with three to four inches of warm water and sit in the water for 10 to 15 minutes. When you are out of the tub, resting with a heating pad on your lower abdominal area can also help, he says.

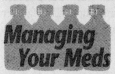

Managing Your Meds

While no medications are believed to make you more prone to urinary tract infections (UTIs), you may already be on medication that can help you avoid UTIs. Estrogen replacement therapy (ERT) reduces the risk of UTIs, says Dorothy M. Barbo, M.D., professor of obstetrics and gynecology and director of the Center for Women's Health at the University of New Mexico in Albuquerque.

The urethra is sensitive to estrogen, explains Dr. Barbo. Lack of estrogen can cause the tissues of the urethra to become dry, thinned out, and more prone to injury and infection, which puts women who are past menopause at increased risk for UTIs. Estrogen improves circulation in all of the tissues of the genital tract and makes them more resilient and less susceptible to infection. This UTI protection is an added benefit of estrogen replacement, she says.

Wear nonrestrictive clothing. Women should avoid clothes that constrict the genital area, says Dr. Barksdale, particularly control-top pantyhose and tight jeans. Clothes with tight crotches put pressure on the inflamed urethral opening, he says, and can force bacteria back up the urine tube. Skirts, loose pants, and knee-highs are far more comfortable and therapeutic when you have a UTI, he says.

Take off that bathing suit. Avoid wearing a wet bathing suit for long periods of time, adds Dr. Barksdale. "Bacteria love to grow in warm, moist areas," he says. "A wet swimsuit provides an ideal environment for bacteria that cause UTI, so you are asking for trouble."

Keep moving. Even though the discomfort of a

UTI may make you want to take to your bed, doctors say it is best to stay active since mobility aids bladder function, says Dr. Barksdale. "Exercise is always beneficial for the bladder, and it helps to get your mind off your discomfort."

Clean with care. Keep infections at bay by cleaning the vaginal area with a front-to-back motion, says Dr. Barbo. Many women were taught to wipe from back to front after a bowel movement, which can spread bacteria from your anus to your urethral opening, she says. Proper wiping can prevent a significant number of UTIs, especially among women who get them recurrently.

Ditch douches and sprays. Give up feminine hygiene sprays and scented douches—both can irritate the urethra and vulva, says Dr. Barbo.

If you feel the need to douche, don't do so any more often than once a month. "Frequent douching can introduce infectious bacteria into the vagina and rinse out the normal 'friendly' noninfectious vaginal bacteria," says Dr. Barbo.

Vaginal Dryness

It's hard to determine which aches more because of this condition—your vagina or your feelings. Sex becomes a lot less fun if you lack the natural lubrication to enjoy lovemaking. In fact, it may get downright painful.

But there's also the self-doubt, depression, and even anger that you and your partner might feel because of it.

Instead of blaming yourself (or him), you might want to point the finger at a lack of estrogen. During menopause, you can expect estrogen to be in short supply. But that's not the only reason for the problem. Other causes might include a low-grade vaginal infection or even the natural aging process. Besides getting estrogen replacement therapy from your doctor, here are some natural ways to make intercourse go more smoothly.

Toss out the cigs. "Smoking destroys estrogen in the body," says Ellen Yankauskas, M.D., director of the Women's Center for Family Health in Atascadero, California. Since the most common cause of vaginal dryness is lack of enough estrogen, smoking only makes the problem worse.

Choose the right lubricant. You can remedy vaginal dryness with a commercial lubricant, but avoid anything scented or oil-based. "You want a lubricant that's water-soluble, unscented, colorless, odorless, and tasteless," says John Willems, M.D., associate clinical professor of obstetrics/gynecology at the University of California, San Diego, and a researcher at the Scripps Clinic and Research Foundation in La Jolla. "After that, it's a matter of personal choice." He and other experts recommend Astroglide, SurgiLube, Lubrin vaginal inserts, Gyne Moisturin, and the more familiar K-Y jelly. Another recommended product is Replens, a moisturizer that can be used on a regular basis. The key is to stay away from oil-based products like petroleum jelly and cocoa butter—or homemade recipes. "Some people use whatever is on the night table—things like suntan oil," says Dr.

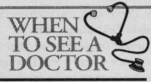

WHEN TO SEE A DOCTOR

"If vaginal dryness leads to bleeding or intense itching, these signs should be looked at by your gynecologist," says Yvonne Thornton, M.D., professor of clinical obstetrics/gynecology at Columbia University College of Physicians and Surgeons in New York City. They could be an indication of more serious problems.

Willems. "But they aren't good for the vagina and can cause problems."

Go for fatty acids. Eating foods that are rich in fatty acids can be a big help. Among the best sources are raw pumpkin, sesame, and sunflower seeds. Also eat fish that contain lots of fatty acids: Salmon, tuna, and mackerel are all good choices, because they help retain estrogen in the body, says Susan Lark, M.D., medical director of the PMS and Menopause Self-Help Center in Los Altos, California.

Don't douche. Most douche products have a drying effect, which contributes to vaginal dryness, adds Dr. Yankauskas. "In general, you shouldn't douche unless you feel it's absolutely necessarily—and it's usually not."

Savor the moment. "Give yourself more time for foreplay," says Dr. Willems. As women age, he points out, their response to sexual stimulus is slower. You don't lose sexual response—it just occurs at a different pace.

Water Retention

W hen you feel as though you're too big for your skin, not to mention your britches, check for some other signs. Perhaps your face is puffy, especially when you first wake up. Your ring may feel tight, and your belly seems bloated. Do your shoes feel like they belong to Minnie Mouse? Does this awful, bloated, uncomfortable feeling seem to come out of the blue? What *is* going on?

It could be water retention, or *edema* (to use the medical name). It happens to all of us to some extent during a normal 24-hour period, says Norman C. Staub, M.D., a professor in the department of physiology at the University of California, San Francisco. "Our bodies are constantly adjusting fluid levels based on what we drink and eat."

Usually our bodies do an admirable job of quickly correcting fluid balance. But sometimes the balance gets temporarily thrown off. Too much salt or alcohol, long periods of inactivity, and, for women, monthly hormone fluctuations can all tip the scale toward fluid retention. A sudden weight gain of several pounds may be your first and only sign that you're retaining fluid. Swollen ankles are a common tip-off, too.

For mild fluid retention, here's what experts suggest.

Get into deep water. As any skin diver knows, water pressure forces fluid out of tissues and, ultimately, into the bladder. You can get similar results by exercising in a swimming pool, according to Vern L. Katz, M.D., associate professor of obstetrics and gynecology at the University of North Carolina Medical School at Chapel Hill. Try a half-hour, three times a week, of gentle water exercise in a pool that's 80° to 90°F, or about skin temperature. "Avoid water above 100° if you're pregnant," Dr. Katz warns.

Avoid using diuretics. While they're very effective at removing excess body fluid for patients who have heart, kidney, or liver disease, diuretics set up the potential for something called rebound edema, says Robert Schrier, M.D., a professor and chairman of the department of medicine at the University of Colorado School of Medicine in Denver. If you're taking them steadily for minor fluid retention, the diuretics turn on a lot of salt- and water-retaining hormones, says Dr. Schrier. "When you stop taking them, the high levels of hormones cause a lot more sodium and water retention, and you get into a vicious cycle."

Shake the salt habit. Too much salt—from hot dogs, popcorn, olives, salted nuts, pickles, or pepperoni pizza—makes your body retain fluid. That fluid stays with you until your kidneys have a chance to excrete the excess salt, which can take about 24 hours. So if you avoid salty foods, you are less likely to have noticeable fluid retention, Dr. Staub says.

While you're at it, shake a leg. Exercise can relieve the body of excess fluid and salt through sweating, increased respiration, and, ultimately, increased urine flow, Dr. Staub says. Walking up and down the hallway or climbing a flight of stairs every hour or so will reduce the fluid retention you develop from sitting for long periods of time. If you must sit still, try this: Point your toes downward, then raise them up as high as you can.

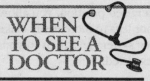

WHEN TO SEE A DOCTOR

Occasionally, your fluid balance can be seriously thrown off. Heart and kidney problems, along with other serious diseases, can cause life-threatening fluid retention. Don't delay seeing your doctor if you have a sudden weight gain, swollen ankles, or difficulty breathing.

If you find that an indentation remains when you press your skin, that's a sign of "pitting edema"—a type of fluid buildup that needs a doctor's attention.

That pumps your calf and your foot muscles. Moving your arms around up over your head will help, too.

Drink plenty of water. Water moves through your kidneys and bladder, diluting the urine. And since urine has some fluid-retaining salt in it, the more it's diluted, the easier it is to remove salt and prevent or decrease edema. "Plain water is definitely the best, because just about every other drink—juices, soda, milk—has sodium in it," Dr. Staub says.

Sip an herbal tea. Several herbs have a mildly diuretic effect, according to William J. Keller, Ph.D., a professor and head of the division of medicinal chemistry and pharmaceutics at Northeast Louisiana University School of Pharmacy in Monroe. Parsley is the best known of these. Try two teaspoons of dried leaves per cup of boiling water. Steep for 10 minutes. Drink up to three cups a day.

Lie down, put up your feet. Sometimes this is the simplest and best thing to do, Dr. Staub says. If you recline with your feet in a raised position, you allow fluid that has pooled in your legs to more easily make its way into the circulatory system and then to your kidneys, where it can be excreted.

Windburn

It seems so unfair. Right in the middle of winter, you find yourself suffering from something as painful as summer's sunburn. But how can you possibly have a burn when you can hardly see the sun at all and the temperature hovers well below 32°F? The reason: windburn.

Despite its name, windburn is actually a skin irritation. But it looks like a burn because your skin appears red and slightly swollen on some exposed areas of your body. "Wind causes the loss of the oil layer on your skin," explains Norman Levine, M.D., professor and chief of dermatology at the University of Arizona Health Sciences Center in Tucson. "And when your skin dries out excessively, you get an irritation that looks and feels like a real burn. To reverse the effect of windburn, you need to add that oil layer back to your skin."

So here are some ways to make winter weather less damaging and to take the burn out of windburn.

Put out the flame with moisturizers. "Any type of injury to the skin causes an inflammatory reaction," says John P. Heggers, M.D., director of clinical microbiology at the Shriners Burns Institute in Galveston, Texas. "A moisturizer such as Dermaid Aloe is a good anti-inflammatory." It restores oil to your skin but allows water to evaporate as usual.

Wash on the mild side. Go for mild soaps and cleansers that have moisturizers, suggests Dr. Levine. They leave necessary oils in the skin. Dr. Levine warns against strong soaps that don't contain moisturizers. "The more effective a soap is as a cleanser, the more drying it is," he says.

Gently rewarm the skin. If you treat damaged skin gently, it is more likely to heal quickly, according to Dr. Heggers. Avoid exposing your skin to extreme temperature changes, he warns, and when you come indoors, allow the heat of the room to defrost your body. Don't turn on the heat lamp or stand next to a roaring fire.

Add a little oil. If the burning sensation is too much to bear, rub an oily skin medication on the windburned area, advises Murray Hamlet, D.V.M., director of the Plans and Operations Division at the U.S. Army Research Institute of Environmental Medicine in Natick, Massachusetts. "Vaseline is good because it is heavy," he says. "Chap Stick will work, too."

Elevate it. Occasionally, there is noticeable swelling in windburned areas. Dr. Heggers recommends elevating wind-burned hands and feet while they are being rewarmed to minimize the swelling.

Wrap things up. Your nose, lips, and ears are particularly susceptible to windburn, notes W. Steven Pray, Ph.D., R.Ph., professor of nonprescription drug products at Southwestern Oklahoma State University in Weatherford. So wear earmuffs or a woolly hat, with a scarf or face mask to cover your nose and lips.

Block the wind. "The best way to protect yourself from the wind is with a barrier," says Carol Frey, M.D., chief of the Foot and Ankle Service and associate clinical professor of orthopedic surgery at the University of Southern California School of Medicine in Los Angeles. She recommends wearing a shell made from Gore-Tex or other synthetics. Zipping it high over the chin and pulling the hood around your face will shield your skin from that parching arctic breeze.

Know the wind chill factor. The wind chill factor is sometimes more of an indication of the weather conditions than the temperature. As the wind chill sends the temperature plummeting, the chance of injury rises, says Dr. Frey. So check the weather report before you head outdoors for those bracing winter activities.

Yeast Infections

It takes very little to get the normally docile *Candida albicans* fungus that lives in a woman's vagina to turn into a rampant troublemaker. Candida is encouraged by many things, including taking antibiotics or using spermicides or birth control pills.

Yeast infections are not dangerous, but they can be painful and embarrassing. The most common symptoms include a bothersome itch and burning that can become maddening. Often there's a white discharge that resembles cottage cheese, sometimes accompanied by a yeasty or fishy smell. Here's how to cease the yeast.

Watch your sweet tooth. Sugar can cause chronic yeast infections—which is one reason why women who binge on sweets are particularly prone. "Avoid candy, cakes, and pies—anything with refined, white, or powdered sugar," says Jack Galloway, M.D., clinical professor of obstetrics and gynecology at the University of Southern California School of Medicine in Los Angeles. If you must indulge your sweet tooth, use brown sugar or honey. Since these take longer to break down in your body, you'll lessen the amount of circulating blood sugars, which can trigger yeast infections.

And watch the rest of your diet. Take heed of the connection between yeast infections and yeasty foods. "Avoid things such as bread, mushrooms, and alcoholic beverages," says Susan Doughty, R.N., a nurse practitioner at Women to Women, a clinic in Yarmouth, Maine. She says that patients with chronic yeast infections who avoid these foods for three to six months will often notice a significant improvement.

"C" an improvement. Eat plenty of foods that are high in vitamin C, such as potatoes, citrus fruits, and broccoli, adds Dr. Galloway. Vitamin C helps boost your immune system, and "if your immunity is down, you're a prime candidate for a yeast infection."

Wear baggy clothing. Tight-fitting clothing doesn't allow for good air circulation in the vaginal area. So stay away from clingy polyester, Lycra spandex, leather, and other fabrics that don't "breathe." "Yeast love it when it's moist, dark, and

Take Yeast Infections to the Cleaners

Perhaps the best weapons for treating yeast infections are in your laundry room. But you have to use special tactics to conquer *Candida albicans*, which can survive regular wash-and-dry cycles. Here are the basics.

Go soak. Soak panties in water for 30 minutes or more before washing them.

Scrub-a-dub. After soaking, scrub the crotch of your panties with unscented detergent before putting them into the washing machine, advises candida specialist Marjorie Crandall, Ph.D., of Yeast Consulting Services in Torrance, California.

Double-rinse. Make sure panties are rinsed thoroughly, since residues from soaps and detergents can intensify vaginitis, according to John Willems, M.D., associate clinical professor of obstetrics/gynecology at the University of California, San Diego, and a researcher at the Scripps Clinic and Research Foundation in La Jolla.

Get 'em hot. Studies have found that the heat-sensitive candida die when panties are touched up with a hot iron.

warm," says John Willems, M.D., associate clinical professor of obstetrics/gynecology at the University of California, San Diego, and a researcher at the Scripps Clinic and Research Foundation in La Jolla.

If you must wear tight clothing or Lycra, do it for only a few hours—and then change into loose-fitting garb made from cotton and other natural fibers. Avoid panty hose when you can, because they're too restrictive in the vaginal area, suggests Dr. Willems.

Change wet clothing fast. Lounging around in a wet bathing suit? You're wearing a perfect environment for yeast growth, adds Dr. Galloway. So once you're out of the pool, change into a dry outfit.

Heal with yogurt. Most experts point to yogurt as *the* natural healer of yeast infections (though it shouldn't be used for other types of vaginitis). Yogurt's lactobacillus cultures fight the candida, says Eileen Hilton, M.D., an infectious disease specialist at Long Island Jewish Medical Center in New Hyde Park, New York, who has studied yogurt's effect on yeast infections. While some experts recommend inserting yogurt into the vaginal area, an easier way is to simply eat at least ½ cup of yogurt containing live cultures each day to prevent and treat infections. (Nearly all yogurt *does* contain live cultures.)

"If you don't like the taste of yogurt, you can get a dose of the same helpful bacteria by drinking milk containing live lactobacillus," suggests Ellen Yankauskas, M.D., director of the Women's Center for Family Health in Atascadero, California. (This type of milk will be identified on the container as cultured milk, acidophilus milk, or kefir milk.)

Sit in a sitz. Frequent douching should be avoided, since it can be too irritating to those with yeast infections. But there's an easy cleansing solution for your vaginal area. Fill the bathtub to hip height with warm water, then add ½ cup of salt (enough to make the water taste salty) and ½ cup of vinegar. Stay in this sitz for about 20 minutes.

Go for a nonprescription medication. "The best way to treat this infection is with an over-the-

Is It Another Yeast Infection?

You've consulted a doctor for a previous yeast infection, and now you seem to be getting the same symptoms again. You may be able to save the time and expense of a return visit to the doctor by going to the drugstore and buying a strip of pH paper—litmus paper.

Moisten the paper with a small amount of vaginal discharge. (The discharge *must* be wet for the paper to react.) "If you have a yeast infection, your pH will be between 4 and 4.5 or less," says Ellen Yankauskas, M.D., director of the Women's Center for Family Health in Atascadero, California. "With other types of vaginitis, the pH tends to be higher."

If the litmus test confirms your suspicions, you may simply want to resume treatment with an over-the-counter cream. But if it's not effective after three days, Dr. Yankauskas says, you should definitely see your doctor again.

counter anti-yeast vaginal cream," according to Dr. Yankauskas. The creams are available in most pharmacies. Just follow the directions on the package.

Give applicators a hot scrub. If you use an anti-yeast cream, you're probably reusing the applicator. "Wash the reusable applicators in hot soapy water," says Dr. Galloway.

Try no-frills toiletries. Avoid bubble baths, colored toilet paper, and other products with dyes, perfumes, and other chemicals that can irritate vaginal tissue, says Dr. Willems. White toilet paper is your best bet.

Index

Boldface page references indicate primary discussions.
<u>Underscored</u> references indicate boxed text.

ASPIRIN
  affect on
    asthma, <u>36</u>
    bleeding, in cuts, <u>104</u>
    bruising, 56-57
    colds, 83
    colitis, 90
    dizziness, <u>124</u>
    gums, 193-94
    mouth, when applied
      topically, 415
    muscle pain, 286, <u>289</u>
    senses of taste and
      smell, <u>251</u>
    tinnitus, 412
    ulcers, <u>418</u>, 420
  ginkgo and, 185
  Reye's syndrome and, 83,
    159
  for treating
    angina, 18
    backache, 39
    burns, 59
    calluses, when applied
      topically, 98
    cataracts, 72
    earache, 142
    fever, 159
    gum pain, 193
    joint pain, <u>4</u>
    phlebitis, 332-33
    rheumatoid arthritis, 31
    sciatica, <u>363</u>
    stiff neck, 389-90
    toothaches, 415
ASTEMIZOLE, 343
ASTHMA, 32–37
  dietary advice for, 34
  medications and, <u>36</u>
  triggers, 32-33, 35, 37
  when to see a doctor for, 33

ATTAPULGITE, <u>121</u>
AURANOFIN, <u>320</u>

B

BACKACHE, 37–42
  pain relief for, 39-42
  when to see a doctor for,
    <u>40</u>
BACK EXTENSIONS, 323
BAG BALM, 348
BAKING SODA, FOR
  bad breath, <u>134</u>
  gum pain, 194
  psoriasis, 348
  quitting smoking, 308
BATHS
  sitz, for
    hemorrhoids, 208
    rectal itching, 355
    yeast infection, 445
  warm, for
    fever, 160-61
    fragile skin, 176-77
    muscle pain, 287-88
    muscle spasms, 295
    psoriasis, 348
    quitting smoking, 308
    restless legs syndrome,
      358
    stress, 405
BECLOMETHASONE
  denture pain and, <u>111</u>
  night vision and, <u>314</u>
  for asthma, <u>36</u>
BEDSORES, 42–46
  dietary advice for, 43-45
  pressure-relief for,
    43, 45
  when to see a doctor for,
    <u>44</u>
  wound care for, 45-46

452

MILK
compress, for eczema,
146–47
products, avoiding, for
colitis, 90
constipation, 94
nausea, 297
ulcers, 420
for treating seasonal
affective disorder,
368–69
MINERALS, FOR
colitis, 89
osteoporosis, 325
MOBILITY, 274–78
exercises for, 277–78
medications and, 277
when to see a doctor for, 275
MOISTURIZATION, FOR
cuts and scrapes, 105
dry eyes, 129–31
dry skin, 136–39
eczema, 145
fragile skin, 177–78
psoriasis, 346–47
windburn, 440–41
MOLESKIN, FOR
corns, 99
foot blisters, 49
MONTEZUMA'S REVENGE.
SEE DIARRHEA
MORNING ACHES AND
PAINS, 279–85
medications and, 282
preventing, 283–85
when to see a doctor for, 280
MORPHINE, DIVERTICULOSIS
AND, 120
MOUTH, DRY, 132–35
bad breath and, 134
causes of, 132–33

dietary advice for, 133–34
gum pain and, 194
relief of, 134–35
MOVEMENT MEDITATION,
75, 76–77
MULTIVITAMIN
SUPPLEMENTS, FOR
bruise prevention, 56
colitis, 89
nerve health, 321
shingles, 374
slow healing, 386–87
MUSCLE PAIN, 285–93
exercise tips for, 289–91
medications for, 286, 289
stretching exercises for,
291–93
when to see a doctor for,
287
MUSCLE SPASMS, 293–96
dietary advice for,
295–96
when to see a doctor for,
294

N

NAPROXEN
affect on
bleeding, in cuts, 104
colitis, 90
muscle pain, 286, 289
ulcers, 418
underweight, 426
side effects of, 170
for treating
night pain, 282
sciatica, 363
NAUSEA, 296–99
relief of, 296–99
when to see a doctor for,
298

462